Pediatric Endoscopy

Editor

JENIFER R. LIGHTDALE

GASTROINTESTINAL ENDOSCOPY CLINICS OF NORTH AMERICA

www.giendo.theclinics.com

Consulting Editor
CHARLES J. LIGHTDALE

January 2016 • Volume 26 • Number 1

ELSEVIER

1600 John F. Kennedy Boulevard • Suite 1800 • Philadelphia, Pennsylvania, 19103-2899

http://www.theclinics.com

GASTROINTESTINAL ENDOSCOPY CLINICS OF NORTH AMERICA Volume 26, Number 1
January 2016 ISSN 1052-5157, ISBN-13: 978-0-323-41451-7

Editor: Kerry Holland
Developmental Editor: Donald Mumford

Photocopying
Single photocopies of single articles may be made for personal use as allowed by national copyright laws. Permission of the Publisher and payment of a fee is required for all other photocopying, including multiple or systematic copying, copying for advertising or promotional purposes, resale, and all forms of document delivery. Special rates are available for educational institutions that wish to make photocopies for non-profit educational classroom use. For information on how to seek permission visit www.elsevier.com/permissions or call: (+44) 1865 843830 (UK)/(+1) 215 239 3804 (USA).

Derivative Works
Subscribers may reproduce tables of contents or prepare lists of articles including abstracts for internal circulation within their institutions. Permission of the Publisher is required for resale or distribution outside the institution. Permission of the Publisher is required for all other derivative works, including compilations and translations (please consult www.elsevier.com/permissions).

Electronic Storage or Usage
Permission of the Publisher is required to store or use electronically any material contained in this periodical, including any article or part of an article (please consult www.elsevier.com/permissions). Except as outlined above, no part of this publication may be reproduced, stored in a retrieval system or transmitted in any form or by any means, electronic, mechanical, photocopying, recording or otherwise, without prior written permission of the Publisher.

Notice
No responsibility is assumed by the Publisher for any injury and/or damage to persons or property as a matter of products liability, negligence or otherwise, or from any use or operation of any methods, products, instructions or ideas contained in the material herein. Because of rapid advances in the medical sciences, in particular, independent verification of diagnoses and drug dosages should be made.

Although all advertising material is expected to conform to ethical (medical) standards, inclusion in this publication does not constitute a guarantee or endorsement of the quality or value of such product or of the claims made of it by its manufacturer.

Gastrointestinal Endoscopy Clinics of North America (ISSN 1052-5157) is published quarterly by Elsevier Inc., 360 Park Avenue South, New York, NY 10010-1710. Months of issue are January, April, July, and October. Business and Editorial Offices: 1600 John F. Kennedy Blvd., Suite 1800, Philadelphia, PA, 19103-2899. Periodicals postage paid at New York, NY and additional mailing offices. Subscription prices are $335.00 per year for US individuals, $538.00 per year for US institutions, $100.00 per year for US students and residents, $370.00 per year for Canadian individuals, $637.00 per year for Canadian institutions, $465.00 per year for international individuals, $637.00 per year for international institutions, and $245.00 per year for Canadian and foreign students/residents. To receive student/resident rate, orders must be accompanied by name of affiliated institution, date of term, and the *signature* of program/residency coordinator on institution letterhead. Orders will be billed at individual rate until proof of status is received. Foreign air speed delivery is included in all *Clinics* subscription prices. All prices are subject to change without notice. **POSTMASTER:** Send address change to *Gastrointestinal Endoscopy Clinics of North America*, Elsevier Health Sciences Division, Subscription Customer Service, 3251 Riverport Lane, Maryland Heights, MO 63043. **Customer Service: 1-800-654-2452 (US). From outside the United States, call 1-314-447-8871. Fax: 1-314-447-8029. E-mail: JournalsCustomerService-usa@elsevier.com (for print support) or JournalsOnlineSupport-usa@elsevier.com (for online support).**

Reprints. For copies of 100 or more, of articles in this publication, please contact the Commercial Reprints Department, Elsevier Inc., 360 Park Avenue South, New York, NY 10010-1710. Tel. 212-633-3874; Fax: 212-633-3820; E-mail: reprints@elsevier.com.

Gastrointestinal Endoscopy Clinics of North America is covered in *Excerpta Medica, MEDLINE/PubMed (Index Medicus), and MEDLINE/MEDLARS.*

Contributors

CONSULTING EDITOR

CHARLES J. LIGHTDALE, MD
Department of Medicine, Columbia University Medical Center, New York, New York

EDITOR

JENIFER R. LIGHTDALE, MD, MPH
Division Chief, Pediatric Gastroenterology, Hepatology and Nutrition; Chief Quality Officer, UMass Memorial Children's Medical Center; Professor of Pediatrics, University of Massachusetts Medical School, Worcester, Massachusetts

AUTHORS

BRADLEY A. BARTH, MD, MPH, FASGE
Associate Professor of Pediatrics, Division of Pediatric Gastroenterology, University of Texas Southwestern Medical Center, Dallas, Texas

SAMUEL BITTON, MD
Division of Pediatric Gastroenterology and Nutrition, Steven and Alexandra Cohen Children's Medical Center of New York; Assistant Professor of Pediatrics, Hofstra North Shore-LIJ School of Medicine, North Shore – Long Island Jewish Health System, New Hyde Park, New York

DAVID E. BRUMBAUGH, MD
Assistant Professor, Department of Pediatrics, Digestive Health Institute, Children's Hospital Colorado, University of Colorado, Aurora, Colorado

JOEL A. FRIEDLANDER, DO, MA-Bioethics
Associate Professor of Pediatrics, Digestive Health Institute, Children's Hospital Colorado, University of Colorado School of Medicine, Aurora, Colorado

ROBERT E. KRAMER, MD, FASGE
Associate Professor, Department of Pediatrics, Digestive Health Institute, Children's Hospital Colorado, University of Colorado, Aurora, Colorado

ARATHI LAKHOLE, MD
Division of Gastroenterology, Hepatology and Nutrition, Children's Hospital Los Angeles, Los Angeles, California

KRISTINA LEINWAND, DO
Department of Pediatrics, Digestive Health Institute, Children's Hospital Colorado, University of Colorado, Aurora, Colorado

DIANA G. LERNER, MD
Assistant Professor, Section of Gastroenterology, Hepatology, and Nutrition, Department of Pediatrics, Medical College of Wisconsin, Milwaukee, Wisconsin

CHRIS A. LIACOURAS, MD
Professor of Pediatrics, Division of Gastroenterology, Hepatology, and Nutrition, The Children's Hospital of Philadelphia; Department of Pediatrics, Perelman School of Medicine, University of Pennsylvania, Philadelphia, Pennsylvania

JENIFER R. LIGHTDALE, MD, MPH
Division Chief, Pediatric Gastroenterology, Hepatology and Nutrition; Chief Quality Officer, UMass Memorial Children's Medical Center; Professor of Pediatrics, University of Massachusetts Medical School, Worcester, Massachusetts

TOM K. LIN, MD
Assistant Professor of Clinical Pediatrics, Cincinnati Children's Hospital Medical Center, Cincinnati, Ohio

RICHARD A. LIRIO, MD
Division of Pediatric Gastroenterology, Hepatology and Nutrition; Assistant Professor, Department of Pediatrics, UMass Memorial Children's Medical Center University Campus, University of Massachusetts Medical School, Worcester, Massachusetts

QUIN Y. LIU, MD
Director of Endoscopy, Division of Gastroenterology, Hepatology, and Nutrition, Children's Hospital Los Angeles, Assistant Professor of Clinical Pediatrics, Keck School of Medicine of USC, Los Angeles, California

MICHAEL A. MANFREDI, MD
Co-Director, Esophageal Atresia and Airway Treatment Center, Boston Children's Hospital; Instructor of Pediatrics, Harvard Medical School, Boston, Massachusetts

MAIREADE E. McSWEENEY, MD, MPH
Attending in Pediatric Gastroenterology, Division of Gastroenterology and Nutrition, Department of Medicine, Boston Children's Hospital; Instructor in Pediatrics, Harvard Medical School, Boston, Massachusetts

JAMIE MERVES, MD
Assistant Professor of Pediatrics, Division of Gastroenterology, Hepatology, and Nutrition, The Children's Hospital of Philadelphia; Department of Pediatrics, Perelman School of Medicine, University of Pennsylvania, Philadelphia, Pennsylvania

AMANDA B. MUIR, MD
Assistant Professor of Pediatrics, Division of Gastroenterology, Hepatology, and Nutrition, The Children's Hospital of Philadelphia; Department of Pediatrics, Perelman School of Medicine, University of Pennsylvania, Philadelphia, Pennsylvania

HARPREET PALL, MD
Associate Professor, Section of Gastroenterology, Hepatology, and Nutrition, St. Christopher's Hospital for Children; Department of Pediatrics, Drexel University College of Medicine, Philadelphia, Pennsylvania

BENJAMIN SAHN, MD, MS
Division of Pediatric Gastroenterology and Nutrition, Steven and Alexandra Cohen Children's Medical Center of New York; Assistant Professor of Pediatrics, Hofstra North Shore-LIJ School of Medicine, North Shore – Long Island Jewish Health System, New Hyde Park, New York

C. JASON SMITHERS, MD
Assistant in Surgery, Department of General Surgery, Boston Children's Hospital;
Instructor in Surgery, Harvard Medical School, Boston, Massachusetts

DAVID M. TROENDLE, MD
Assistant Professor of Pediatrics, Division of Pediatric Gastroenterology, University of
Texas Southwestern Medical Center, Dallas, Texas

CATHARINE M. WALSH, MD, MEd, PhD, FAAP, FRCPC
Division of Gastroenterology, Hepatology and Nutrition, The Learning Institute and the
Research Institute, Hospital for Sick Children; Department of Paediatrics and the Wilson
Centre, University of Toronto, Toronto, Canada

Contents

As pediatric gastrointestinal endoscopy continues to develop and evolve, pediatric gastroenterologists are more frequently called on to develop and direct a pediatric endoscopy unit. Lack of published literature and focused training in fellowship can render decision making about design, capacity, operation, equipment purchasing, and staffing challenging. To help guide management decisions, we distributed a short survey to 18 pediatric gastroenterology centers throughout the United States and Canada. This article provides practical guidance by summarizing available expert opinions on the topic of setting up a pediatric endoscopy unit.

A key aspect of pediatric gastroenterology practice is the ability to perform endoscopy procedures safely, effectively, and efficiently. Similar to adult endoscopy, performance of pediatric endoscopy requires the acquisition of related technical, cognitive, and integrative competencies to effectively diagnose and manage gastrointestinal disorders in children. However, the distinctive requirements of pediatric patients and their families and the differential spectrum of disease highlight the need for a pediatric-specific training curriculum and assessment framework to ensure endoscopic procedures are performed safely and successfully in children. This review outlines the current state of evidence as it pertains to pediatric endoscopy training and assessment.

Informed consent and refusal for pediatric procedures involves a process in which the provider, child, and parents/guardians participate. In pediatric gastroenterology, many procedures are considered elective and the process generally begins with an office visit and ends with the signing of the consent document. If the process is emergent then this occurs more expeditiously and a formal consent may not be required. Information about the procedure should be shared in a way that allows a decision-making process to occur for both the parent/guardian and the child, if of assenting age.

Measuring quality in endoscopy includes the assessment of appropriateness of a procedure and the skill with which it is performed. High-quality pediatric endoscopy is safe and efficient, used effectively to make proper diagnoses, is useful for excluding other diagnoses, minimizes adverse events, and is accompanied by appropriate documentation from beginning through end of the procedure. There are no standard quality metrics for pediatric endoscopy, but proposed candidates are both process and outcomes oriented. Both are likely to be used in the near future to increase transparency about patient outcomes, as well as to influence payments for the procedure.

Upper gastrointestinal (UGI) bleeding is generally defined as bleeding proximal to the ligament of Treitz, which leads to hematemesis. There are several causes of UGI bleeding necessitating a detailed history to rule out comorbid conditions, medications, and possible exposures. In addition, the severity, timing, duration, and volume of the bleeding are important details to note for management purposes. Despite the source of the bleeding, acid suppression with a proton-pump inhibitor has been shown to be effective in minimizing rebleeding. Endoscopy remains the interventional modality of choice for both nonvariceal and variceal bleeds because it can be diagnostic and therapeutic.

This article provides an overview of the evaluation and management of lower gastrointestinal bleeding (LGIB) in children. The common etiologies at different ages are reviewed. Conditions with endoscopic importance for diagnosis or therapy include solitary rectal ulcer syndrome, polyps, vascular lesions, and colonic inflammation and ulceration. Diagnostic modalities for identifying causes of LGIB in children include endoscopy and colonoscopy, cross-sectional and nuclear medicine imaging, video capsule endoscopy, and enteroscopy. Pre-endoscopic preparation and decision-making unique to pediatrics is highlighted. The authors conclude with a summary of current and emerging therapeutic hemostatic techniques that can be used in pediatric patients.

Gastrointestinal injuries secondary to button battery ingestions in children have emerged as a dangerous and difficult management problem for pediatricians. Implementation of a multidisciplinary team approach, with rapid and coordinated care, is paramount to minimize the risk of negative outcomes. In addition to providing a comprehensive review of the topic, this article outlines the authors' referral center's experience with patients with severe battery ingestion, highlighting the complications, outcomes, and important lessons learned from their care. The authors also propose an algorithm for clinical care that may be useful for guiding best management of pediatric button battery ingestion.

Endoscopic retrograde cholangiopancreatography is a technically challenging endoscopic technique that provides a minimally invasive way of evaluating and treating pathologic abnormality in the bile ducts and pancreas. Its utilization in children is increasing rapidly, broadening the understanding of its pediatric indications, clinical utility, and technical limitations. This article updates providers about specific considerations of endoscopic retrograde cholangiopancreatography in children as they relate to appropriate indications, patient preparation, available equipment, as well as expected technical and clinical outcomes following the procedure in pediatric populations.

The application of endoscopic ultrasound (EUS) in children is growing, with studies demonstrating a positive impact of EUS in the management of childhood diseases. EUS has shown to be useful in the evaluation and management of a spectrum of childhood diseases including pancreaticobiliary disease, congenital anomalies, submuocsal lesions, biliary stones disease, inflammatory bowel disease, and eosinophilic esophagitis. Its diagnostic capabilities with fine-needle aspiration and core-needle biopsy are shown to be technically successful, safe, and effective in several pediatric studies. Therapeutic EUS procedures include endoscopic cystgastrostomy, celiac plexus neurolysis, and biliary access. This article discusses the role of EUS for diagnostic and therapeutic purposes in pediatrics.

Technological advances for visualizing the small bowel have significantly grown over the past few decades. Balloon-assisted enteroscopy has come to the forefront of these innovations, and has been found to be safe and effective in children with small bowel ailments. The expanding body of research into balloon-assisted enteroscopy will continue to refine the current knowledge base of this technique, along with a growing assessment of the long-term benefits of such interventions.

Placement of gastrostomy tubes in infants and children has become increasingly commonplace. A historical emphasis on use of open gastrostomy has been replaced by less invasive methods of placement, including percutaneous endoscopic gastrostomy and laparoscopically assisted gastrostomy procedures. Various complications, ranging from minor to the more severe, have been reported with all methods of placement. Many pediatric patients who undergo gastrostomy tube placement will require long-term enteral therapy. Given the prolonged time pediatric patients may remain enterally dependent, further quality improvement and education initiatives are needed to improve long-term care and outcomes of these patients.

Eosinophilic esophagitis (EoE) is a chronic allergic (immune-mediated) disease that leads to esophageal dysfunction and feeding disorders in children. Foods, and possibly environmental triggers, cause an inflammatory response in the esophagus, leading to esophageal inflammation, eosinophilic infiltration, and esophageal dysmotility, which may progress to dysphagia, food impaction, and esophageal stricture. Endoscopy with biopsy and histologic evaluation is currently the only method to diagnose EoE. Once diagnosed with EoE, children undergo follow-up endoscopy after therapy initiation and adjustments to ensure remission. Furthermore, children with food impactions or strictures may require endoscopic intervention such as foreign body removal and/or esophageal dilation.

The reported incidence of anastomotic stricture after esophageal atresia repair has varied in case series from as low as 9% to as high as 80%. The cornerstone of esophageal stricture treatment is dilation with either balloon or bougie. The goal of esophageal dilation is to increase the luminal diameter of the esophagus while also improving dysphagia symptoms. Once a stricture becomes refractory to esophageal dilation, there are several treatment therapies available as adjuncts to dilation therapy. These therapies include intralesional steroid injection, mitomycin C, esophageal stent placement, and endoscopic incisional therapy.

GASTROINTESTINAL ENDOSCOPY CLINICS OF NORTH AMERICA

THE CLINICS ARE AVAILABLE ONLINE!
Access your subscription at:
www.theclinics.com

GASTROINTESTINAL ENDOSCOPY CLINICS
OF NORTH AMERICA

FORTHCOMING ISSUES

April 2016

July 2016

October 2016

RECENT ISSUES

Foreword

Pediatric Gastrointestinal Endoscopy: A Mature Subspecialty

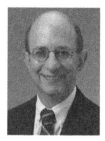

Charles J. Lightdale, MD
Consulting Editor

The burden of gastrointestinal disease affecting infants and children is high and increasing. Fortunately, there are a growing number of specialists trained in both pediatrics and pediatric gastroenterology: enough to be available to most general pediatricians for evaluation and management of gastrointestinal illness. As in adults, gastrointestinal endoscopy has become a key element in the diagnosis and therapy of many diseases affecting children. It is certainly preferable to have endoscopies in children carried out by pediatric gastroenterologists who have specific knowledge and understanding of children's diseases. There is more availability of such specialists for the performance of the most common upper and lower GI endoscopies. In addition, there is an increasing cadre of pediatric gastroenterologists who have been trained in advanced procedures, including enteroscopy, endoscopic retrograde cholangiopancreatography, and endoscopic ultrasonography.

It has been nearly 15 years since the last issue of *Gastrointestinal Endoscopy Clinics of North America* was devoted to pediatric endoscopy, and of course, there has been tremendous progress in the field. This is remarkably well documented in this terrific issue, which offers critical basic information needed to ensure the safety and success of GI endoscopy in children, including how to set up a pediatric endoscopy unit, how to train and assess pediatric endoscopy specialists, how to properly obtain informed consent for procedures in children, and how to measure the quality of endoscopic procedures, so critical in the current era. The emphasis in children's endoscopy is different than in much of adult gastroenterology: much less relating to cancer and much more relating to congenital abnormalities, inflammatory diseases, and allergic diseases. A good example in this issue of a particular problem in young children is the proper management of button battery ingestion, a situation uncommon in adults, which requires specific understanding and is seen as a paradigm for management of severe pediatric

Gastrointest Endoscopy Clin N Am 26 (2016) xiii–xiv
http://dx.doi.org/10.1016/j.giec.2015.10.002
1052-5157/16/$ – see front matter © 2016 Published by Elsevier Inc.

giendo.theclinics.com

foreign body ingestion. Endoscopic placement of gastrostomy feeding tubes can be essential, allowing continued growth and development in seriously ill young patients. It is common for certain pediatric GI diseases to continue into adult life, and adult gastroenterologists should be interested in topics covered in this issue: eosinophilic esophagitis and small bowel imaging in celiac disease and inflammatory bowel disease.

From a personal perspective, this is an extraordinarily special issue of the *Gastrointestinal Endoscopy Clinics of North America*. You might blink a few times when you see the cover, since the name Lightdale appears twice. You are not seeing double. There was no doubt in my mind that my daughter, Dr Jenifer R. Lightdale, should be the editor of this issue. Much to my delight, she has become a widely recognized leader in the field of pediatric endoscopy and has selected the topics and the outstanding authors for this remarkable issue. I believe there was a critical tipping point during her pediatric residency, when I invited her to accompany me on a trip to Japan. There, we had the opportunity to witness the actual hand manufacture of endoscopes and some spectacular new endoscopic procedures. It wasn't long after that trip when Jen amazed me by joining a fellowship program in pediatric gastroenterology, and she continues to amaze me at all she has accomplished and continues to do. Every pediatric gastroenterologist should read this timely issue. Needless to say, it has my strongest recommendation for everyone interested in the field.

Charles J. Lightdale, MD
Department of Medicine
Columbia University Medical Center
161 Fort Washington Avenue
New York, NY 10032, USA

E-mail address:
CJL18@columbia.edu

Preface

Pediatric Endoscopy

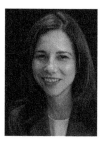

Jenifer R. Lightdale, MD, MPH
Editor

My father and I have been frequent visitors to the US Open Tennis tournament in New York City since the early 1980s, when the women's championship was festooned by the Virginia Slims slogan, "You've come a long way, baby." Times have changed; cigarette companies no longer sponsor professional sports, and I now call Boston home. But the certainly dated slogan has always stuck with me. And as I contemplate the current state of pediatric endoscopy, its sentiment seems wildly appropriate.

Pediatric endoscopy has indeed come a long way since the early 1980s, when reports of its feasibility and diagnostic potential were just emerging from a few small centers. In 2016, gastrointestinal endoscopy is a fundamental component of health care for infants and children. Both upper and lower procedures are regularly performed, for elective and urgent indications, by thousands of certified pediatric endoscopists, in family-friendly environments specifically designed to ensure patient safety of children during endoscopy, as well as procedural quality and efficiency.

Every day, worldwide, thousands of parents provide informed consent for pediatric endoscopists to help diagnose or treat their children's digestive disorders. These include congenital conditions of the gastrointestinal tract, such as biliary atresia and tracheoesophageal fistula, as well as disorders characterized by mucosal inflammation, including celiac disease, inflammatory bowel disease, and eosinophilic esophagitis. Unfortunately, many digestive diseases in children are not rare, and it has become an imperative for medical providers to recognize indications for referral. Just as critical may be timely recognition by pediatric gastroenterologists of indications for performing endoscopic procedures, which may be invaluable in helping children to thrive, and even saving lives.

I feel extremely fortunate to have assembled an impressive and passionate group of colleagues to provide this comprehensive review of important, current topics in pediatric endoscopy. Many are first-time authors for the *Gastrointestinal Endoscopy Clinics of North America*, signifying a new generation of experts. A bird's-eye view of the list of articles demonstrates broad contributions from across North America, while also

Gastrointest Endoscopy Clin N Am 26 (2016) xv–xvi
http://dx.doi.org/10.1016/j.giec.2015.10.001
1052-5157/16/$ – see front matter © 2016 Published by Elsevier Inc.

giendo.theclinics.com

attesting to the increasing access that children have to advanced endoscopic procedures, should they require them. Fortunately, fewer children have conditions that call for the most technically advanced procedures, including deep enteroscopy, endoscopic ultrasound, and endoscopic retrograde cholangiopancreatography, leaving us still much to learn about how best to ensure their quality of care. Future studies in pediatric endoscopy will undoubtedly reflect rigorous design and big data across multicenters. We've come a long way, but we still have a ways to go.

I would like to thank all of the authors for their outstanding contributions to this issue of *Gastrointestinal Endoscopy Clinics of North America*, as well as Kerry Holland and Donald Mumford from Elsevier for their careful assistance and infinite patience in assembling it. Finally, I want to thank my father for believing that I have come far enough to take on the honor of editing it, as well as for always being willing to mentor and brainstorm, with love, about where I might go next.

Jenifer R. Lightdale, MD, MPH
Pediatric Gastroenterology and Hepatology
UMass Memorial Children's Medical Center
University of Massachusetts Medical School
55 Lake Street North
Worcester, MA 01655, USA

E-mail address:
jenifer.lightdale@umassmemorial.org

Setting up the Pediatric Endoscopy Unit

Diana G. Lerner, MD[a], Harpreet Pall, MD[b],*

KEYWORDS

- Pediatric endoscopy • Staff • Design • Equipment

KEY POINTS

- Gastrointestinal endoscopy in children can be performed in a variety of settings, but each should ensure a child-friendly design and pediatric-trained staff.
- Determining the capacity for a pediatric endoscopy suite depends on unit efficiencies such as procedure and turnover times.
- Having some flexibility in the unit's schedule can help accommodate more urgent cases and lead to better patient satisfaction.
- Endoscopies are performed in children of all ages and sizes and the pediatric endoscopy suite should stock appropriate equipment sizes to accommodate all patients.
- Data from 18 centers around the country are summarized to help guide design, operational, and equipment management decisions.

INTRODUCTION

As pediatric gastrointestinal endoscopy continues to develop and evolve, pediatric gastroenterologists are more frequently called on to develop and direct a dedicated pediatric endoscopy unit. Lack of published literature and focused training in fellowship has rendered decision making around procedural unit design, operation, equipment purchasing, and staffing challenging.

To help guide management decisions, we distributed a short survey to 18 pediatric gastroenterology (GI) centers throughout the United States and Canada. The survey was sent to members of the North American Society of Pediatric Gastroenterology Hepatology and Nutrition Endoscopy and Clinical Practice Committee. Eighteen

Disclosures: The authors have nothing to disclose.
[a] Section of Gastroenterology, Hepatology, and Nutrition, Department of Pediatrics, Medical College of Wisconsin, 8701 West Watertown Plank Road, Milwaukee, WI 53226, USA;
[b] Section of Gastroenterology, Hepatology, and Nutrition, St. Christopher's Hospital for Children, Department of Pediatrics, Drexel University College of Medicine, 160 East Erie Avenue, Philadelphia, PA 19134, USA
* Corresponding author.
E-mail address: harpreet.pall@drexelmed.edu

Gastrointest Endoscopy Clin N Am 26 (2016) 1–12
http://dx.doi.org/10.1016/j.giec.2015.08.008
1052-5157/16/$ – see front matter © 2016 Elsevier Inc. All rights reserved.

members from unique programs responded. Sixty-six percent of the respondents described themselves as performing procedures in centers that also trained pediatric GI fellows. In turn, responses to the survey were representative of both academic and community-based units, contributing to our intention to provide practical information that may be of help to those responsible for setting up and managing pediatric endoscopy units.

UNIT DESIGN

Pediatric endoscopy procedures are currently performed in a variety of settings, including general operating rooms (ORs), procedure/sedation rooms, dedicated endoscopy suites, and stand-alone surgical centers (**Fig. 1**). Some design elements should be incorporated regardless of location. In particular, all settings where pediatric endoscopy is performed should aim to provide a calming atmosphere. Less preprocedure anxiety in children has been shown to decrease postoperative pain and increase satisfaction scores.[1] Achieving a calming atmosphere can be accomplished by creating a play area for both younger and older children, with a variety of age-appropriate entertainment, including gaming systems, books, children's furniture, toys, and TV screens with child-appropriate programming.

The layout of all types of units should ideally feature a physical and obvious separation between the check-in/waiting area and the clinical and procedural areas in terms of design and feel. Patients and medical staff movement should be directed so as to limit encounters of preprocedure with postprocedure patients. Design of patient flow is crucial to envision before building the unit. Expected duration of time that patients will spend in the most relaxing and family-centered environments should be maximized. Facilities should offer easily accessible and private bathrooms at all stages of the procedure, as well as a refreshments station for parents, who are likely

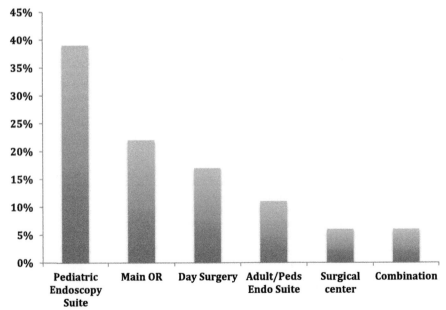

Fig. 1. Endoscopy unit design reported by surveyed pediatric endoscopy centers. Endo, endoscopy; Peds, pediatric.

to spend most of their time in the waiting area. One more recent option has featured patient monitoring screens, which allow family members to stay updated on the patient's progress while in surgery.

There are clear benefits and drawbacks for various models of endoscopy settings. For example, a combined adult/pediatric unit can offer cost savings in terms of equipment and facilities, as well as close proximity for pediatric endoscopists to therapeutic endoscopists performing procedures in adults. However, this model may lack in the pediatric-specific design and pediatric-trained nursing staff.

Results of our survey suggest that 40% of centers currently perform procedures in a dedicated pediatric endoscopy suite. The rooms can be customized for endoscopic procedures and equipment reprocessing. In addition, the unit can include a pediatric-specific motility suite, capsule endoscopy viewing room, and an advanced endoscopy room for fluoroscopic procedures.

To save space and costs, some centers have opted to have their pediatric endoscopy unit function within the broader practice of a multispecialty day surgery department within a hospital. Staffing of day surgery centers, although vital for GI procedures, involves a profit loss because staff cannot be billed directly. This model can allow departments to share the cost associated with using waiting room and recovery staff. At present, outpatient centers and open center endoscopy models are popular in adult GI practice, but are not commonly used in pediatrics. This model likely offers high efficiency throughput because of limited delays often associated with inpatients, trainees, and emergent cases. To make this model profitable for a pediatric group, it needs to be a high volume or be shared with other subspecialties. In contrast, sharing space with other subspecialties may also decrease the potential to customize rooms for endoscopy and may present limitations for procedure scheduling and expansion options.

GENERAL ENDOSCOPY UNIT AREAS

All endoscopy units are required to meet the same periprocedural needs of patients and staff, and should have areas that are dedicated to specific parts of the procedure. In particular, all units should have a clear reception and waiting room, where patients are greeted when they first arrive for a procedure. Once escorted into the unit, patients require a clear area to be prepared for the procedure. This space needs to be appropriate for private examination. It is common to have a television with child programming in the room as well as a computer for accessing the electronic medical records. From this area the patient is transferred directly to a procedure room. After the procedure, a dedicated area for immediate and/or final recovery is needed, whereas a separate, private space for consultation with parents is desirable. Some facilities may choose to play easy-listening music in this area. To facilitate efficient procedures, an area for cleaning and reprocessing of endoscopes is necessary, as well as dedicated space for endoscope storage. In addition, if staff members are to be comfortable, dedicated changing rooms and specific spaces for conferences as well as breaks should be made available. Allocating offices for unit leaders, including the medical endoscopy director and/or the nurse manager, allows them to work throughout the day and be easily accessible to unit staff.

UNIT SIZE AND CAPACITY

An endoscopy suite with a minimum of 2 endoscopy rooms is preferable if at least 2 endoscopists will be performing procedures. Two rooms allow for concurrent examinations and the ability to perform emergent procedures. Three endoscopy rooms are recommended if the goal is to perform 3000 or more procedures per year. Adult teaching hospitals are generally expected to do 1000 endoscopic procedures per room per year.[2] A nonteaching institution generally aims to be 30% to 40% more productive, and may set as a goal 1300 to 1500 procedures per room per year.[3] Plans for designing a pediatric endoscopy unit should originate with anticipated volume, procedural complexity and growth of the unit over time. Mulder et al. have proposed equations to estimate the daily projected volume (DV), room capacity (RC) and number of endoscopy rooms needed (ER)

Daily Projected Volume (DV) = (annual projected volume ÷ working days per year)

RC = number of working hours ÷ (average procedure time + turnabout time)

ER Needed = DV ÷ (RC) × 0.7 (activity factor)

Based on our survey, including turnover time, an esophagogastroduodenoscopy (EGD) is on average allocated 43 minutes, colonoscopy 58 minutes, and the two procedures combined 76 minutes (**Fig. 2**). It is important to recognize that an endoscopy unit should not target 100% efficiency, because this leads to less patient satisfaction and more scheduling conflicts.[4] Instead, standard efficiency rates should be considered to be 70% to 85%.[5,6] The suggested procedure times can be multiplied by the efficiency factor (0.7–0.85) to estimate yearly procedure volumes. It may be important to discuss this point with administrators when considering more OR time or space planning.

In pediatric endoscopy, turnover time, or the room time between procedures, clearly varies from center to center. In our survey, most respondents reported turning over a room in 16 to 20 minutes, with 1 center reporting an average turnover time of more than 30 minutes (**Fig. 3**). Optimizing turnover time should be a target for quality improvement initiatives because it has direct impact on unit productivity.

REPROCESSING

A major decision that must be made regarding any space used for pediatric endoscopy is where and how endoscopes will be reprocessed between cases. High Level

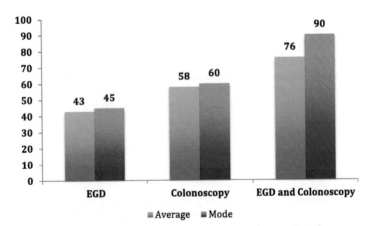

Fig. 2. Percentage of pediatric endoscopy centers surveyed reporting the average scheduling time including turnover time in minutes for EGD, colonoscopy, and EGD/colonoscopy.

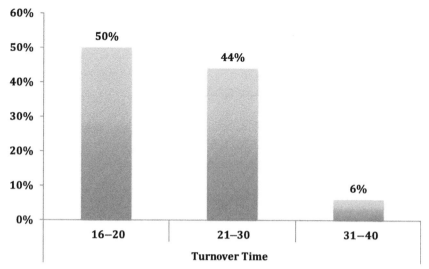

Fig. 3. Percentage of pediatric endoscopy centers surveyed reporting turnover time (minutes) after endoscopy procedures.

Disinfection (HLD) is considered the standard of care for flexible endoscopes and is defined as a 106 reduction in bacteria. In general, the risk of infection from cross-contamination between patients is estimated to be very low at 1 in 1.8 million.[7,8] However, cross-contamination between patients undergoing endoscopic procedures may be underreported. Endoscopy staff should be well trained in disinfection procedures and skills should be assessed on an annual basis. Step-by-step guidelines on appropriate scope disinfection can be found in the multi-society guidelines published in 2011.[9] To improve adherence to protocols, all technicians and nurses should receive training. Scope processing can be manual or automated. There are benefits and drawbacks to both, which are further discussed in **Table 1**.[7,10]

General principles of scope disinfection include the need to perform bedside cleaning and aspiration of enzymatic detergent, as well as subsequent manual washing and brushing of accessible channels in a dedicated "dirty utility room" space. Scopes will also require disinfection, including rinsing and alcohol flush. They will then need appropriate space to dry and to be stored.

There are many different commercially available automated flexible endoscope reprocessors. In turn, there are a number of potential questions to ask prior to purchasing a reprocessor beyond cost (**Box 1**). The American Society of Gastrointestinal

Table 1	
Benefits and drawbacks of automatic endoscope reprocessors	
Benefits	**Drawbacks**
• Limit chemical exposure of endoscopy staff • More consistent disinfection • Reprocess multiple endoscopes simultaneously	• Require regular maintenance • Increased cost • May increase turnaround time • Not all channels disinfected • Does not replace initial manual cleaning and flushing

---

Box 1
Potential questions to ask before purchasing an automated flexible endoscope reprocessor

- Cost
  - Initial and per procedure
  - Training
  - Accessories
  - Water filters
  - Chemical indicators
  - Liquid chemical germicide (LCG) disposal costs
- Space requirements (table top, floor standing, cart mounted)
- Any history of endoscope contamination or damage
- Model-specific options:
  - Detergent cleaning, alcohol flush, and forced-air drying cycles
  - Variable cycle times
  - LCG vapor recovery systems
  - Automated leak testing
  - Automated detection of channel obstruction
  - Documentation of reprocessing parameters
  - Number of scopes that can be reprocessed simultaneously

Endoscopy (ASGE) regularly reviews and discusses details about available models in their technical reports.[11] However, gaining an understanding of how a specific reprocessor might be integrated into a unit under design is critical to avoiding any last minute space refitting, as well as potential breaches in patient safety once procedures are being performed.

STAFFING THE ENDOSCOPY UNIT

The Society of Gastroenterology Nurses and Associates has published guidelines suggesting the minimum number of qualified personnel who should be allocated to various positions during endoscopic procedures (**Table 2**).[12,13] A qualified endoscopy assistant may be a registered nurse (RN), a licensed practical nurse (also known as a registered practical nurse in Canada), or nursing assistive personnel or technician. Each of these personnel can assist with procedures, equipment maintenance, new hire training, record keeping, and electrical safety.[14] The Nurse Practice Act of each state is a good resource to consult for determining the scope of practice of each position. This information can be found at https://www.ncsbn.org.

Based on our survey, more than 70% of centers use an endoscopy RN and an endoscopy technician in the room during the performance of each procedure, and 100% of centers use dedicated anesthesia staff (**Fig. 4**).

AFTER-HOURS COVERAGE

Plans for endoscopy room coverage should be determined for weekend and after-hour emergencies. The availability of an on-call and weekend endoscopy nurse is associated with earlier upper endoscopy for evaluation of bleeding[6] and is cost-effective for patient discharge.[15,16] Based on current survey results, 66% of centers currently have a system in which a GI technician, a dedicated GI RN, or both are available on call for all weekend and evening procedures (**Fig. 5**). This arrangement supports the endoscopist by ensuring trained personnel who can transport the endoscopy cart, set up the procedure, as well as perform bedside cleaning and/or

Table 2 Suggestions for staffing the various positions in an endoscopy suite		
Work Area	**Minimum Staff Requirements**	**Duties**
Preprocedure area	One RN per 2 patients	Patient assessment before sedation and IV start
Procedure room	One RN Extra member of endoscopy team should be present for: • Unstable patients • Pediatric patients • Complex procedures (ERCP, percutaneous endoscopic gastrostomy (PEG), emergency cases)	Monitor patient during procedure. When anesthesia provider is providing sedation, RN assists health care team
Postprocedure area	One RN per 2 patients	Patient assessment during recovery from analgesia and sedation
Reprocessing room	One appropriately trained staff member	Equipment care and disinfection
Medical staff office/ physician affairs	Medical administrator	Credentialing, privileging, maintenance/oversight of professional standards
Human resources	Nursing administrator	Nursing care plans, hiring, credentialing, privileging, training, staffing, and maintenance of competencies for nurses and other allied health staff[8]
Management	Medical director	Manage doctors and nurses, plan unit expansion and use, make financial decisions, assess equipment needs and purchasing, and oversee quality improvement activities. Should also maintain relationships with other departments, such as radiology, surgery, and pathology

Abbreviations: ERCP, endoscopic retrograde cholangiopancreatography; IV, intravenous; RN, registered nurse.

scope reprocessing. On-call staff should be cross-trained so that they are qualified to function independently in all aspects of the procedure and in all unit areas. The remaining centers report using general OR staff to help with after-hours procedures, whereas some of the training programs have required that fellows set up and take down equipment.

In our experience, it is optimal to have GI specialized staff on call because of the ever-increasing complexity of pediatric endoscopic procedures, which may include endoscopic retrograde cholangiopancreatography (ERCP), endoscopic ultrasonography (EUS), enteroscopy, variceal banding, hemostasis, and foreign body removal. Having well-trained staff reprocess endoscopic equipment could increase proper handling and prolong shelf life. If the fellows are responsible for equipment reprocessing, a formal training program and competency testing should be part of the orientation.

In institutions where after-hours endoscopy nurses are not available, the OR staff can be used to assist with urgent procedures, which means that procedures are likely

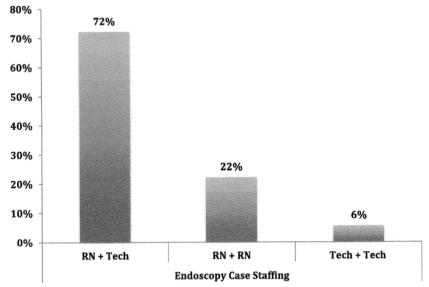

Fig. 4. Percentage of surveyed centers reporting staffing during pediatric endoscopy procedures.

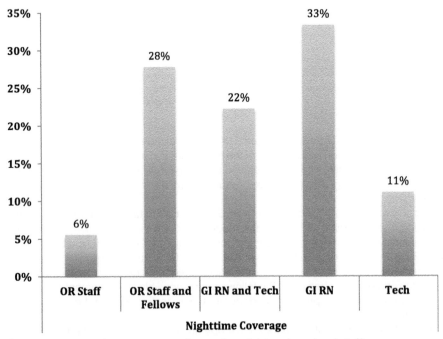

Fig. 5. Percentage of centers surveyed reporting night and weekend staff coverage.

to be performed with the assistance of nurses and/or technicians who may not be trained in endoscopic procedures. Cost, efficiency, and volumes must be considered when designing the after-hours strategy for an endoscopy unit.

EQUIPMENT

Purchasing or leasing endoscopic equipment and accessories represents a significant capital budget item for any setting in which pediatric endoscopy will be performed. There are 3 manufacturers: Olympus, Pentax, and Fujinon.[17] Comparison of the brands is beyond the scope of this article. However, there are a few factors that can help in the initial purchasing decision, including the projected number of endoscopists who are likely to be performing procedures concurrently on any given day, as well as the number of concurrent endoscopy rooms. Fewer endoscopes may be necessary to run concurrent rooms in smaller centers, compared with larger centers that feature more endoscopists and more endoscopy rooms. It may also be useful to consider scope reprocessing time, because manufacturers may differ in this regard, as well as the anticipated time required for equipment upgrades and repairs. In addition, it may be helpful to discuss anticipated endoscope equipment purchases with other groups in an institution that also uses scopes and related equipments (eg, carts, light sources), because coordinating a large purchase of equipment with other services such as otolaryngology, pulmonology, or general surgery may allow for better value in contracts around purchasing and/or technical support.

There are no data to help guide how many scopes should be on hand at any endoscopy unit. To maximize efficiency, 1 light source and processor should be available per endoscopy room and 1 scope reprocessor allocated for each 1000 procedures per year. For adult units, 1 colonoscope and gastroscope per 350 procedures per year has been suggested as ideal numbers,[12] but this general recommendation may not generalize to the practice of pediatric endoscopy, in which there may be a need for endoscopes of various insertion diameters to accommodate infants and children. This issue was evident in our survey, which suggests that smaller centers own less equipment, but relatively more scopes per endoscopist than larger centers (**Fig. 6**). The results of our survey also suggest significant variability across pediatric endoscopy centers in numbers of endoscopes purchased. Given that upper GI endoscopy is performed more commonly in children than colonoscopy, it seems logical that centers would own more upper endoscopes than lower scopes. However, as **Fig. 6** shows, the opposite finding was seen in our survey results, which may reflect the requirement of colonoscopies for more frequent upgrades or maintenance.

The frequency of anticipated endoscope upgrades is also a major factor in determining how many endoscopes should be purchased. In our survey, most centers reported replacing the endoscopes every 6 to 7 years, with the second peak at 4 to 5 years. More than 20% of centers reported only upgrading their endoscopes when they broke or needed replacement, or had no specific plan for regular equipment updates in place at the time of the survey (**Fig. 7**).

An optimal endoscopy unit offers diagnostic endoscopy, including capsule endoscopy, small bowel enteroscopy, pH impedance testing, and motility testing. Therapeutic endoscopies, including control of bleeding, percutaneous endoscopic gastrostomy tube (PEG) placement, foreign body removal, stricture management, and ERCP/EUS should be available at pediatric centers or offered by an adult gastroenterologist in the area. **Table 3** summarizes some of the equipment needed for a fully operational suite. If trained endoscopy personnel are not always available to participate in emergent cases, having specific tool kits, such as a bleeding kit or a foreign body removal kit,

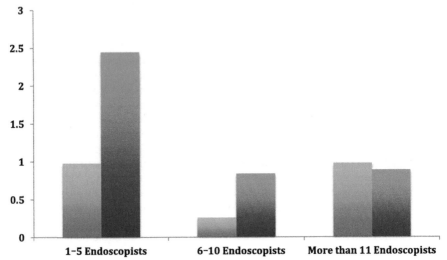

Fig. 6. Average number of upper and lower endoscopes owned by the surveyed center based by size of practice.

can ensure that the correct endoscopic accessories are available. Offering PEG tube placement would also require stocking tubes and accessories of various sizes.

SUMMARY/DISCUSSION

Well-designed pediatric endoscopy units are critical to ensuring effective diagnosis and management of gastrointestinal disorders in children. When developing an endoscopy unit for a pediatric GI group, special consideration should be made to identify a unit director. This person leads process improvement initiatives, and plays a critical

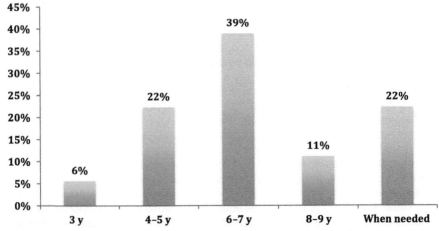

Fig. 7. Frequency of endoscope replacement reported by percentage of surveyed centers.

Table 3
Suggested equipment for an endoscopy suite

Equipment	Control of Bleeding/ Polypectomy	Foreign Body Removal/ Stricture Management
Video processor/light source	Electrosurgical generator units (±argon beam coagulator)	Graspers (rat tooth, alligator) Retrieval net
Gastroscope Neonatal, diameter 4.9–6 mm Pediatric, diameter 7.8–9 mm Adult, diameter 9–10 mm	Multipolar electrocautery probes	Overtube
Colonoscope Pediatric, diameter 9.8– 11.8 mm Adult, diameter 12–14 mm	Noncontact thermal devices/ argon plasma coagulation	McGill forceps
Enteroscope[a] Single/double balloon	Endoscopic clipping devices Through the scope Over the scope	Snare
Capsule endoscopy deployment device Sensing system with pad/belt Data recorder and battery pack Personal computer Software	Injection needles	Wire basket
ERCP[a]	Variceal band ligator	Foreign body protector hood
CO$_2$ insufflator[a]	Epinephrine	Transparent caps
EUS[a]	Hemostatic graspers[a]	Balloon dilators[a]
Manometry[a] Esophageal, antroduodenal, anorectal, colonic	Polypectomy snare	Bougie dilators[a]
Smart pill[a]	Sclerosants	Triamcinolone
pH impedence	—	Stents[a]
Endoscopy software	—	—

[a] Not available at all centers. Care must be taken to have an endoscopic partner who can offer these services to children.
Data from Refs.[11,18–22]

role in ensuring that equipment and services remain competitive. Designing and guiding the construction of a new unit can be challenging given the ever-changing frontiers in pediatric endoscopy. The survey we conducted offers valuable perspective on unit setup, equipment, and staffing by institutions of various sizes. Further research should focus on the best model of pediatric endoscopy units, operational excellence, unit efficiency, and equipment management.

REFERENCES

1. Yacavone RF, Locke GR, Gostout CJ, et al. Factors influencing patient satisfaction with GI endoscopy. Gastrointest Endosc 2001;53(7):703–10.

2. Beilenhoff U, Neumann CS. Quality assurance in endoscopy nursing. Best Pract Res Clin Gastroenterol 2011;25(3):371–85.
3. Mulder CJJ, Jacobs MAJM, Leicester RJ, et al. Guidelines for designing a digestive disease endoscopy unit: Report of the World Endoscopy Organization. Dig Endosc 2013;25(4):365–75.
4. Sonnenberg A. Waiting lines in the endoscopy unit. Gastrointest Endosc 2000; 52(4):517–24.
5. Cotton PB, Williams CB. Practical gastrointestinal endoscopy. 5th edtion. Hobeken (NJ): Wiley-Blackweel Publishing; 2008.
6. da Silveira EB, Lam E, Martel M, et al. The importance of process issues as predictors of time to endoscopy in patients with acute upper-GI bleeding using the RUGBE data. Gastrointest Endosc 2006;64(3):299–309.
7. Kovaleva J, Peters FTM, van der Mei HC, et al. Transmission of infection by flexible gastrointestinal endoscopy and bronchoscopy. Clin Microbiol Rev 2013; 26(2):231–54.
8. Kimmery MB, Burnett DA, Carr-Locke DL, et al. Transmission of infection by gastrointestinal endoscopy. Gastrointest Endosc 1993;39(6):885–8.
9. Petersen BT, Chennat J, Cohen J, et al. Multisociety guideline on reprocessing flexible GI endoscopes: 2011. Infect Control Hosp Epidemiol 2011;32(6):527–37.
10. Muscarella LF. Advantages and limitations of automatic flexible endoscope reprocessors. Am J Infect Control 1996;24(4):304–9.
11. ASGE Technology Committee, Desilets D, Kaul V, et al. Automated endoscope reprocessors. Gastrointest Endosc 2010;72(4):675–80.
12. Petersen BT, Ott B. Design and management of gastrointestinal endoscopy units. Cotton/advanced digestive endoscopy: practice and safety. Oxford (United Kingdom): Blackwell publishing, Ltd; 2009. p. 3–32.
13. Committee SP. SGNA position statement on minimal registered nurse staffing for patient care in the gastrointestinal endoscopy unit. Gastroenterol Nurs 2002; 25(6):269–70.
14. Larson DE, Ott BJ. The structure and function of the outpatient endoscopy unit. Gastrointest Endosc 1986;32(1):10–4.
15. Davies AHG, Ishaq S, Brind AM, et al. Availability of fully staffed GI endoscopy lists at the weekend for inpatients: does it make a difference? Clin Med 2003; 3(2):189–90.
16. Muthiah KC, Enns R, Armstrong D, et al. A survey of the practice of after-hours and emergency endoscopy in Canada. Can J Gastroenterol 2012;26(12):871–6.
17. ASGE Technology Committee. High-definition and high-magnification endoscopes. Gastrointest Endosc 2014;80(6):919–27.
18. ASGE Technology Committee, Tokar JL, Barth BA, et al. Electrosurgical generators. Gastrointest Endosc 2013;78(2):197–208.
19. ASGE Technology Committee, Conway JD, Adler DG, et al. Endoscopic hemostatic devices. Gastrointest Endosc 2009;69(6):987–96.
20. Cohen SA. Pediatric capsule endoscopy. Tech Gastrointest Endosc 2013;15(1): 32–5.
21. Barth BA, Banerjee S, Bhat YM, et al. Equipment for pediatric endoscopy. Gastrointest Endosc 2012;76(1):8–17.
22. ASGE Technology Committee, Siddiqui UD, Banerjee S, et al. Tools for endoscopic stricture dilation. Gastrointest Endosc 2013;78(3):391–404.

Training and Assessment in Pediatric Endoscopy

Catharine M. Walsh, MD, MEd, PhD, FAAP, FRCPC

KEYWORDS

- Endoscopy, gastrointestinal/education • Endoscopy, gastrointestinal/standards
- Endoscopy, pediatric • Clinical competence • Educational measurement
- Education, medical, graduate/standards • Patient simulation • Assessment

KEY POINTS

- Given its unique nature, training in pediatric gastrointestinal endoscopy requires an approach that is tailored to pediatric practice to ensure delivery of high-quality endoscopic care in children.
- There remains a need for a comprehensive pediatric-specific endoscopy curriculum that incorporates best evidence in procedural skills education and reflects the current competency-based model of training.
- Current evidence supports the use of endoscopy simulation–based training for novice endoscopists to help speed up the early learning curve and reduce patient burden, although pediatric-specific data are limited.
- Assessment is an essential component of pediatric endoscopy education that drives both teaching and learning.
- Structured direct observational assessment tools, such as the $GiECAT_{KIDS}$, provide a framework for teaching, facilitate feedback provision, and can be used to generate aggregate assessment data across training programs to help gauge trainees' progress toward specific competency-based milestones.

INTRODUCTION

A key aspect of pediatric gastroenterology practice is the ability to perform endoscopy procedures safely, effectively, and efficiently. Similar to adult endoscopy, performance of pediatric endoscopy requires the acquisition of related technical, cognitive, and integrative competencies to effectively diagnose and manage gastrointestinal disorders in children. However, the distinctive requirements of pediatric patients and their

Conflict of Interest: The author reports no conflicts of interest and has nothing to declare.
Division of Gastroenterology, Hepatology and Nutrition, Department of Paediatrics, The Learning Institute, The Research Institute, The Wilson Centre, Hospital for Sick Children, University of Toronto, 555 University Avenue, Room 8409, Black Wing, Toronto, Ontario M5G 1X8, Canada
E-mail address: catharine.walsh@utoronto.ca

Gastrointest Endoscopy Clin N Am 26 (2016) 13–33
http://dx.doi.org/10.1016/j.giec.2015.08.002
1052-5157/16/$ – see front matter © 2016 Elsevier Inc. All rights reserved.

families and the differential spectrum of disease highlight the need for a pediatric-specific training curriculum and assessment framework to ensure endoscopic procedures are performed safely and successfully in children. This review outlines the current state of evidence as it pertains to pediatric endoscopy training and assessment.

TRAINING

Training in pediatric gastrointestinal endoscopy largely occurs during formalized pediatric gastroenterology training programs that generally last 2 to 3 years in duration. Duty-hour restrictions and an increasing focus on patient quality, safety, and accountability have resulted in a paradigm shift across postgraduate medical education toward a competency-based system that defines desired training outcomes.[1] Resultantly, there is increasing focus on the determination of when an individual is truly competent to perform a procedure independently, how much training is required to reach this skill level, and how to optimally train.

Any practitioner wishing to perform endoscopic procedures should receive formal training in the principles and practice of safe endoscopy. To date, training in endoscopy continues to be predominantly based on the apprenticeship model with trainees learning fundamental skills under the supervision of experienced endoscopists in the clinical setting. Although adult and pediatric endoscopic practice are similar in many regards, there are key dissimilarities, such as differing procedural indications, the need for ileal intubation, and the importance of routine tissue sampling.[2] The unique nature of pediatric endoscopy dictates the need for endoscopists who wish to perform procedures on children to train under the supervision of certified pediatric endoscopists, as there is a steep learning curve even for fully trained adult endoscopists.[2]

Pediatric endoscopy training programs are obliged to ensure learners are competent to deliver high-quality endoscopic care at completion of training. To help guide and enhance training, endoscopy skills curricula have been outlined for surgical[3,4] and adult gastroenterology[5] trainees. However, there remains a need for a comprehensive pediatric-specific endoscopy curriculum that has been designed from a background of scientific research to ensure it is valid, efficient, and reflects the current competency-based training model. This section discusses a framework of procedural skill acquisition, describes commonly available training aids designed to enhance endoscopy education, and outlines the value of trainer education.

Endoscopy Skill Acquisition

The road to acquiring competency, and potentially expertise, in performing endoscopic procedures requires a combination of innate ability, dedicated trainers, and many hours of deliberate practice. With regard to procedures, skill acquisition has been described by Fitts and Posner[6] as a sequential process involving 3 major phases: cognitive, associative, and autonomous. In the *cognitive* stage, learners begin to develop a mental understanding of the procedure through instructor explanation and demonstration. Performance during this stage is often erratic and error filled. Feedback during this phase should focus on explanation of how the procedure is performed correctly and identifying common errors to increase learners' understanding of the tasks. Subsequently, in the *associative* phase, learners begin to translate the knowledge acquired in the cognitive stage into appropriate motor behaviors so that tasks are gradually executed more efficiently, with fewer errors and interruptions. Feedback is essential for learning during this stage, as has been demonstrated by the study by Mahmood and Darzi,[7] which showed no performance improvement in learners who received no feedback despite substantial training on a virtual reality colonoscopy simulator. Feedback during the cognitive stage should aim to help learners identify errors and corresponding corrective actions, as this has been shown to enhance skills acquisition within the surgical domain.[8] Finally, with ongoing practice and feedback, learners transition to the *autonomous* stage in which motor performance becomes automated such that skills are performed without significant cognitive or conscious awareness devoted to performance. Ongoing lifelong learning and practice are then required to ensure maintenance of skills.[9]

Endoscopy Training Aids

The increased focus on quality of training and patient safety has prompted educators to seek alternative methods of teaching endoscopy. Novel instructional aids are increasingly being integrated into training curricula with the aim of speeding up the learning curve, facilitating instruction, and helping to ensure trainees attain some degree of proficiency before performing real-life procedures. The following section discusses 2 commonly used aids designed to enhance endoscopy education: magnetic endoscopic imagers and simulation.

Magnetic endoscopic imagers

Magnetic endoscopic imaging is a nonradiographic technique that provides real-time 3-dimensional views of the colonoscope shaft configuration and its position within the abdomen during a procedure.[10] Imagers have been shown to be safe and beneficial for removing loops during colonoscopy in the clinical setting.[11] A recent meta-analysis of 13 randomized studies found that use of magnetic endoscopic imaging during real-life colonoscopy is associated with lower risk of procedure failure, lower patient pain scores, and shorter time to cecum compared with conventional endoscopy.[12] Regarding training, research indicates that use of an imager may enhance learners' understanding of loop formation and loop-reduction maneuvers.[13] For novice endoscopists, there has been shown to be no detrimental effects with regard to performance or workload with use of an imager during clinical training.[14] Additionally, imagers potentially allow trainers to better guide learners without having to take over the procedure. They have also been shown to potentially enhance simulation-based colonoscopy training, although research is limited.[15] Magnetic endoscopic imaging is a promising new training aide for endoscopy; however, studies to date have largely been carried out within the adult clinical context. Further research is required to establish its efficacy for pediatric endoscopy and to determine how best to maximize its effectiveness during training.

Simulation-based endoscopy training

Several factors have contributed to the shift toward incorporation of simulation into pediatric endoscopy training curricula. First, recent guidelines have encouraged the use of simulation-based training, as it is now mandated by accreditation organizations in certain jurisdictions such as the United States.[16] Second, although the "ideal" platform for training has traditionally been considered the patient, endoscopy is uniquely challenging to teach in the clinical setting, as supervisors are required to relinquish complete control of the endoscope to allow trainees to gain adequate experience. Additionally, clinical demands can limit a trainers' capacity to provide detailed instruction and feedback, and training on patients occurs through chance encounters, which may limit exposure to particular pathologies. Finally, with regard to pediatric endoscopy specifically, parents and trainers are often very protective of children; a factor that can limit case availability and training exposure.

Simulation-based training is steadily gaining grounds as a means of teaching the cognitive, technical, and integrative competencies related to pediatric endoscopy in a safe setting. The simulated setting is an optimal learning environment in many ways, as learners can build a framework of basic techniques through sustained deliberate practice in a setting in which they can make mistakes without causing patient harm. Additionally, learners can rehearse key aspects of procedures at their own pace, training can be structured to maximize learning, and errors can be allowed to progress to allow trainees to learn from their mistakes.[17] The use of simulation also permits educators to systematically vary training tasks; an instructional design feature that enhances learning.[18] Furthermore, faculty do not have to juggle teaching and clinical demands, thus creating a learner-centered educational experience.

The reasons to integrate simulation into endoscopy training are many. Additionally, it has been shown to be efficacious as a means to supplement the apprenticeship model of training for novice adult endoscopy trainees.[19,20] A systematic review of 13 randomized controlled trials (278 participants) revealed that simulation-based training, before patient-based training, enhanced novice endoscopist performance within the clinical setting as compared with untrained controls as measured by independent procedure completion, time, insertion depth, overall rating of performance, error rate, and visualization.[19] Another systematic review of 39 studies (21 randomized controlled trials, 1181 participants) found that simulation-based training, as compared with no intervention, is associated with improved patient outcomes in the clinical environment (procedure completion and major complications).[20] With regard to pediatric endoscopy, computer-based simulators have been shown to have face validity even through most models do not have pediatric-specific training cases.[21] Additionally, simulation-based training has been shown to increase pediatric endoscopic trainees' confidence and technical skills as measured by self-report.[21]

Evidence suggests that simulation-based endoscopy training is effective and learning outcomes transfer to the clinical setting; however, simply providing trainees with access to simulators does not guarantee their effective use. Educators must decide how to apply simulation-based technology to achieve optimal learning. Reviews examining principles of effective instructional design and selection of simulation modalities broadly have identified a number of best practices in simulation-based education, including feedback, repetitive practice, distributed practice, mastery learning, interactivity, and range of difficulty.[18,22–24] As mentioned, feedback is a major motivator for leaners and one of the most crucial determinants in ensuring successful procedural mastery within both the clinical and simulated settings.[23,24] The simulated setting provides an optimal environment for feedback provision, as learners can work through errors independently and feedback can be structured to enhance learning without compromising patient safety. For example, our educational research team has found that the timing of feedback provision is an important factor influencing skill acquisition in novice endoscopists in the simulated setting.[25] Terminal feedback that is given at task completion is more effective as compared with feedback given during task performance, because constant feedback may lead to an overreliance on feedback and suboptimal learning.[25] Concerns for patient safety do not permit use of terminal feedback within the clinical setting, pointing to the idea that simulation technology allows educators to use strategies shown to enhance learning, such as terminal feedback, which are not possible to use when teaching in the clinical setting.

Recent research has begun to assess characteristics of curriculum design and instruction required to enhance acquisition of broader endoscopic competencies, such as cognitive and integrative skills. A recently published study by Grover and colleagues[26] provides validity evidence for a structured comprehensive curriculum consisting of 6 hours of didactic lectures interlaced with 8 hours of virtual reality simulation-based training with expert feedback.[26] The curriculum improved technical, cognitive, and integrative skill acquisition for novice endoscopists and skill transfer to the clinical environment, as compared with self-regulated learning on simulators.[26] Building on this work, Grover and colleagues[27] found that a simulation-based training curriculum of progressive fidelity and task complexity improves colonoscopy skill acquisition and transfer to the clinical setting as compared with a curriculum using high-fidelity simulation in isolation. This finding is commensurate with the challenge point framework, which postulates that learners must be appropriately challenged for optimal and efficient learning to occur.[28] Learning is postulated to be enhanced when task difficulty is matched to a trainees' skill level and progressively increased as the individual acquires new skills to continually challenge them in an optimal manner. Additionally, the results provide support for the idea that less expensive, part-task simulators may be more appropriate for teaching very basic skills, as the information content of virtual reality simulators may impede novice learning by overwhelming learners' cognitive capacities.[28]

Based on current evidence, endoscopy simulation has been shown to be useful in the early training phase in helping to speed up trainees' learning curve and reduce patient burden, although pediatric-specific data are limited. To date, simulation has primarily been examined as a means to train novice endoscopists. An evidence base needs to be further developed with respect to optimal use of simulation for nontechnical skills training and more advanced endoscopic skills. Specifically, studies are needed that assess the use of simulation to teach higher-level competencies, such as crisis management, that require the integration of both technical and nontechnical skills for successful management.

Training the Pediatric Endoscopy Trainer

Effective endoscopy instruction requires the skillful application of evidence-based educational principles. There is increasing recognition that training should be provided by individuals with the skills and behaviors required to teach endoscopy, including an awareness of principles of adult education, best practices in procedural skills education, and appropriate use of beneficial educational strategies (eg, feedback).[29] The ability to teach endoscopy is an important skill that can be improved with instruction. "Train the trainer" courses have been developed to heighten trainers' awareness with regard to educational approaches that can be used to enhance endoscopy teaching. These courses are now mandatory for adult gastroenterology endoscopy trainers in the United Kingdom and are increasingly being implemented across other jurisdictions, such as Canada. Pediatric gastroenterology societies should strongly consider adapting the content of "train the trainer" courses to pediatric endoscopy practice.

ASSESSMENT

Endoscopic procedures are an integral component of pediatric gastroenterology practice, and training programs strive to ensure learners are competent to perform procedures independently at completion of training. Assessment is required to support training and subsequent practice to optimize learners' and practitioners' capabilities through the provision of motivation and direction for future learning, to ensure competency before performing procedures independently (ie, certification), and to protect society from substandard care.[30] The unique nature of pediatric endoscopy highlights the need for an assessment approach tailored to pediatric endoscopy practice and the use of pediatric-specific assessment methods and measures. The subsequent section examines how endoscopic competence is conceptualized, outlines the importance of integrating assessment throughout the endoscopy learning cycle, and discusses currently available assessment methods and measures for pediatric endoscopy.

Endoscopic Competence

Endoscopic competence has been defined as the minimum level of skill, knowledge, and/or expertise, derived through training and experience, required to safely and proficiently perform a task or procedure.[31] Skills required to perform endoscopic procedures have traditionally been classified into 2 skill domains: technical and cognitive. Examples of technical or psychomotor skills include strategies for scope advancement (eg, torque steering) and loop-reduction techniques.[32,33] Cognitive competencies are reflective of knowledge and the application of endoscopically derived information to clinical practice. Examples include knowledge of procedural indications and contraindications, equipment selection, and pathology identification.[32,33]

In addition to technical and cognitive competencies, there are nontechnical skills that are required to perform endoscopic procedures safely and proficiently that are outlined explicitly within general competency-based frameworks from accreditation bodies such as the Accreditation Council of Graduate Medical Education in the United States[34] and the Royal College of Physicians and Surgeons of Canada.[35] Additionally, the importance of assessing nontechnical skills is recognized by pediatric gastroenterology-focused organizations such as the North American Society for Pediatric Gastroenterology, Hepatology, and Nutrition (NASPGHAN).[33] Although no studies have investigated the role of nontechnical skills within the pediatric context specifically, literature from adult practice suggests they play a central role in high-quality care. For example, the vast majority of recommendations stemming from a report by the National Confidential Enquiry into Patient Outcomes and Death,[36] which investigated deaths occurring within 30 days of therapeutic endoscopy procedures in the United Kingdom, highlight failings in nontechnical skills, such as communication and teamwork, as opposed to technical skills.

A well-defined understanding of the competencies required to carry out pediatric endoscopic procedures is fundamental to the development of an assessment framework. The literature highlights that technical and cognitive skills are necessary but not sufficient to ensure acquisition and maintenance of competency in gastrointestinal endoscopy. Nontechnical skills are an integral facet of competent endoscopic practice and an important contributor to patient safety and clinical outcomes. It has, therefore, been proposed that endoscopic competence should be conceptualized as encompassing 3 core competency domains: technical, cognitive, and integrative competencies (**Table 1**).[37] Integrative competencies are defined as higher-level competencies required to perform an endoscopic procedure that complement an individual's technical skills and clinical knowledge to facilitate effective delivery of safe and effective care in varied contexts.[38] Examples of integrative competencies include teamwork and professionalism. Reflective of this framework of endoscopic competence, assessment methods and measures should ideally reflect the full scope of technical, cognitive and integrative competencies required to perform pediatric endoscopic procedures.

Intent of Assessment: Formative Versus Summative

From an educational perspective, assessment can be broadly classified as formative or summative. Formative assessment is process focused. It aims to provide trainees with informative, timely feedback and benchmarks to enable leaners to reflect on their

Table 1
Examples of technical, cognitive, and integrative competencies required for performance of endoscopic procedures

Competency Domain	Example Skills
Technical	• Correct hand position to hold scope • Use of scope controls • Torque steering • Tip control • External pressure • Withdrawal • Visualization of mucosa
Cognitive	• Anatomy • Pathology identification • Principles for safe sedation and monitoring • Procedural indications and risks • Equipment selection
Integrative	• Communication • Team work • Situational awareness • Professionalism • Patient safety awareness • Interpretation and management of findings • Patient education

performance and guide future learning to foster their progress from novice to competent (and beyond).[30,39] Summative assessment, alternatively, is outcome focused. It aims to produce an overall judgment to determine competence, readiness for independent practice or qualification for advancement, and, therefore, must have sufficient psychometric rigor.[30] Although summative assessment provides professional self-regulation and accountability, it may not provide adequate feedback to direct learning.[30,40] Assessment must be an ongoing process throughout the endoscopy learning cycle, from training to accreditation to independent practice, and thoughtful integration of both formative and summative assessment is essential to simultaneously optimize the learning and certification functions of assessment (**Table 2**).

Table 2
Framework for the integration of assessment throughout the endoscopy learning cycle from training to independent practice

Stage of Learning	Assessment Goals	Assessment Type
Training or retraining	• Monitor progress • Provision of focused feedback • Optimize learning capabilities • Enhance motivation • Guide instruction	Formative
Accreditation (certification)	• Establish competence	Summative
Independent practice	• Quality improvement • Ensure maintenance of competence (recertification) • Ensure provision of high-quality patient care	Formative Summative

Assessment Aims

The Miller pyramid provides a framework that can be used to help guide selection of assessment methods to target specific facets of clinical competence, including "knows," "knows how," "shows how," and "does."[41] This framework, which moves from a focus on learner's cognition at the lower end of the pyramid and toward a focus on learner's behaviors, has heightened educators' awareness that competence can and should be evaluated at multiple levels. It also highlights the importance of assessments conducted in the authentic clinical environment. **Table 3** outlines each of the 4 levels of the Miller pyramid matched to assessment methods of relevance to pediatric endoscopy.

Current State of Assessment of Pediatric Endoscopy

Over the past 2 decades, we have seen a profound shift in training as a result of several factors, including an increased focus on learner centeredness, quality, outcomes, and accountability. Postgraduate medical education has shifted from a process-based framework that delineates the time required to "learn" specified content (eg, 3-year gastroenterology fellowship) to a competency-based model that defines desired training outcomes (eg, perform upper and lower endoscopic evaluation of the luminal gastrointestinal tract for screening, diagnosis, and intervention[42]) that are organized around competencies derived from an analysis of societal and patient needs.[43–45] Assessment is an integral component of competency-based education, as it is required to monitor progression throughout training, document trainees' competence before entering unsupervised practice, and ensure maintenance of competence. Despite the shift toward competency-based assessment and training, procedural assessment in pediatric gastroenterology still focuses predominately on the number of procedures and a "gestalt" view of the supervising physician.[46] This type of informal global assessment is fraught with bias inherent to subjective assessment and is not designed to aid in the early identification of trainees requiring remediation. To support high-quality pediatric endoscopic care, assessment is required to monitor learners' progress, provide focused and informative feedback, document competency to practice, ensure practitioners maintain competence, and monitor

Table 3
Relationship between the Miller pyramid[41] and potential methods of assessment of pediatric endoscopy skills

Level of Miller Pyramid		Assessment Construct	Assessment Approach
Professional authenticity	Does	Knowledge, skills, and attitudes integrated into context	Performance integrated into practice (eg, direct observation, practice portfolio, workplace-based assessments, narratives)
	Shows how	Integrated knowledge, skills, and attitudes	Demonstration of learning (eg, simulation, standardized patient-based tests, objective structured clinical examination)
	Knows how	Applied knowledge	Interpretation and/or application (eg, problem-based scenarios, extended matching, case-based multiple-choice questions)
	Knows	Knowledge	Fact gathering (eg, multiple-choice questions, short answers)

training quality. Assessment methods and measures that are commonly used in the context of pediatric colonoscopy and upper endoscopy procedures are reviewed later in this article.

Procedural numbers

Within the traditional apprenticeship model of training, the number of endoscopic procedures performed under supervision sufficed as a surrogate for demonstration of competent performance.[47–49] However, research on adult endoscopists has shown that there is wide variation in the rate at which trainees acquire skills.[50,51] Furthermore, in addition to procedural volume, there are many other factors that affect skill acquisition, including training intensity,[50] presence of disruptions in training,[52] use of training aids (eg, simulation[19,20]), quality of teaching and feedback received, and a trainees' innate ability.[53] Procedural number requirements, therefore, do not ensure competence. Additionally, the accuracy and objectivity of logbooks, which have been traditionally used by endoscopists to record their experience, has been questioned.[54,55] Logbooks also do not provide learners and educators with specific information about the nature of learning achieved.

Reflective of these concerns, current pediatric credentialing guidelines outline "competency thresholds," as opposed to absolute procedural number requirements that ensure attainment of competence. A "competence threshold" is the minimum recommended number of supervised procedures a trainee is required to perform before competence can be assessed.[56] As seen in **Table 4**, there is variability with regard to current credentialing guidelines that outline competence thresholds for pediatric upper endoscopy and colonoscopy. Guidelines for upper endoscopy are principally based on expert opinion due to the lack of high-quality data. Two adult studies have examined competency in upper endoscopy. Cass and colleagues[47] demonstrated an 80% success rate of esophageal intubation after 100 procedures, whereas Vassiliou and colleagues[57] concluded that 50 procedures are required to achieve a plateau in skills as measured using the Global Assessment of Gastrointestinal Endoscopic Skills tool.

There is a paucity of literature with regard to endoscopic skill learning curves among pediatric endoscopists; therefore, current guidelines for colonoscopy have largely been extrapolated from adult data. Current guidelines are principally based on the study by Cass and colleagues[58] that assessed 135 adult gastroenterology trainees from 14 programs and showed it took, on average, 140 colonoscopies to achieve a 90% cecal intubation rate. More recent studies that have attempted to validate adult procedural volume recommendations indicate that published requirements may significantly underestimate the amount of training required to achieve competence.[59] Two recent studies, involving 41 and 93 trainees, found that competency thresholds were achieved, on average, by 275 and 250 procedures when using criteria including cecal intubation rate, time to intubation, and competency benchmarks on the Mayo Colonoscopy Skills Assessment Tool[60] and the newer Assessment of Competency in Endoscopy[61] tool, respectively. However, it took upwards of 400 procedures for some trainees to achieve competence. The largest study to date that prospectively analyzed 297 trainees over 1 year in the United Kingdom found that it took, on average, 233 colonoscopies to achieve a 90% cecal intubation rate.[50] Additionally, a regression analysis of 10 adult studies, including 189 trainees, estimated 341 colonoscopies are required to achieve a 90% cecal intubation rate.[62]

Further research is required to help clearly delineate appropriate competence thresholds for both pediatric colonoscopy and upper endoscopy. However, as mentioned, pediatric endoscopy training guidelines (see **Table 4**) emphasize

Table 4
Training requirement recommendations from pediatric endoscopy professional organizations

Organization	Country	Colonoscopy		Upper Endoscopy	
		Minimum No. of Cases	Other Training Requirements	Minimum No. of Cases	Other Training Requirements
North American Society for Pediatric Gastroenterology, Hepatology, and Nutrition[33]	North America	120	• Cecal intubation rate: ≥90% • 10 snare polypectomies	100	• 10 foreign body removals • 15 with control of bleeding (variceal or nonvariceal) with various methods[b] and/or colonoscopy with control of bleeding
Joint Advisory Group Pediatric Certification (BSPGHAN Endoscopy Working Group)[64]	United Kingdom	100	• Terminal ileal intubation rate: >60% • Cecal intubation rate: >90% • Formative DOPS: >90% 3s and 4s (>10 DOPS assessments) • Serious complications: <0.5%[a] • Completed "Basic Skills Course Lower GI Endoscopy" • Summative assessment (≥2 assessors, ≥2 procedures)	100	• D2 intubation rate: >95% • Retroflexion rate: >95% • Unassisted physically: >95% • Formative DOPS: >90% 3s and 4s (minimum 10 DOPS) • Completed "Basic Skills Course in Upper GI Endoscopy" • Summative assessment (≥2 assessors, ≥2 procedures)
Conjoint Committee[119]	Australia	100	• To the cecum (ileum preferable) • Cecal intubation rate: >90% excluding patients with severe colitis (preferably ileum) • ≥75 in pediatric patients under supervision of recognized pediatric supervisor • Some polypectomy experience	200	• Unassisted, complete examination • ≥100 in pediatric patients under supervision of recognized pediatric supervisor • ≥10 therapeutic procedures of which ≥5 involve control of upper GI hemorrhage

Abbreviations: DOPS, Direct Observation of Procedure or Skills; GI, gastrointestinal.

[a] Serious complications defined as death, perforation, significant bleeding requiring a two or more unit transfusion, unplanned post-procedure hospital stay of over 24 hours (related to the procedure) or admission to hospital due to a complication of the procedure following discharge from the endoscopy Unit.

[b] Methods to control bleeding may include injection, band ligation, electrocautery (eg, heater probe, multipolar probe, argon plasma coagulator, loop application, hemostatic clips), or additional methods as they become available.

procedural numbers as "competence thresholds"; promoting the idea that numbers in isolation do not guarantee competence. The question still remains: how can we best assess learning and performance to determine when a trainee displays clinical performance commensurate with competent, independent practice?

Tools for Assessment

Assessment is reliant on the existence of tools and measures that are reliable and valid. Reliability is a measure of the consistency or reproducibility of assessment data or scores.[63] The validity of a test reflects the degree to which an assessment measures what it is purported to measure.[63] The following section outlines tools that can be used to aid in the assessment of endoscopic competence. Ultimately, competence is best assessed using objective criteria such as quality metrics and direct observation of performance, an idea supported by pediatric gastroenterology-focused organizations such as NASPGHAN[33] and the Joint Advisory Group on gastrointestinal endoscopy.[64]

Written knowledge tests

Knowledge relevant to endoscopy (eg, anatomy, scope selection) is essential to the development of clinical competence and should be tested alongside other competency domains. With regard to adult endoscopy, the Fundamentals of Endoscopic Surgery Program developed by Society for Endoscopic and Gastrointestinal Surgeons uses a multiple-choice examination to assess cognitive knowledge.[65] Additionally, in the United Kingdom, assessment of colonoscopy-specific knowledge is part of the accreditation process for the UK Bowel Cancer Screening Program.[66]

The core cognitive skills underpinning safe pediatric endoscopy practice have been outlined by organizations such as NASPGHAN[33]; however, corresponding assessments with good reliability and validity evidence have yet to be formally developed for pediatric endoscopy. There are many ways of assessing knowledge, such as multiple-choice or short-answer questions (see **Table 3**). However, for cognitive skills, educational best practice supports the use of assessments that test trainees' ability to apply knowledge to problem solving or clinical reasoning in specific clinical contexts at the "knows how" level of the Miller pyramid.[41,67] For example, testing pathology recognition skills through the use of clinical vignettes linked with images or videos.

Simulation-based assessment

Simulation technology is increasingly being integrated into medical education as a means to assess performance across a variety of domains[68]; however, the validity evidence for simulation-based assessment of endoscopic skills remains limited.[68,69] Simulation-based assessments are attractive to educators, as they offer a proxy for clinical observations and are capable of providing objective, reproducible assessments at the "shows-how" level of the Miller pyramid.[41] Simulation allows for standardization of scenarios, anatomy, and pathology across trainees. The controlled nature of the simulated learning environment also permits assessment of trainees as they perform tasks independently in a risk-free environment, thus removing considerations of patient safety. Additionally, simulation enables assessment of integrative (nontechnical) competencies, such as situational awareness and teamwork. For example, through use of an endoscopy-based Integrated Procedural Performance Instrument[70] format assessment scenario, during which a learner is assessed performing a simulated endoscopy procedure while interacting with team members (eg, endoscopic assistant, anesthesiologist) and an actor portraying a patient in a naturalistic setting.

Although simulation-based assessment of endoscopic competence is an attractive idea, before widespread implementation, more research is required to ensure assessments can reliably distinguish individuals with a range of levels of endoscopic skill and can accurately predict performance within the clinical setting.[71] Simulator metrics, motion analysis, and direct observational assessment tools are commonly used to assess simulated endoscopy performance.[72] High-fidelity virtual reality simulators typically provide learners with objective computer-generated performance metrics, such as completion time and patient discomfort.[73] However, research assessing the validity evidence of these measures has yet to demonstrate that they are capable of meaningfully discriminating between endoscopists across skill levels.[74–86] Metrics generated from tasks performed on part-task endoscopy simulators that reflect speed and precision also are being studied as a potential tool to assess technical skills[87,88]; however, further validity evidence is required before widespread adoption. Assessments based on motion analysis aim to quantify performance using parameters produced by motion-tracking hardware and/or software that are extracted from movements of an endoscopists' hands and/or procedural instrument(s) (eg, path length).[89] Research to date is limited and further validity evidence of the technology as an assessment tool within the simulated and/or clinical setting must be gathered before implementation.[90–94] Direct observational assessment tools depend on an external rater who scores learners using predefined criteria that are built around an assessment framework (see the section "Direct observational assessment tools," later in this article). Such assessments are advantageous, as compared with simulator-generated metrics and motion analysis, because they are capable of providing trainees with informative feedback. To date, however, no studies have been carried out to examine reliability and validity evidence of a direct observational tool for simulated pediatric endoscopy.

Endoscopic simulation has recently been integrated into the board-certification process for general surgery in the United States through the Fundamentals of Endoscopic Surgery Program.[95] The performance-based manual skills assessment is composed of 5 individual tasks on a virtual reality simulator designed to assess fundamental technical skills.[95] The hands-on component has good test-retest reliability and scores have been shown to vary across skill levels (discriminative validity).[95] Scores also correlate moderately with clinical colonoscopy performance; however, assessors were not blinded to the endoscopists' skill level.[96] Although this is a promising first step in the application of simulation to the assessment of endoscopic skills, additional research is still required to determine whether passing scores are a reliable and valid marker of competency in performing endoscopy within the clinical setting. Reliability and validity evidence of the assessment in the context of pediatric endoscopy has not been assessed.

Quality metrics in pediatric endoscopy
In line with the current health care systems' focus on delivery of effective, safe, equitable, and high-quality care, current pediatric endoscopy credentialing guidelines emphasize the importance of using evidence-based endoscopy quality metrics to help determine competency. Endoscopy training programs are increasingly requiring learners to monitor quality measures, such as independent terminal ileal intubation rate and patient comfort, so that they can be used as part of a summative assessment of trainees. Additionally, quality metrics are being used by practicing endoscopists as a formative assessment tool to help promote improvement in care delivery. Although quality metrics reflect trainees' performance at the "does" level of the Miller pyramid[41] (see **Table 3**), they do not provide trainees with detailed feedback to help pinpoint

deficiencies. Additionally, although there is evidence in adult practice to show that these metrics can be used to authenticate provision of high-quality endoscopic care,[97–99] research is required to provide validity evidence for their use as objective measures of competence in performing endoscopy during training.

In adult practice, the introduction of cancer screening programs has fostered the development and validation of evidenced-based quality and safety indicators.[98,99] However, given the unique nature of pediatric practice, quality and safety indicators derived from adult practice are not always directly applicable to the specific needs of children and their families.[2,100] Currently, there are limited data on the applicability of adult-derived quality metrics to pediatric practice and their impact on clinically relevant outcomes. For example, with regard to cecal intubation rate, the reported successful completion rate for pediatric endoscopists varies from 48% to 96%.[101–106] Terminal ileum intubation rate is a potential quality indicator specific to pediatric colonoscopy, given the differential indications for pediatric colonoscopy as compared with adults. The reported ileum intubation rate varies from 11.0% to 87.5%,[101,103–107] and the independent success rates of pediatric trainees at various stages of training have not been reported. Given the paucity of literature, additional research is required to further delineate and define pediatric-specific quality indicators that can be used for assessment and quality assurance purposes, and validate them in a longitudinal prospective fashion.[100]

Direct observational assessment tools

In recent years, accreditation bodies and endoscopy training and credentialing guidelines have been placing greater emphasis on the continuous assessment of trainees as they progress toward competence. Direct observational assessment tools are one such method to support ongoing skills assessment. Additionally, direct observational tools can be used to support a competency-based education model that defines desired training milestones and outcomes and necessitates the use of psychometrically sound assessment tools to document achievement. Typically, the acquisition of procedural proficiency in endoscopy has been based on an apprenticeship model, in which supervising staff make a subjective global judgment at the end of training as to whether a learner is prepared to perform procedures independently. However, without a structured schema on which to base such observations, these assessments are largely unreproducible and unreliable.[108,109] These global assessments also do not allow for the timely identification of learners in difficulty. Increasingly in medical education, it is recognized that the addition of structure to components of the assessment process makes it more objective, valid, and reliable.[110–112] Additionally, there has been an augmented focus on assessment of real-world events, such as procedures, through direct observation, as it allows for assessment of clinical competence at the "does" level of the Miller pyramid.[41,113]

Although a number of endoscopy assessment tools have been developed and validated within the adult setting, until recently there has been limited research outlining the development or validation of tools designed to assess competence in performing pediatric endoscopy. Key practice differences between adult and pediatric endoscopy emphasize the need for pediatric-specific procedural assessment tools. The NASPGHAN training guidelines[33] outline endoscopy scorecards; however, the psychometric properties of these instruments have not been evaluated. Additionally, although pediatric trainees were included in a study assessing validity evidence for the Global Assessment of Gastrointestinal Endoscopic Skills tools for upper endoscopy and colonoscopy, these tools were developed in the adult context, they focus on technical skills, and only a handful of procedures from one pediatric institution were included.[114]

The Gastrointestinal Endoscopy Competency Assessment Tool for pediatric colonoscopy (GiECAT$_{KIDS}$)

Our team recently developed the Gastrointestinal Endoscopy Competency Assessment Tool for pediatric colonoscopy (GiECAT$_{KIDS}$), a task-specific 7-item global rating scale that assesses holistic aspects of pediatric colonoscopy skill and a structured 18-item checklist that outlines key steps required to complete the procedure.[37] Using Delphi methodology, the GiECAT$_{KIDS}$ was developed by 41 pediatric endoscopy experts from 28 North American hospitals and thus is reflective of endoscopic practice across institutions. A recent prospective study that examined 116 colonoscopies performed by 56 pediatric endoscopists (25 novice, 21 intermediate, and 10 experienced) from 3 North American academic hospitals provides reliability and validity evidence of the GiECAT$_{KIDS}$ for use in the authentic clinical context in a formative manner throughout training, including evidence of strong interrater reliability; excellent test-retest reliability; evidence of content, response process, and internal structure validity; discriminative validity (ability to detect differences in skill level); validity evidence of associations with other variables thought to reflect endoscopic competence (eg, ileum intubation rate); and educational usefulness.[38] As an assessment measure, the GiECAT$_{KIDS}$ has a number of strengths. In particular, it has been designed to assess the broad array of competencies required to perform pediatric colonoscopy (including cognitive, integrative, and technical skill components) in an integrated manner that is known to facilitate learning.[115] Additionally, it addresses performance of all components of the procedure, including preprocedural, intraprocedural, and postprocedural aspects of care.

Assessment is an essential component of endoscopy education, as it drives both teaching and learning.[115,116] The GiECAT$_{KIDS}$ represents a critical step in the development of a robust pediatric-specific program of assessment to support pediatric endoscopy training and practice. The integration of rigorously developed assessment tools, such as the GiECAT$_{KIDS}$, with strong reliability and validity evidence throughout the training cycle, is essential because they can support trainees' learning through the provision of instructive feedback, allow program directors to monitor skill acquisition to ensure trainees are progressing, facilitate identification of skill deficits, and help ensure readiness for independent practice.[117] Looking to the future, the universal adoption of robust assessment tools, such as the GiECAT$_{KIDS}$, by pediatric gastroenterology training programs across jurisdictions would be useful, as it would generate aggregate data that could be used to develop average learning curves of pediatric endoscopists. These data could then be used to define milestones for pediatric endoscopists at different levels of training and to help to establish minimal performance-based benchmark criteria for competence in pediatric endoscopy procedures to support competency-based training.

SUMMARY

Endoscopy is an important diagnostic and therapeutic tool for gastrointestinal disorders in children. Differences between pediatric and adult practice highlight the need for pediatric-specific training and assessment approaches to ensure safe and effective endoscopy in pediatric populations. The ultimate goal of pediatric endoscopy training is to ensure trainees are competent to perform procedures independently. Over the past decade a lot of effort has been made to more clearly define the competencies required to carry out pediatric endoscopic procedures and develop tools to support the assessment of competency in performing pediatric endoscopy. In addition, novel methods of instruction, such as simulation, have been developed and introduced with the aim of accelerating the endoscopy learning curve and ensuring trainees attain some degree of proficiency before performing real-life procedures. Ultimately, assessment goals and goals for teaching and curriculum development should be fully intertwined, as assessment is known to drive learning.[118] Reflective of this, there remains a need for a comprehensive evidence-based pediatric endoscopy training curricula and a complementary assessment system that integrates multiple assessment methods to examine the technical, cognitive, and integrative domains of endoscopic competence longitudinally from training to independent practice to ensure achievement and maintenance of competence.

Although great strides have been made in recent years with regard to pediatric endoscopy training and assessment, looking to the future, additional research is required to examine best practices with regard to the use of novel instructional aids, such as simulation, that are designed to accelerate the endoscopy learning curve. In addition, studies are required to help further delineate instructional design features (eg, mastery learning, feedback) that optimize pediatric endoscopy skill acquisition. There also remains a need to systematically integrate common pediatric-specific gastrointestinal endoscopy competency assessment tools, such as the GiECAT$_{KIDS}$, across training programs to help systematically define milestones for pediatric endoscopists and subsequently, to monitor trainees' progress to support competency-based training.

REFERENCES

1. Leung W. Competency based medical training: review. BMJ 2002;325(7366): 693–6.
2. Lightdale JR, Acosta R, Shergill AK, et al. Modifications in endoscopic practice for pediatric patients. Gastrointest Endosc 2014;79(5):699–710.
3. Bell RH. Surgical council on resident education: a new organization devoted to graduate surgical education. J Am Coll Surg 2007;204(3):341–6.
4. Poulose BK, Vassiliou MC, Dunkin BJ, et al. Fundamentals of endoscopic surgery cognitive examination: development and validity evidence. Surg Endosc 2014;28(2):631–8.
5. Sedlack RE, Shami VM, Adler DG, et al. Colonoscopy core curriculum. Gastrointest Endosc 2012;76(3):482–90.
6. Fitts A, Posner M. Human performance. Belmont (CA): Brooks/Cole; 1967.
7. Mahmood T, Darzi A. The learning curve for a colonoscopy simulator in the absence of any feedback: no feedback, no learning. Surg Endosc 2004;18(8): 1224–30.
8. Rogers DA, Regehr G, MacDonald J. A role for error training in surgical technical skill instruction and evaluation. Am J Surg 2002;183(3):242–5.
9. Ericsson KA. Deliberate practice and the acquisition and maintenance of expert performance in medicine and related domains. Acad Med 2004;79(10 Suppl): S70–81.
10. Shah SG, Brooker JC, Williams CB, et al. Effect of magnetic endoscope imaging on colonoscopy performance: a randomised controlled trial. Lancet 2000; 356(9243):1718–22.
11. Saunders BP, Bell GD, Williams CB, et al. First clinical results with a real time, electronic imager as an aid to colonoscopy. Gut 1995;36(6):913–7.

12. Mark-Christensen A, Brandsborg S, Iversen LH. Magnetic endoscopic imaging as an adjuvant to elective colonoscopy: a systematic review and meta-analysis of randomized controlled trials. Endoscopy 2015;47(3):251–61.
13. Shah SG, Thomas-Gibson S, Lockett M, et al. Effect of real-time magnetic endoscope imaging on the teaching and acquisition of colonoscopy skills: results from a single trainee. Endoscopy 2003;35(5):421–5.
14. Coderre S, Anderson J, Rikers R, et al. Early use of magnetic endoscopic imaging by novice colonoscopists: improved performance without increase in workload. Can J Gastroenterol 2010;24(12):727–32.
15. Kaltenbach T, Leung C, Wu K, et al. Use of the colonoscope training model with the colonoscope 3D imaging probe improved trainee colonoscopy performance: a pilot study. Dig Dis Sci 2011;56(5):1496–502.
16. Accreditation Council for Graduate Medical Education. ACGME Program Requirements for Graduate Medical Education in Gastroenterology. Intern Med 2013. Available at: http://www.acgme.org/acgmeweb/Portals/0/PFAssets/Program Requirements/144_gastroenterology_int_med_2016.pdf.
17. Ziv A, Wolpe PR, Small SD, et al. Simulation-based medical education: an ethical imperative. Acad Med 2003;78(8):783–8.
18. Cook DA, Hamstra SJ, Brydges R, et al. Comparative effectiveness of instructional design features in simulation-based education: systematic review and meta-analysis. Med Teach 2013;35(1):e867–98.
19. Walsh C, Sherlock M, Ling S, et al. Virtual reality simulation training for health professions trainees in gastrointestinal endoscopy. Cochrane Database Syst Rev 2012;(6):CD008237.
20. Singh S, Sedlack RE, Cook DA. Effects of simulation-based training in gastrointestinal endoscopy: a systematic review and meta-analysis. Clin Gastroenterol Hepatol 2014;12(10):1611–23.e4.
21. Lightdale JR, Newburg AR, Mahoney LB, et al. Fellow perceptions of training using computer-based endoscopy simulators. Gastrointest Endosc 2010;72(1):13–8.
22. Cook DA, Brydges R, Zendejas B, et al. Mastery learning for health professionals using technology-enhanced simulation: a systematic review and meta-analysis. Acad Med 2013;88(8):1178–86.
23. Hatala R, Cook DA, Zendejas B, et al. Feedback for simulation-based procedural skills training: a meta-analysis and critical narrative synthesis. Adv Health Sci Educ Theory Pract 2014;19(2):251–72.
24. Issenberg SB, McGaghie WC, Petrusa ER, et al. Features and uses of high-fidelity medical simulations that lead to effective learning: a BEME systematic review. Med Teach 2005;27(1):10–28.
25. Walsh CM, Ling SC, Wang CS, et al. Concurrent versus terminal feedback: it may be better to wait. Acad Med 2009;84(10 Suppl):S54–7.
26. Grover SC, Garg A, Scaffidi MA, et al. Impact of a simulation training curriculum on technical and nontechnical skills in colonoscopy: a randomized trial. Gastrointest Endosc 2015. http://dx.doi.org/10.1016/j.gie.2015.04.008.
27. Grover SC, Scaffidi MA, Garg A, et al. A simulation-based training curriculum of progressive fidelity and complexity improves technical and non-technical skills in colonoscopy: a blinded, randomized trial. Gastrointest Endosc 2015;81(5S): AB324–5 [abstract: Su 1550].
28. Guadagnoli M, Morin M-P, Dubrowski A. The application of the challenge point framework in medical education. Med Educ 2012;46(5):447–53.
29. Coderre S, Anderson J, Rostom A, et al. Training the endoscopy trainer: from general principles to specific concepts. Can J Gastroenterol 2010;24(12):700–4.

30. Epstein RM. Assessment in medical education. N Engl J Med 2007;356(4): 387–96.
31. Eisen GM, Baron TH, Dominitz JA, et al. Methods of granting hospital privileges to perform gastrointestinal endoscopy. Gastrointest Endosc 2002;55(7):780–3.
32. Sedlack RE. Colonoscopy. In: Cohen J, editor. Successful training in gastrointestinal endoscopy. 1st edition. Oxford (United Kingdom): Wiley-Blackwell; 2011. p. 42–72.
33. Leichtner AM, Gillis LA, Gupta S, et al. NASPGHAN guidelines for training in pediatric gastroenterology. J Pediatr Gastroenterol Nutr 2013;56(Suppl 1): S1–8.
34. Swing SR. The ACGME outcome project: retrospective and prospective. Med Teach 2007;29(7):648–54.
35. Frank JR, Snell L, Sherbino J, editors. The draft CanMEDS 2015 physician competency framework–series IV. Ottawa (Canada): The Royal College of Physicians and Surgeons of Canada; 2015.
36. Cullinane M, Gray A, Hargraves C, et al. Scoping our practice. The 2004 report of the national confidential enquiry into patient outcome and death. London: 2005. Available at: http://www.ncepod.org.uk/2004report/. Accessed June 1, 2015.
37. Walsh CM, Ling SC, Walters TD, et al. Development of the gastrointestinal endoscopy competency assessment tool for pediatric colonoscopy (GiECAT-KIDS). J Pediatr Gastroenterol Nutr 2014;59(4):480–6.
38. Walsh CM, Ling SC, Mamula P, et al. The gastrointestinal endoscopy competency assessment tool for pediatric colonoscopy. J Pediatr Gastroenterol Nutr 2015;60(4):474–80.
39. Shute VJ. Focus on formative feedback. Rev Educ Res 2008;78(1):153–89.
40. Govaerts MJB, van der Vleuten CPM, Schuwirth LWT, et al. Broadening perspectives on clinical performance assessment: rethinking the nature of in-training assessment. Adv Health Sci Educ Theory Pract 2007;12(2):239–60.
41. Miller GE. The assessment of clinical skills/competence/performance. Acad Med 1990;65(9 Suppl):S63–7.
42. Rose S, Fix OK, Shah BJ, et al. Entrustable professional activities for gastroenterology fellowship training. Gastrointest Endosc 2014;80(1):16–27.
43. Frank JR, Mungroo R, Ahmad Y, et al. Toward a definition of competency-based education in medicine: a systematic review of published definitions. Med Teach 2010;32(8):631–7.
44. Long DM. Competency-based residency training: the next advance in graduate medical education. Acad Med 2000;75(12):1178–83.
45. Iobst WF, Sherbino J, Ten Cate O, et al. Competency-based medical education in postgraduate medical education. Med Teach 2010;32(8):651–6.
46. Coyle WJ, Fasge F. Developing tools for the assessment of the learning colonoscopist. Gastrointest Endosc 2014;79(5):808–10.
47. Cass OW, Freeman ML, Peine CJ, et al. Objective evaluation of endoscopy skills during training. Ann Intern Med 1993;118(1):40–4.
48. Chak A, Cooper GS, Blades EW, et al. Prospective assessment of colonoscopic intubation skills in trainees. Gastrointest Endosc 1996;44(1):54–7.
49. Parry BR, Williams SM. Competency and the colonoscopist: a learning curve. Aust N Z J Surg 1991;61(6):419–22.
50. Ward ST, Mohammed MA, Walt R, et al. An analysis of the learning curve to achieve competency at colonoscopy using the JETS database. Gut 2014;63: 1–9.

51. Dafnis G, Granath F, Påhlman L, et al. The impact of endoscopists' experience and learning curves and interendoscopist variation on colonoscopy completion rates. Endoscopy 2001;33(6):511–7.
52. Jorgensen JE, Elta GH, Stalburg CM, et al. Do breaks in gastroenterology fellow endoscopy training result in a decrement in competency in colonoscopy? Gastrointest Endosc 2013;78(3):503–9.
53. Cohen J. Training and credentialing in gastrointestinal endoscopy. In: Cotton PB, editor. Digestive endoscopy: practice and safety. Oxford (United Kingdom): Blackwell Publishing; 2008. p. 289–362.
54. Sidhu R, Grober E, Musselman L, et al. Assessing competency in surgery: Where to begin? Surgery 2004;135(1):6–20.
55. Klasko SK, Cummings RV, Glazerman LR. Education resident data collection: do the numbers add up? Am J Obstet Gynecol 1995;172(4 Pt 1):1312–6.
56. Armstrong D, Enns R, Ponich T, et al. Canadian credentialing guidelines for endoscopic privileges: an overview. Can J Gastroenterol 2007;21(12):797–801.
57. Vassiliou MC, Kaneva PA, Poulose BK, et al. How should we establish the clinical case numbers required to achieve proficiency in flexible endoscopy? Am J Surg 2010;199(1):121–5.
58. Cass O, Freeman M, Cohen J, et al. Acquisition of competency in endoscopic skills (ACES) during training: A multicenter study. Gastrointest Endosc 1996; 43(4):308.
59. Shahidi N, Ou G, Telford J, et al. Establishing the learning curve for achieving competency in performing colonoscopy: a systematic review. Gastrointest Endosc 2014;80(3):410–6.
60. Sedlack RE. Training to competency in colonoscopy: assessing and defining competency standards. Gastrointest Endosc 2011;74(2):355–66.e1-e2.
61. Sedlack RE, Coyle W. Colonoscopy learning curves and competency benchmarks in GI fellows. Gastrointest Endosc 2015;81(5S):AB34 [Abstract: Su 1550].
62. Cass OW. Training to competence in gastrointestinal endoscopy: a plea for continuous measuring of objective end points. Endoscopy 1999;31(9):751–4.
63. Cook DA, Beckman TJ. Current concepts in validity and reliability for psychometric instruments: theory and application. Am J Med 2006;119(2):166.e7–16.
64. BSPGHAN Endoscopy Working Group. JAG paediatric endoscopy certification, version 2.1. 2014. Available at: http://www.thejag.org.uk/downloads%5CJAG%20certification%20for%20paediatric%20trainees%5CJAG%20Paediatric%20Certification%202.1%20300513.pdf. Accessed September 1, 2015.
65. Vassiliou MC, Dunkin BJ, Marks JM, et al. FLS and FES: comprehensive models of training and assessment. Surg Clin North Am 2010;90(3):535–58.
66. Thomas-Gibson S, Saunders BP. Development and validation of a multiple-choice question paper in basic colonoscopy. Endoscopy 2005;37(9):821–6.
67. Case SM, Swanson DB. Item content: testing application of clinical scientific knowledge. In: Case SM, Swanson DB, editors. Constructing written test questions for the basic and clinical sciences. 3rd edition. Philadelphia: National Board of Medical Examiners; 2002. p. 51–68.
68. Cook DA, Brydges R, Zendejas B, et al. Technology-enhanced simulation to assess health professionals: a systematic review of validity evidence, research methods, and reporting quality. Acad Med 2013;88(6):872–83.
69. Haycock A. Moving from training to competency testing. Tech Gastrointest Endosc 2011;13(2):155–60.
70. Kneebone RL, Nestel D, Moorthy K, et al. Learning the skills of flexible sigmoidoscopy—the wider perspective. Med Educ 2003;37(Suppl 1):50–8.

71. Cohen J, Thompson CC. The next generation of endoscopic simulation. Am J Gastroenterol 2013;108(7):1036–9.
72. Palter VN, Grantcharov TP. Simulation in surgical education. CMAJ 2010; 182(11):1191–6.
73. Sedlack RE. Competency assessment: it's time to expect more from our simulator. Dig Liver Dis 2012;44(7):537–8.
74. Elvevi A, Cantù P, Maconi G, et al. Evaluation of hands-on training in colonoscopy: is a computer-based simulator useful? Dig Liver Dis 2012;44(7):580–4.
75. McConnell RA, Kim S, Ahmad NA, et al. Poor discriminatory function for endoscopic skills on a computer-based simulator. Gastrointest Endosc 2012;76(5): 993–1002.
76. Plooy AM, Hill A, Horswill MS, et al. Construct validation of a physical model colonoscopy simulator. Gastrointest Endosc 2012;76(1):144–50.
77. Verdaasdonk EGG, Stassen LPS, Schijven MP, et al. Construct validity and assessment of the learning curve for the SIMENDO endoscopic simulator. Surg Endosc 2007;21(8):1406–12.
78. Felsher JJ, Olesevich M, Farres H, et al. Validation of a flexible endoscopy simulator. Am J Surg 2005;189(4):497–500.
79. Fayez R, Feldman LS, Kaneva P, et al. Testing the construct validity of the Simbionix GI Mentor II virtual reality colonoscopy simulator metrics: module matters. Surg Endosc 2010;24(5):1060–5.
80. Koch AD, Buzink SN, Heemskerk J, et al. Expert and construct validity of the Simbionix GI Mentor II endoscopy simulator for colonoscopy. Surg Endosc 2008;22(1):158–62.
81. Sedlack RE, Kolars JC. Validation of a computer-based colonoscopy simulator. Gastrointest Endosc 2003;57(2):214–8.
82. Mahmood T. Darzi a. A study to validate the colonoscopy simulator. Surg Endosc 2003;17(10):1583–9.
83. Grantcharov TP, Carstensen L, Schulze S. Objective assessment of gastrointestinal endoscopy skills using a virtual reality simulator. JSLS 2005;9(2):130–3.
84. Sedlack RE, Coyle WJ, Obstein KL, et al. ASGE's assessment of competency in endoscopy evaluation tools for colonoscopy and EGD. Gastrointest Endosc 2014;79(1):1–7.
85. Sedlack RE, Baron TH, Downing SM, et al. Validation of a colonoscopy simulation model for skills assessment. Am J Gastroenterol 2007;102(1):64–74.
86. Haycock AV, Bassett P, Bladen J, et al. Validation of the second-generation Olympus colonoscopy simulator for skills assessment. Endoscopy 2009; 41(11):952–8.
87. Jirapinyo P, Kumar N, Thompson CC. Validation of an endoscopic part-task training box as a skill assessment tool. Gastrointest Endosc 2015;81(4):967–73.
88. Thompson CC, Jirapinyo P, Kumar N, et al. Development and initial validation of an endoscopic part-task training box. Endoscopy 2014;46(9):735–44.
89. Mason JD, Ansell J, Warren N, et al. Is motion analysis a valid tool for assessing laparoscopic skill? Surg Endosc 2013;27(5):1468–77.
90. Mohankumar D, Garner H, Ruff K, et al. Characterization of right wrist posture during simulated colonoscopy: an application of kinematic analysis to the study of endoscopic maneuvers. Gastrointest Endosc 2014;79(3):480–9.
91. Appleyard MN, Mosse CA, Mills TN, et al. The measurement of forces exerted during colonoscopy. Gastrointest Endosc 2000;52(2):237–40.
92. Shergill AK, Asundi KR, Barr A, et al. Pinch force and forearm-muscle load during routine colonoscopy: a pilot study. Gastrointest Endosc 2009;69(1):142–6.

93. Obstein KL, Patil VD, Jayender J, et al. Evaluation of colonoscopy technical skill levels by use of an objective kinematic-based system. Gastrointest Endosc 2011;73(2):315–21, 321.e1.
94. Ende AR, Shah PM, Chandrasekhara V, et al. Quantitative force application during simulated colonoscopy is significantly different between novice and expert endoscopists. Gastrointest Endosc 2014;79(5S):AB217 [abstract: Su 1568].
95. Vassiliou MC, Dunkin BJ, Fried GM, et al. Fundamentals of endoscopic surgery: creation and validation of the hands-on test. Surg Endosc 2014;28(3):704–11.
96. Mueller CL, Kaneva P, Fried GM, et al. Colonoscopy performance correlates with scores on the FESTM manual skills test. Surg Endosc 2014;28(11):3081–5.
97. Tinmouth J, Kennedy E, Baron D, et al. Guideline for colonoscopy quality assurance in Ontario. Toronto (ON): Cancer Care Ontario; 2013. Program in evidence-based care evidence-based series No: 15-5 Version 2.
98. Armstrong D, Barkun A, Bridges R, et al. Canadian association of gastroenterology consensus guidelines on safety and quality indicators in endoscopy. Can J Gastroenterol 2012;26(1):17–31.
99. Cohen J, Pike IM. Defining and measuring quality in endoscopy. Gastrointest Endosc 2015;81(1):1–2.
100. Forget S, Walsh CM. Pediatric endoscopy: need for a tailored approach to guidelines on quality and safety. Can J Gastroenterol 2012;26(10):735.
101. Poerregaard A, Wewer AV, Becker PU, et al. Pediatric colonoscopy. Ugeskr Laeger 1998;160(14):2105–8.
102. Hassall E, Barclay GN, Ament ME. Colonoscopy in childhood. Pediatrics 1984;73(5):594–9.
103. Dillon M, Brown S, Casey W, et al. Colonoscopy under general anesthesia in children. Pediatrics 1998;102(2 Pt 1):381–3.
104. Stringer MD, Pinfield A, Revell L, et al. A prospective audit of paediatric colonoscopy under general anaesthesia. Acta Paediatr 1999;88(2):199–202.
105. Israel DM, McLain BI, Hassall E. Successful pancolonoscopy and ileoscopy in children. J Pediatr Gastroenterol Nutr 1994;19(3):283–9.
106. Mamula P, Markowitz JE, Neiswender K, et al. Success rate and duration of paediatric outpatient colonoscopy. Dig Liver Dis 2005;37(11):877–81.
107. Thakkar KH, Holub JL, Gilger MA, et al. Factors affecting ileum intubation in pediatric patients undergoing colonoscopy. Gastrointest Endosc 2014;79(5S):AB279–80 [abstract: Su1739].
108. Darzi A, Smith S, Taffinder N. Assessing operative skill. Needs to become more objective. BMJ 1999;318(7188):887–8.
109. Reznick RK. Teaching and testing technical skills. Am J Surg 1993;165(3):358–61.
110. Ilgen JS, Ma IWY, Hatala R, et al. A systematic review of validity evidence for checklists versus global rating scales in simulation-based assessment. Med Educ 2015;49:161–73.
111. Winckel CP, Reznick RK, Cohen R, et al. Reliability and construct validity of a structured technical skills assessment form. Am J Surg 1994;167(4):423–7.
112. Regehr G, MacRae H, Reznick RK, et al. Comparing the psychometric properties of checklists and global rating scales for assessing performance on an OSCE-format examination. Acad Med 1998;73(9):993–7.
113. Epstein RM, Hundert EM. Defining and assessing professional competence. JAMA 2002;287(2):226–35.

114. Vassiliou MC, Kaneva PA, Poulose BK, et al. Global assessment of gastrointestinal endoscopic skills (GAGES): a valid measurement tool for technical skills in
flexible endoscopy. Surg Endosc 2010;24(8):1834–41.
115. Beard JD, Marriott J, Purdie H, et al. Assessing the surgical skills of trainees in
the operating theatre: a prospective observational study of the methodology.
Health Technol Assess 2011;15(1):i–xxi, 1–162.
116. Kromann CB, Jensen ML, Ringsted C. The effect of testing on skills learning.
Med Educ 2009;43(1):21–7.
117. Beard JD. Assessment of surgical competence. Br J Surg 2007;94(11):1315–6.
118. Pangaro L, ten Cate O. Frameworks for learner assessment in medicine: AMEE
Guide No. 78. Med Teach 2013;35(6):e1197–210.
119. Conjoint Committee for the Recognition of Training in Gastrointestinal Endoscopy. Information for applicants - requirements for CCRTGE Recognition. Available at: http://www.conjoint.org.au/applicants.html#procedural. Accessed June
1, 2015.

Informed Consent for Pediatric Endoscopy

Joel A. Friedlander, DO, MA-Bioethics*, David E. Brumbaugh, MD

KEYWORDS

- Informed consent • Endoscopy • Shared decision making
- Pediatric gastroenterology • Enteroscopy • Esophagogastroduodenoscopy
- Endoscopic retrograde cholangiopancreatography • Pediatrics

KEY POINTS

- Pediatric informed consent is a unique process that involves the provider, the parent/guardian, and the mature adolescent, if appropriate.
- Pediatric assent, in particular obtaining permission from an adolescent, is highly recommend for pediatric endoscopy.
- Each procedure has a general list of indications, methods, risks, benefits, and alternatives that should be discussed with the decision maker. The provider obtaining consent should evaluate a general sense of understanding from the parent/guardian, as well as from the patient, when appropriate.
- Endoscopic providers should be aware of relevant procedural risks and the specific frequencies with which each occur.

INTRODUCTION

Procedural or surgical informed consent is the process by which a practitioner obtains permission from an autonomous decision maker to allow a procedure or invasive test to be done on a patient or subject.[1] This concept is used frequently in the practice of pediatric gastroenterology as it is relates to procedures, transfusions, and transplants.

The general concept of informed consent most commonly finds its origins in ideas stemming from the Nuremberg Trials after World War II.[2] The term was greatly expanded subsequently based on laws relating to assault and battery.[1–3] The 1969 case of Canterbury v. Spence highlights the modern-day concept of informed consent and the more familiar discussion of risks, benefits, alternatives, indications, and methods. The case highlights the failure of Dr Spence to disclose the possible ramifications of back surgery and subsequent paralysis.[3] The patient was not informed of the risk of complications and

Digestive Health Institute, Children's Hospital Colorado, University of Colorado School of Medicine, 13123 E 16th Ave, B290, Aurora, CO 80045, USA
* Corresponding author.
E-mail address: joel.friedlander@childrenscolorado.org

Gastrointest Endoscopy Clin N Am 26 (2016) 35–46
http://dx.doi.org/10.1016/j.giec.2015.08.005
1052-5157/16/$ – see front matter © 2016 Elsevier Inc. All rights reserved.

a lawsuit ensued. Such cases and history highlight the need for practitioners to share information with a rational, informed, and noncoerced decision maker, or else with a surrogate/proxy. This process is known as respect for autonomy.

Informed consent is part of the continual process of shared decision making that encompasses the transfer of information between practitioner and patient or patient surrogate/parents.[4,5] Informed consent is the finalization and obtaining of permission with probable documentation of the process that leads to a procedure or test. This consent process accompanies the right of that individual to make an informed refusal. Pediatric assent, a unique component to the care of children, is the process by which a consent modality is applied to an adolescent decision maker.[6]

In contrast, variations to this process in an emergent setting allow for deviations from this routine. One such an example is a life-threatening gastrointestinal bleeding event in which the family was not available. Because of the uniqueness of the pediatric setting and the legal interest of protecting children, formal consent is not always needed in emergency circumstances.[3]

Components of Informed Consent

There are several necessary components to informed consent (**Box 1**). Some of these are implicit or assumed in routine interactions between the provider and family, whereas others must be specifically transferred as information. Assumed components of the informed consent process include assessment of the decision-making capacity of the decision maker, as well as their voluntariness. Decision-making capacity is the ability to understand and process information and come to a decision. Voluntariness is the understanding of a decision maker that they are intended to make a decision that is free from pressure or coercion by the provider. Both assessments are informal and rarely documented.[1] These issues are not as problematic in pediatrics because of the presence of parental proxies, but can play a role in older adolescents or parents

---

Box 1
Components of pediatric informed consent

Preconditions: provider assessed:

1. Competence: decision-making capacity

2. Voluntariness: free from coercion, pressure

Information elements: provider disclosed:

1. Disclosure
   a. Indications
   b. Methods
   c. Risks
   d. Benefits
   e. Alternatives

2. Recommendation

3. Understanding

Consent achieved

1. Decision by parent/adolescent

2. Authorization/documentation

Form Beauchamp TL, Childress JF. Principles of biomedical ethics. New York: Oxford University Press, 2009.

---

of limited mental capacity. Even with the use of parents, comprehension and understanding can still be limited.[7,8]

The transfer of information is the next component with which most providers are familiar, and includes a discussion of the risks, benefits, indications, methods, and alternatives of the procedure. Transfer of information usually contains a clinical recommendation by the provider. In addition, in this component of informed consent, the provider needs to obtain a decision and authorization from the patient, guardian, or proxy.[1]

Pediatric Assent

Pediatric assent is similar to consent as noted earlier, but the presentation and discussion are focused on the nonlegal bound adolescent patient rather than the legal guardian or decision maker. Assent is usually obtained in patients 11 years of age and older, but assessment of maturity level may influence the age at which this is practical.[6] Some states allow adolescents to give informed consent for specific abortion or sexual reproductive health procedures, although not for other standard procedures, such as pediatric endoscopy.[9]

Although assent is not legally binding, it is imperative in pediatrics for the patient to be involved in the consent process. For example, in pediatric gastroenterology the adolescent may not want an elective endoscopy to be performed.[10] If an endoscopy were to be performed against the adolescent's wishes, this could be considered battery and is neither ethically nor legally recommended.[1,11] In the case of unsedated or procedures with minimal sedation, for which a cooperative patient is necessary, following the patient's wishes is absolutely necessary. Examples of such procedures include unsedated transnasal/transoral endoscopy and capsule endoscopy.[12–14]

Methods of Consent

Regarding methods of consent, there is significant research showing that all methods generally fail to achieve a complete consent. A recent meta-analysis done by Cochrane confirms that further research and new techniques for implementing the consent process are needed urgently.[7,8,15–21] Specifically regarding gastrointestinal endoscopy, studies have shown that there is a general understanding by families and patients of the procedure and basic risks, but there are deficiencies in understanding the voluntariness and alternatives of most procedures.[7,8,22–25] Most of the current research into consent processes focuses on paper-based or electronic form–based techniques, but video, decision-aid assistance, and interactive Web-based methods have also been investigated.

Several companies in the United States sell video or Web-based decision-aid and information videos for endoscopy, although few are pediatric focused. Milwaukee Children's Hospital recently published an informative video regarding pediatric endoscopy, but it has not been studied specifically as a decision aid for obtaining consent.[26] One commercial video by Epic Systems Inc has been studied and has been shown to improve consent attainment as based on understanding the risks, benefits, alternatives, indications, and methods using the Consent-20 instrument.[7]

Expertise in the Procedure

In order to obtain consent and provide information transfer to families, technical and nontechnical expertise in the procedure being performed is necessary. Individuals obtaining consent should also be familiar with their own expertise, and be able to provide personal information about general past procedural numbers, and their experience with complications if asked by the consenter. This recommendation may present challenges in training environments, in which fellows are learning to engage in procedural consent.[27] In that there is yet to be a method of consent that has shows significant and complete success, it is important to recognize that teaching consent is difficult. Further research is needed to improve education around the process of consenting for pediatric endoscopy.

Individuals obtaining consent and performing transfer of information must also be familiar with both general and unique components of each procedure, including potential outcomes and risks, of various types and categories of pediatric gastrointestinal procedure. Because of a paucity of data on the specific outcomes in pediatric procedures, some of this information is anecdotal and vague. The Endoscopy and Procedure Committee of the North American Society of Pediatric Gastroenterology, Hepatology and Nutrition (NASPGHAN) is currently working on an agenda to better populate information about risks in pediatric procedures. With this agenda ongoing, even the best data are limited by the experience of each endoscopist and should be interpreted with caution. For example, a single-center risk of perforation quoted at 1:10,000 for diagnostic endoscopy may vary by endoscopist and by risk profile of the patient selection (ie, disease process or comorbidity). One physician may have a complication rate of 1:5000, whereas another may be 1:15,000. In addition, the nature and type of procedure may augment risk, as discussed later.

DIAGNOSTIC ESOPHAGOGASTRODUODENOSCOPY AND COLONOSCOPY

There is limited pediatric literature on the safety of esophagogastroduodenoscopy (EGD)/colonoscopy in pediatrics, but some of the generally accepted norms for the most significant adverse events can be derived from several large recent studies by the PEDS-CORI (Pediatric Endoscopy Database Sysem-Clinical Outcomes Research Initiative) consortium and Hsu and colleagues,[28] and are listed in **Box 2**.[29,30] EGD/colonoscopy has common risks, adverse events, and more significant risks of complications that should be addressed at the least with the patient's parent/guardian. If the patient is mature enough, these considerations are also important to address with the patient undergoing the procedure.

There is common debate among practitioners of what qualifies as expected experience versus an adverse event or complication of the procedure, but such information and the relative risk of each should be disclosed. There is also variation in the risk for adverse events based on a patient's known medical conditions, as well as the

---

Box 2
Adverse events and percentages associated with complications in pediatric sedated diagnostic EGD/colonoscopy

1. Hypoxia (36.8%/37.2%)

2. Bleeding (29.4%/38.6%)

3. Respiratory distress (7.4%/NR)

4. Wheezing (8.8%/NR)

5. Nausea/vomiting (4.4%/NR)

6. Rash (1.5%/NR)

7. Perforation (NR/0.01%)

Abbreviation: NR, not reported recently.
    Data from Refs.[28–30]

procedural sedation plan. For example, EGD/colonoscopy that is to be performed with anesthesia may have a different set of potential adverse events than EGD/colonoscopy that is performed with endoscopist-administered procedural sedation or nonsedation.[13,14] It is important to differentiate risks and expectations of the procedure from the risks associated with the form of sedation. For detailed risk information on forms of sedation, the reader is referred to existing pediatric sedation guidelines.[31,32]

Common postprocedure symptoms after EGD/colonoscopy may include sore throat lasting minutes to a couple days, fatigue, and abdominal pain. A pediatric study reviewing complaints after outpatient diagnostic EGD found the following frequency of symptoms: sore throat, 34.6%; fatigue, 6.6%; cough, 4.1%; headache, 3.3%; nausea, 2.5%; gas/burping, 2.8%; nausea, 2.5%; abdominal pain, 2%; and fever, 2%.[33] This same study showed that 6% of subjects sought medical assistance for such events.[33] Post-EGD emesis events may be blood tinged or contain coffee ground–type material because of the biopsies. If biopsies are not obtained, the risks of discomfort or bleeding may be less. However, this distinction is largely academic because EGD without biopsy is not as common in pediatrics as it is in adults.[34,35] In any case, such postprocedure complaints are not considered adverse events, but should be disclosed to the patient as common expectations.

After discussing expected postprocedural symptoms, the endoscopist should review the risk for more serious adverse events after EGD/colonoscopy. The 2 main risks are bleeding/hematoma from the biopsy sites or scope trauma; and risk for esophageal, gastric, small bowel, or large bowel perforation, and need for repair. Although these events are exceedingly rare in pediatrics (some studies note <1 per 5000–10,000 endoscopies), it has become common practice to disclose these rare risks to patients and their families.[28,30]

Infection from diagnostic forward-viewing EGD/colonoscopy is even more rare than bowel perforation, and the American Hospital Association has consistently recommended against the use of antibiotic prophylaxis for diagnostic endoscopic procedures.[36]

As more pediatric centers are favoring anesthesia administered by an anesthesiologist, risk for hypoxemia should be disclosed by the sedation physician or provider rather than the gastroenterologist. Likewise, if sedation is administered, then disclosure of risks such as aspiration pneumonia, airway trauma, tooth trauma, allergic reaction, hypotension, death, and allergy to medication should also be disclosed.[32] In contrast, if procedural sedation is administered by a pediatric gastroenterologist, the endoscopic provider has responsibility for these disclosures.

Using the PEDS-CORI database, Thakkar and colleagues[30] found that the most common adverse event with sedated EGD was hypoxemia, although it is unclear whether this was attributable to EGD versus sedation practice. Regarding colonoscopy, Thakkar and colleagues[29] reported a 1.1% overall complication rate, with half relating to the gastrointestinal system, including 38.6% with bleeding, 25% with hypoxia, and 1 perforation (0.01%). Hsu and colleagues[28] and Thakkar and colleagues[29] both reported this perforation rate in pediatric diagnostic colonoscopy.

More recently, literature has shown an association between anesthesia exposure and developmental delay in children, but this needs significantly more study and evaluation.[37,38] This association should be considered for disclosure to families undergoing repetitive sedated procedures.

Failure to Disclose

Although an adverse event does not imply physician/provider wrongdoing, a parent whose expected postprocedure symptoms and potential adverse events were not disclosed before the event might think that the provider was negligent in failing to disclose. Failure to disclose potential adverse events prevents patients from being autonomous decision makers with regard to their care, and this issue was at the heart of the Spence case discussed earlier.

A typical disclosure for events linked to diagnostic EGD/colonoscopy may read as follows. The risk of the procedure may include but is not limited to: pain; abdominal pain; sore throat/anus; nausea; vomiting; infection; bleeding; bruising; and rare risk of perforation and need for repair with surgery, antibiotics, and intensive care unit care. Risks of sedation, such as cough, fatigue, hypoxemia, and headache, should be considered as well. Documentation of the consent process using a paper or electronic method is strongly recommended.

INFORMED CONSENT FOR PERFORMING THERAPEUTIC GASTROINTESTINAL PROCEDURES IN CHILDREN

Informed consent for therapeutic EGD/colonoscopy (eg, foreign body removal, dilation, polypectomy, endoscopic hemostasis, treatment of infection) is different from consent for diagnostic procedures because, each specific therapeutic maneuver has inherent postprocedural symptoms and possible adverse events. For example, compared with diagnostic endoscopy, foreign body extraction carries increased risk of gastrointestinal tract damage or perforation.

A recent adult study showed a risk of up to 1.4% risk for perforation but this varies based on type of foreign body, such as a sharp or button battery, and duration of impact.[39] Pediatric literature shows that this risk may be as high as 2%.[28] Esophageal dilation may have up to a 12% to 15% risk of perforation with certain esophageal disorders but could be less when used for other types of stricture.[40–43] Some pediatric literature shows this to be around 0.4%.[28] Polypectomy and hemostatic/bleeding control maneuvers carry increased risk compared with diagnostic endoscopy but that risk varies based on endoscopist experience and polyp type. There are some pediatric reports of perforation after colonoscopy with polypectomy but further data are needed.[44] Two pediatric studies reported more than 300 endoscopies without a single perforation.[28,29]

Ultimately, the true risk may not be appreciated until the endoscopist evaluates the site of intervention and chooses a modality at the time of the procedure. However, a recent large adult study by Rutter and colleagues regarding screening colonoscopy with polypectomy in the United Kingdom quoted risk at 0.6 per 10,000, which is less than for diagnostic endoscopy as noted by Hsu and colleagues.[28,45]

In any case, recently published risk rates for adverse events of therapeutic endoscopy should be familiar to endoscopists performing these procedures. In addition, the informed consent process should include discussion of any factors that may increase risk for adverse events, including small patient size. Some centers have dedicated pediatric gastrointestinal proceduralists who perform interventional or therapeutic endoscopy and thus may be more familiar with risks for these procedures. Other centers may also opt to change the usual preprinted consent forms from their diagnostic procedures.

CONSENT FOR PLACEMENT OF PERCUTANEOUS ENDOSCOPIC GASTROSTOMY

Placement of a percutaneous endoscopic gastrostomy (PEG) involves unique conversations that vary from more traditional interventional endoscopy and also carry increased risks. There is often a need for more focus on the sections of consent that involve the family's understanding of the indications and alternatives of the procedure. A gastrostomy (G) tube is not simply a test or quick procedure, but its placement offers a method to guarantee long-term enteral access in a child who may be unable to survive without it at the end of life or with severe neurologic disability. A recent study showed that feeding tubes are being placed with increased frequency, especially in developmentally delayed children.[46–48] In turn, endoscopists, or primary gastroenterologists in certain circumstances, must discuss the ethical ramifications of tube placement with an emphasis on parental autonomy, child beneficence, and nonmaleficence. That discussion should use the full principles of shared decision making and be focused on each child's circumstances.

For example, a family may choose to place a PEG to prolong a child's life indefinitely by preventing aspiration of oral intake. Another child may also have a similar indication for a G tube but the family prefers oral intake in that child with a progressive neurologic condition. The latter child medically needs nutrition but is slowly dying. In this circumstance, placement of a PEG may be optional, and oral intake may be appropriately recognized as preserving the child's and family's quality of life. Not placing the tube would prevent maleficence by allowing the child to die from poor nutrition as the disease progresses, rather than extending life and having the child die from another cause later in life. The family does have an ethical right to choose such an alternative as long as it is made in the child's best interest.

Because of such possibilities, it is important for endoscopists or primary gastroenterologists to not simply be the proceduralists when placing a PEG tube, but to ensure that the family understands the choice and long-term possibilities they are making for their child. In certain indications the conversation may be simple because the tube may also be used for temporary or supplemental purposes, such as in a treatable but severe illness or esophageal injury.

Regarding the discussion of risks for consent, the primary risk of a PEG includes the EGD items noted earlier, with the more significant possibilities relating to gastric puncture and devices. Depending on the method performed (eg, a traditional full-profile PEG inserted through the mouth; a surgical assisted method; or a primary, newer, low-profile button) the risk of adverse events may vary.

Risks associated with PEGs are both immediate (at the time of placement) and long term, occurring long after the procedure has been performed. Recent studies by McSweeney and colleagues[47,48] in 2015 across 591 pediatric PEG placements showed that up to 24.5% of patients experience an adverse event at some point in the 6 months after the procedure is performed. The investigators also differentiated between a 10.5% risk of major complication (requiring additional hospitalization or surgery) and a 16.4% risk of minor complications associated overall with PEG placement.

Although presumably this rate of complications may vary based on indication, child comorbidity, age, and institutional technique, it may nevertheless be important in the consenting process to discuss long-term risks of complications beyond those experienced during the procedure. In their review, McSweeney and colleagues[48] found a 16.2% risk of infection, 9.3% risk of infection requiring hospitalization, 4.6% risk of tube dislodgement, 1% risk of dehiscence, 0.3% risk of surgery to repair significant granulation tissue, 0.3% risk of perforation of colon/viscera, and 0.1% of pneumoperitoneum and esophageal hematoma. It is also imperative to discuss such risks with the family because they are significant. Future study of various methods is needed, as with other endoscopic procedures, to understand whether these long-term risks can be generalized to all types of PEGs and methods of placement.

CONSENT FOR SMALL BOWEL ENTEROSCOPY IN CHILDREN

Enteroscopy involves similar risks to diagnostic or therapeutic endoscopy but additional discussion regarding pancreatitis, which can occur up to 3% of cases, is required. A recent study in 2014 notes complication rates of up to 5.4% in pediatric small bowel enteroscopy.[49] These risks can include increased risk of pain, hematoma, or perforation compared with standard EGD.

CONSENT FOR PEDIATRIC CAPSULE ENDOSCOPY

There is a broad variation in the methods of obtaining consent for capsule endoscopy. Some centers choose a nursing consent method, others lack a formal consent process, and others use a formal consent document. Regardless of institutional process, documentation of a conversation with the family regarding risks, benefits, alternatives, methods, and indications for capsule endoscopy should occur, either as a chart note or as part of a formal consent process.

Capsule endoscopy generally has limited risks but that risk is not zero. Such risks listed in order of frequency include aspiration of capsule, capsule retention (approximately 1% in pediatric patients), bowel obstruction, abdominal pain, perforation, and vomiting.[12] In addition, it is important for an ordering provider to consider relative contraindications to capsule endoscopy,[50] although a full discussion of these is outside the scope of this article. A consensus statement regarding capsule endoscopy is currently being developed by NASPGHAN.

CONSENT FOR NASAL ENDOSCOPY IN CHILDREN

The use of unsedated transnasal esophagoscopy has recently been described in pediatric patients.[14,51] This method of endoscopy has similar risks to EGD and colonoscopy but does not involve risks of sedation. There remains the possibility of aspiration with the instillation of a topical nasal anesthetic and emesis. In addition, the nasal route introduces the increased risk of nasal trauma, which may result in epistaxis. Further research using this technique in pediatrics is required. Although this technique has been reported extensively in adult literature, the novelty of this technique in pediatrics does not allow for a discussion of absolute rates of risk for adverse events. However, risk of adverse events is likely similar to or safer than for sedated EGD in pediatrics.

CONSENT FOR PEDIATRIC pH/pH IMPEDANCE/WIRELESS pH MONITORING

Similar to capsule endoscopy consent methods, the consent process for these various reflux assessment techniques varies greatly across institutions. This procedure, although considered safe and time tested, also has the potential for nasal trauma, throat trauma, epistaxis, discomfort, and vomiting. Adverse event data are scarce. Wireless pH devices have the risk of device retention and perforation. The manufacturer states that it has additional risks of premature detachment of the pH capsule, failure of the pH capsule to detach from the esophagus within several days after placement, failure to attach to the esophagus, discomfort associated with the pH capsule, tears in the mucosa, capsule aspiration, capsule retention, and bleeding.[52] As with capsule endoscopy, a conversation with the patient and family regarding anticipated symptoms and adverse events is recommended. Who performs that conversation varies based on institution and provider.[53,54] Documentation of that conversation through a formal consent form or e-method, or simply noting it in the chart, is recommended.

CONSENT FOR ENDOSCOPIC RETROGRADE CHOLANGIOPANCREATOGRAPHY IN CHILDREN

Endoscopic retrograde cholangiopancreatography (ERCP) has been performed by only a few pediatric gastroenterologists in the United States but its use has been increasing.[55] Compared with adults, there is less need for this procedure in pediatrics. Hence, the training required for procedural competence has limited the number of pediatric proceduralists performing ERCP. To be able to provide for a proper consent for this procedure, data regarding pediatric adverse events are still needed, although to some extent they have been forthcoming through recent collaborative studies.[56]

Similar to enteroscopy, the primary additive risk of ERCP compared with diagnostic EGD is injury to the pancreatic or biliary system. ERCP data frequently quote up to a 10% risk of pancreatitis in ERCP, but often-asymptomatic increase of pancreatic enzyme levels may occur. A large recent retrospective study in pediatrics noted a 7.7% risk of pancreatitis.[57] Another smaller study in 2013 showed a pancreatitis rate of 4.3% and an overall complication rate of 7.1%.[58] The consent for ERCP as a specialized therapeutic procedure should be comprehensive and done by a pediatric gastroenterologist or other gastroenterologist who is an expert in such a technique. Although pediatric endoscopists perform many ERCPs, many centers continue to work with adult gastroenterologists to perform this procedure in their patients. An adult gastroenterologist performing consent should be familiar with the uniqueness of pediatric consent methods.

SUMMARY

Informed consent for pediatric gastroenterology procedures requires knowledge of each component of the procedure, general common postprocedural expectations, and the more significant adverse events that can occur. Informed consent also requires a full discussion regarding indications, methods, risk, benefits, and alternatives. Because of the specialized nature of pediatric procedures and their overall lower volume, performance of endoscopy by individuals with specific training in pediatric procedures may be necessary to minimize procedural risks to the patient and family. Information about provider experience and training in pediatric procedures should be available for discussion, if the family or practitioner thinks that it is prudent and relevant to the consent process.

At present, there exists variation among pediatric institutions and individuals as to consent methods and style for pediatric gastrointestinal endoscopy. Many of these differences are in large part caused by federal, state, and institutional requirements. Nevertheless, additional research is needed to standardize and improve on best practices for pediatric informed consent processes. As pediatric gastroenterologists continue to improve on the unique pediatric components of their procedures, a better understanding of inherent risks to various procedures, and best practices for specific consent methods, will likely be elucidated.

REFERENCES

1. Beauchamp TL, Childress JF. Principles of biomedical ethics. New York: Oxford University Press; 2009.
2. Vollmann J, Winau R. Informed consent in human experimentation before the Nuremberg code. BMJ 1996;313:1445–9.
3. Menikoff J. Law and bioethics: an introduction. Washington, DC: Georgetown University Press; 2001.

4. Jones JW, McCullough LB, Richman BW. A comprehensive primer of surgical informed consent. Surg Clin North Am 2007;87:903–18, viii.
5. Fiks AG, Jimenez ME. The promise of shared decision-making in paediatrics. Acta Paediatr 2010;99:1464–6.
6. Lee KJ, Havens PL, Sato TT, et al. Assent for treatment: clinician knowledge, attitudes, and practice. Pediatrics 2006;118:723–30.
7. Friedlander JA, Loeben GS, Finnegan PK, et al. A novel method to enhance informed consent: a prospective and randomised trial of form-based versus electronic assisted informed consent in paediatric endoscopy. J Med Ethics 2011;37: 194–200.
8. Jubbal K, Chun S, Chang J, et al. Parental and youth understanding of the informed consent process for pediatric endoscopy. J Pediatr Gastroenterol Nutr 2015;60:769–75.
9. Moon M. Adolescents' right to consent to reproductive medical care: balancing respect for families with public health goals. Virtual Mentor 2012;14:805–8.
10. Palmer R, Gillespie G. Consent and capacity in children and young people. Arch Dis Child Educ Pract Ed 2014;99:2–7.
11. Alessandri AJ. Parents know best: or do they? Treatment refusals in paediatric oncology. J Paediatr Child Health 2011;47:628–31.
12. Cohen SA, Ephrath H, Lewis JD, et al. Pediatric capsule endoscopy: review of the small bowel and patency capsules. J Pediatr Gastroenterol Nutr 2012;54:409–13.
13. Bishop PR, Nowicki MJ, May WL, et al. Unsedated upper endoscopy in children. Gastrointest Endosc 2002;55:624–30.
14. Friedlander JA, Deboer E, Deterding RR, et al. Monitoring pediatric eosinophilic esophagitis using unsedated transnasal esophagoscopy. Gastrointest Endosc 2015;81:AB172–3.
15. Kinnersley P, Phillips K, Savage K, et al. Interventions to promote informed consent for patients undergoing surgical and other invasive healthcare procedures. Cochrane Database Syst Rev 2013;(7):CD009445.
16. Felley C, Perneger TV, Goulet I, et al. Combined written and oral information prior to gastrointestinal endoscopy compared with oral information alone: a randomized trial. BMC Gastroenterol 2008;8:22.
17. Cousino M, Hazen R, Yamokoski A, et al. Parent participation and physician-parent communication during informed consent in child leukemia. Pediatrics 2011;128:e1544–51.
18. Hazen RA, Drotar D, Kodish E. The role of the consent document in informed consent for pediatric leukemia trials. Contemp Clin Trials 2007;28:401–8.
19. Hazen RA, Eder M, Drotar D, et al. A feasibility trial of a video intervention to improve informed consent for parents of children with leukemia. Pediatr Blood Cancer 2010;55:113–8.
20. Wirshing DA, Sergi MJ, Mintz J. A videotape intervention to enhance the informed consent process for medical and psychiatric treatment research. Am J Psychiatry 2005;162:186–8.
21. Pothier DD. Many patients may not understand consent forms. BMJ 2005;330: 1151.
22. Mayberry MK, Mayberry JF. Towards better informed consent in endoscopy: a study of information and consent processes in gastroscopy and flexible sigmoidoscopy. Eur J Gastroenterol Hepatol 2001;13:1467–76.
23. Parmar VN, Mayberry JF. An audit of informed consent in gastroscopy: investigation of a hospital's informed consent procedure in endoscopy by assessing current practice. Eur J Gastroenterol Hepatol 2005;17:721–4.

24. Shepherd HA, Bowman D, Hancock B, et al. Postal consent for upper gastrointestinal endoscopy. Gut 2000;46:37–9.
25. Woodrow SR, Jenkins AP. How thorough is the process of informed consent prior to outpatient gastroscopy? A study of practice in a United Kingdom District Hospital. Digestion 2006;73:189–97.
26. Lerner D. Endoscopy education video. In: Lerner D, editor. Endoscopy education video-pediatrics, vol. 2015. Children's Hospital Wisconsin; 2015.
27. Sherman HB, McGaghie WC, Unti SM, et al. Teaching pediatrics residents how to obtain informed consent. Acad Med 2005;80:S10–3.
28. Hsu EK, Chugh P, Kronman MP, et al. Incidence of perforation in pediatric GI endoscopy and colonoscopy: an 11-year experience. Gastrointest Endosc 2013;77:960–6.
29. Thakkar K, El-Serag HB, Mattek N, et al. Complications of pediatric colonoscopy: a five-year multicenter experience. Clin Gastroenterol Hepatol 2008;6:515–20.
30. Thakkar K, El-Serag HB, Mattek N, et al. Complications of pediatric EGD: a 4-year experience in PEDS-CORI. Gastrointest Endosc 2007;65:213–21.
31. ASGE Standards of Practice Committee, Lightdale JR, Acosta R, et al. Modifications in endoscopic practice for pediatric patients. Gastrointest Endosc 2014;79:699–710.
32. American Academy of Pediatrics, American Academy of Pediatric Dentistry, Coté CJ, et al. Guidelines for monitoring and management of pediatric patients during and after sedation for diagnostic and therapeutic procedures: an update. Pediatrics 2006;118:2587–602.
33. Samer Ammar M, Pfefferkorn MD, Croffie JM, et al. Complications after outpatient upper GI endoscopy in children: 30-day follow-up. Am J Gastroenterol 2003;98:1508–11.
34. Kori M, Gladish V, Ziv-Sokolovskaya N, et al. The significance of routine duodenal biopsies in pediatric patients undergoing upper intestinal endoscopy. J Clin Gastroenterol 2003;37:39–41.
35. Krugmann J, Neumann H, Vieth M, et al. What is the role of endoscopy and oesophageal biopsies in the management of GERD? Best Pract Res Clin Gastroenterol 2013;27:373–85.
36. Wilson W, Taubert KA, Gewitz M, et al. Prevention of infective endocarditis: guidelines from the American Heart Association: a guideline from the American Heart Association Rheumatic Fever, Endocarditis, and Kawasaki Disease Committee, Council on Cardiovascular Disease in the Young, and the Council on Clinical Cardiology, Council on Cardiovascular Surgery and Anesthesia, and the Quality of Care and Outcomes Research Interdisciplinary Working Group. Circulation 2007;116:1736–54.
37. Gleich SJ, Flick R, Hu D, et al. Neurodevelopment of children exposed to anesthesia: design of the Mayo Anesthesia Safety in Kids (MASK) study. Contemp Clin Trials 2015;41:45–54.
38. Gano D, Andersen SK, Glass HC, et al. Impaired cognitive performance in premature newborns with two or more surgeries prior to term-equivalent age. Pediatr Res 2015;78(3):323–9.
39. Yan XE, Zhou LY, Lin SR, et al. Therapeutic effect of esophageal foreign body extraction management: flexible versus rigid endoscopy in 216 adults of Beijing. Med Sci Monit 2014;20:2054–60.
40. Fan Y, Song HY, Kim JH, et al. Evaluation of the incidence of esophageal complications associated with balloon dilation and their management in patients with malignant esophageal strictures. AJR Am J Roentgenol 2012;198:213–8.

41. Kim IO, Yeon KM, Kim WS, et al. Perforation complicating balloon dilation of esophageal strictures in infants and children. Radiology 1993;189:741–4.
42. Jacobs JW Jr, Spechler SJ. A systematic review of the risk of perforation during esophageal dilation for patients with eosinophilic esophagitis. Dig Dis Sci 2010; 55:1512–5.
43. Uygun I, Arslan MS, Aydogdu B, et al. Fluoroscopic balloon dilatation for caustic esophageal stricture in children: an 8-year experience. J Pediatr Surg 2013;48: 2230–4.
44. Mattei P, Alonso M, Justinich C. Laparoscopic repair of colon perforation after colonoscopy in children: report of 2 cases and review of the literature. J Pediatr Surg 2005;40:1651–3.
45. Rutter MD, Nickerson C, Rees CJ, et al. Risk factors for adverse events related to polypectomy in the English Bowel Cancer Screening Programme. Endoscopy 2014;46:90–7.
46. Fox D, Campagna EJ, Friedlander J, et al. National trends and outcomes of pediatric gastrostomy tube placement. J Pediatr Gastroenterol Nutr 2014;59:582–8.
47. McSweeney ME, Jiang H, Deutsch AJ, et al. Long-term outcomes of infants and children undergoing percutaneous endoscopy gastrostomy tube placement. J Pediatr Gastroenterol Nutr 2013;57:663–7.
48. McSweeney ME, Kerr J, Jiang H, et al. Risk factors for complications in infants and children with percutaneous endoscopic gastrostomy tubes. J Pediatr 2015; 166:1514–9.e1.
49. Urs AN, Martinelli M, Rao P, et al. Diagnostic and therapeutic utility of double-balloon enteroscopy in children. J Pediatr Gastroenterol Nutr 2014;58:204–12.
50. Imaging G. PillCam capsule endoscopy-indications/risks, vol. 2015. Given; 2015. Available at: http://www.givenimaging.com/en-us/Innovative-Solutions/Capsule-Endoscopy/Pillcam-SB/Indications-Risks/Pages/default.aspx.
51. Committee AT, Rodriguez SA, Banerjee S, et al. Ultrathin endoscopes. Gastrointest Endosc 2010;71:893–8.
52. Imaging G. Reflux monitoring, Bravo pH, indications and risks, 2015. Available at: http://www.givenimaging.com/en-us/Innovative-Solutions/Reflux-Monitoring/Bravo-pH/Indications-Risks/Pages/default.aspx.
53. Waloszkova J, Avey F, Leahy A. OC-003 Nurse vs doctor consent within endoscopy: are they equal? Gut 2012;61:A1–2.
54. Burrows A, Asare J. Nurse-led consent in endoscopy. Gastrointest Nurs 2014;12: 24–8.
55. Pant C, Sferra TJ, Barth BA, et al. Trends in endoscopic retrograde cholangiopancreatography in children within the United States, 2000-2009. J Pediatr Gastroenterol Nutr 2014;59:57–60.
56. Troendle DM, Liu Q, Kim KM, et al. ERCP in younger vs older children: initial report from the multicenter pediatric ERCP database initiative. Gastrointest Endosc 2015;81:AB173.
57. Giefer MJ, Kozarek RA. Technical outcomes and complications of pediatric ERCP. Surg Endosc 2015. [Epub ahead of print].
58. Halvorson L, Halsey K, Darwin P, et al. The safety and efficacy of therapeutic ERCP in the pediatric population performed by adult gastroenterologists. Dig Dis Sci 2013;58:3611–9.

Measuring Quality in Pediatric Endoscopy

Jenifer R. Lightdale, MD, MPH

KEYWORDS

- Quality • Metrics • Pediatric endoscopy • Pediatric colonoscopy • Training
- GiECAT$_{KIDS}$ • Benchmarks • Quality improvement

KEY POINTS

- Quality measurements in pediatric endoscopy can be used to increase transparency about patient care processes and outcomes.
- Although the definition of quality for pediatric endoscopy is yet to be fully developed, it can be promoted by adhering to various established metrics for procedural documentation.
- The Gastrointestinal Endoscopy Competency Assessment Tool for Pediatrics Colonoscopy (GiECAT$_{KIDS}$) is a rigorously developed quality measure of procedural competence.
- Continuous quality improvement initiatives that engage trainees, as well as established pediatric endoscopists, to examine their own procedural processes and outcomes can be considered to be valuable at both the individual provider and endoscopy unit level.

INTRODUCTION

Measuring procedural quality should be expected to become an increasingly standard component of performing gastrointestinal endoscopy in children in the twenty-first century. Quality measurements in endoscopy, as in all aspects of medical practice, are increasingly being used to appraise clinical care processes, as health care in the United States and beyond continues down its current path of reformation.[1] Such metrics are also likely to be used to increase transparency about patient outcomes, as well as to influence payments for the procedure.[2–4] In turn, pediatric gastroenterologists must be open to defining aspects of high-quality endoscopy, as well as to begin to self-identify opportunities for improvement. The risk to not engage in the quality movement is that others (including regulatory boards, administrative agencies, or third-party payers) will define these measures for us.

Disclosure Statement: The author serves as a consultant for Medtronic, Perrigo, and Norgine.
Division of Pediatric Gastroenterology, Hepatology and Nutrition, UMass Memorial Children's Medical Center, University of Massachusetts Medical School, University Campus, 55 Lake Avenue North, Worcester, MA 01655, USA
E-mail address: jenifer.lightdale@umassmemorial.org

Box 1 lists candidate quality metrics for pediatric endoscopy, which can be either process or outcomes oriented.[4,5] Regardless of their origin or intended use, it is reasonable to mandate that all metrics devised to assess quality of pediatric endoscopy be accurate, meaningful, and practical. Measuring quality in endoscopy involves assessing 2 dimensions of care: (1) appropriateness of a procedure and (2) the skill with which the procedure is performed.[6] It also should encompass the 6 domains of quality put forth by the Institute of Medicine, by ensuring that procedures are effective, patient-centered, safe, efficient, timely, and equitable.[7] The definition of pediatric endoscopic quality is still to be fully developed; however, when viewed at the societal level, it is plausible to assume that endoscopy should be recommended and performed, when indicated, in an expeditious, skillful, successful, safe, and comfortable manner. Performance of pediatric endoscopy also should be of high value, providing the best quality for the least cost.

To date, there are limited measures of endoscopic quality that have been universally accepted when treating either adult or pediatric patients. However, a number of high-stake interest groups, including the American Society of Gastrointestinal Endoscopy (ASGE), have put forward individual and multisociety consensus statements on the

---

Box 1
Elements of pediatric endoscopic quality that reflect individual processes of care, as well as clinical outcomes

Endoscopic Procedures
  Procedure volume by type
  Appropriateness of indications
  Absence of contraindications
  Patient comfort
  Adverse events
  Technical performance (eg, ileal intubation)
  Therapeutic success (eg, esophageal dilation, polyp removal)
  Accuracy of endoscopic diagnosis
  Completeness of documentation

Patient Based
  Waiting room time
  Patient satisfaction (eg, with discharge instructions, procedures, sedation)
  Parental satisfaction
  Family/patient complaints
  Rescheduled or canceled procedures
  Waiting time for transfer, transport, admission

Nursing/Support Staff
  Intravenous access difficulties
  Adequacy of bowel preparation
  Completeness of preprocedure assessments
  Completeness of sedation/anesthesia records
  Mislabeled specimens
  Follow-up care documented
  Room turnover time

Environment and safety
  Universal precautions use
  Emergency equipment readiness
  Safe stretcher use
  Expired drug disposal
  Radiation drug use
  Storage and disposal of chemicals/toxins
  Room turnover time

Infection Control
  Scope disinfection procedure followed
  Accessory reprocessing procedure followed
  Bacteremia following procedures
  Proper specimen handling
  Needle disposal

Other
  Procedure report sent to referring physician
  Specimen loss
  Missing consent forms
  Endoscope repairs (type, frequency, turnover)
  Missing prior authorization
  Billing rejection

Adapted from Brown RD, Goldstein JL. Quality assurance in the endoscopy unit. Gastrointest Endosc Clin N Am 1999;9(4):596; with permission.

topic.[4,8,9] In short, there is good agreement that a quality endoscopic procedure is safe and efficient, is used effectively to make proper diagnoses, can essentially exclude other diagnoses, minimizes adverse events, and is accompanied by appropriate documentation from beginning through the end of the procedure. This includes the documentation of timely communication of all results, including pathologic analysis of tissue sampling.

Common methods for improving quality in health care include the identification of threshold standards, below which care can be considered to be inadequate; benchmarking personal practice with that of peers; the provision of additional training and education; the performance of self-evaluation and reporting; as well as engagement in continuous quality improvement processes. The process of identifying a standard, and then evaluating whether all practice meets that standard, can be considered quality assurance. Although quality assurance is critical to all procedures, it only targets improvement or elimination of performance below the set threshold. In contrast, quality improvement assumes that there is variability in practice that can be used to motivate all performers on a "bell-shaped curve" to improve toward the highest levels.

MEASURING QUALITY THROUGH PROCEDURAL DOCUMENTATION

Quality in endoscopy can be promoted by adhering to various established metrics for procedural documentation.[10] **Box 2** lists recommendations for endoscopic procedure documentation that were proposed by the ASGE in a monograph on quality in 1998

Box 2
Recommendations from the American Society of Gastrointestinal Endoscopy (ASGE) for standard elements of endoscopic procedure documentation

Procedure Report
  Date of procedure
  Patient identification data (eg, Medical record number, account number, encounter number)
  Procedure type
  Indication for procedure
  Patient medical history/comorbidities
  Physical Status (American Society of Anesthesiology)
  Endoscopic instrument identification data
  Medications used (eg, general anesthesia, sedatives, antibiotics)
  Anatomic extent of examination
  Limitations of examination
  Tissue or fluid samples obtained (number, location)
  Findings
  Diagnostic impression
  Results of therapeutic intervention
  Adverse events (immediate vs delayed)
  Disposition
  Recommendations for further care

Endoscopic Unit Record
  (In addition to Procedure Report Data)
  Duration of procedure
  Presence of informed consent document
  Evidence of preprocedural and postprocedural evaluation
  Procedure Sedation Record
  Evidence of postprocedure recovery (ie, Aldrete score)

Adapted from Brown RD, Goldstein JL. Quality assurance in the endoscopy unit. Gastrointest Endosc Clin N Am 1999;9(4):599; with permission.

---

that reviewed recommendations of various regulatory bodies, including the Department of Health and Human Services' Agency for Healthcare Research and Quality, as well as the Joint Commission.[5] Many of these key elements of documentation have since been supported by adult and pediatric studies as appropriate for universal application across endoscopic procedures.[9,10] Generally speaking, pediatric procedural documentation of endoscopy is intended to maintain standards upheld in documentation of surgeries, as well as procedures in adults. Whenever possible, such standards should be evidenced-based.

Endoscopic quality should be assessed at each time point of a procedure, including before, during, and after its performance.[9] Strictly speaking, the process of performing endoscopy often begins in the clinic with referral for the procedure, and ends after patients have left the procedural unit. Documentation that reflects the quality of each time point in the procedure is an imperative and must relate to critical elements.

Preprocedural elements that can be used to assess the quality of documentation of pediatric gastrointestinal endoscopy include clear mention of the procedural indication; discussion of informed consent, including discussion of risks, benefits, and alternatives to the procedure; evidence that the endoscopist performed a preprocedure assessment, either by documentation of a physical examination and/or by noting the patient's physical status; as well as evidence that the endoscopist established a plan for how sedation would be achieved, even if that routinely involves an anesthesiologist-administered regimen.

Major intraprocedural elements should include a full description of the procedure performed, delineation of any findings with specific mention of anatomic landmarks, quantification of estimated blood loss, and note of any complications. Ideally, standard language is used to describe findings.[11] Postprocedural elements that should be clearly documented to ensure reflection of procedural quality include cataloging of any patient recommendations postprocedure. There also should be clear documentation of communications that ensued regarding results of the procedure, including immediately after the procedure in terms of endoscopic impressions, and later, after processing and review of tissue samples.

Large multicenter studies of quality of endoscopy reports have shown clear gaps in documentation quality that may benefit from improvement.[12-14] In particular, investigators examining data from the Clinical Outcomes Research Initiative or CORI project of more than 400,000 procedures over a 2-year period found tremendous variation in reporting, with many basic elements of procedural reports found to simply be missing.[14] In similar findings using different methodology, Robertson and colleagues[12] reviewed 122 separate endoscopy centers for adherence to ASGE guidelines for reporting. They set a threshold for adequate performance for any criterion at 70% compliance, and found that colonoscopy reporting practices were widely variable and often suboptimal, even with this low standard.

Endoscopy reports by pediatric gastroenterologists may similarly suffer from inconsistencies and significant provider variation. One recent study by Thakkar and colleagues[10] examined more than 21,000 records from 14 pediatric centers in the pediatric endoscopy database system - clinical outcomes research initiative (PEDS-CORI) network for adherence to key quality indicators and found that more than half of pediatric endoscopy notes analyzed were missing at least one element. Key indicators included documentation of bowel preparation, ileal intubation rate, American Society of Anesthesiologists physical status, and procedure time. This study underscores the importance of focusing on standardizing documentation as a starting point for engaging in discussions of quality, even as we continue to explore best measures for pediatric procedures.

QUALITY AND ENDOSCOPIC TRAINING

Training in pediatric endoscopy may represent the most critical time to teach best practices around not only performing procedures, but also their documentation. The goals of training in endoscopy are to perform procedures, safely, completely, independently, and expeditiously; to accurately interpret and describe findings; to integrate endoscopic findings into the management plan; to recognize and manage complications; and to effectively communicate both the endoscopic and pathologic results of procedures to patients and to other clinical providers.[15] Recent pediatric guidelines stipulate that trainees must aim to know appropriate indications, contraindications, and alternatives to procedures; appearances of both normal and abnormal findings; and how to select and apply appropriate sedation strategies and equipment.[16] High-quality documentation of a procedure from both trainees and experienced endoscopists should routinely reflect attainment of each of these goals.

Of course, beyond learning to document, it is paramount that trainees develop procedural competence during their fellowship years. In this regard, the Gastrointestinal Endoscopy Competency Assessment Tool for Pediatric Colonoscopy (GiECAT$_{KIDS}$) should be recognized as the most rigorously developed quality measure to date for pediatric gastrointestinal procedures.[17,18] The GiECAT$_{KIDS}$ was developed by Dr Catharine Walsh at the University of Toronto to support a competency approach to training and assessment of pediatric colonoscopy. Dr Walsh used a Delphi method involving more than 40 expert endoscopists from a variety of practice settings across North America. Through this process, 3 major domains of colonoscopy competency were developed: (1) technical (psychomotor skill), (2) cognitive (knowledge), and (3) integrative (judgment, clinical reasoning).[17]

A final score on the GiECAT$_{KIDS}$ is calculated from 2 components. The first is an 18-item highly structured checklist, which outlines key steps required to complete the procedure. This checklist is modeled after validated versions used in general surgery and is scored dichotomously, where 1 = done correctly and 0 = not done or done incorrectly. The second component of the GiECAT$_{KIDS}$ score is a 7-domain Global Rating Scale (GRS), which is designed to assess holistic aspects of skill in terms of provider autonomy, including technical skill, strategies for scope advancement, visualization of mucosa, independent procedure completion (vs need for assistance), knowledge of procedure, interpretation and management of findings, and patient safety. Each domain of the GRS is scored on a 5-point Likert scale, with higher scores reflective of better performance (more autonomy demonstrated) by the endoscopist (**Box 3**).

Box 3
Likert anchors used in scoring the Global Rating Scale component of the Gastrointestinal Endoscopy Competency Assessment Tool for Pediatric Colonoscopy, which differentiates between levels of procedural competency, as defined by degree of provider autonomy

1. Unable to achieve tasks despite significant verbal and/or hands-on guidance

2. Achieves some of the tasks but requires significant verbal and/or hands-on guidance

3. Achieves most of the tasks independently, with minimal verbal and/or manual guidance

4. Competent for independent performance of all tasks without the need for any guidance

5. Highly skilled advanced performance of all tasks

The GiECAT$_{KIDS}$ has excellent reliability and validity and should be regarded as a mature quality indicator that can be used in training programs.[17] In particular, it has been shown to have high interrater, as well as test-retest, reliability. Total scores can be used to discriminate among novice, intermediate, and advanced endoscopists. Higher scores are also significantly associated with more procedural experience (**Fig. 1**), as well as higher cecal and ileal intubation rates.[18] In turn, although the GiE-CAT is currently only recommended for training, it is plausible to assume future studies may find it can be useful in granting procedural privileges or in monitoring continued competence, for practicing clinicians.

QUALITY IMPROVEMENT AND MAINTENANCE OF CERTIFICATION

As endoscopists transition from trainee to faculty, competencies in procedural performance should be maintained. Identifying gaps in procedural quality is critical to improving pediatric endoscopic practices at all levels of expertise. Continuous quality improvement (CQI) initiatives that engage trainees, as well as practicing endoscopists, to examine their own procedural processes and outcomes can be considered to be valuable at the individual and endoscopy unit level.[19] Not only may CQI help in maintenance of competence certification for providers, but it can also help in identifying areas of process vulnerabilities across a clinical practice.[20]

For example, systematic examination of peri-procedural records of multiple providers within a practice may reveal lack of standardized documentation around informed consent. This may leave open the possibility that a patient could undergo endoscopy without clear documentation that consent was obtained, should the consent form be misplaced. It also creates the potential for omission of particular risks, which could be cited later by a patient or a family who could state they were not prepared in the event of a complication. Identifying and mitigating such vulnerabilities could facilitate the determination of a best practice within the unique practice environment engaged in the CQI activity to ensure that consent is obtained by all providers in a standardized manner, and that the process is invariably documented in a specific location in the medical record.

Although the current process for maintaining subspecialty board certification in pediatric gastroenterology is controversial, the American Board of Pediatrics has pledged support for efforts by the North American Society for Pediatric Gastroenterology, Hepatology, and Nutrition (NASPGHAN) and other societies to host quality improvement maintenance of certification (MOC) activities.[21] NASPGHAN, specifically, has offered

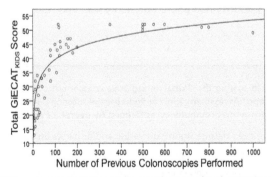

Fig. 1. Total GiECAT$_{KIDS}$ scores increase in line with procedural experience, with a notable plateau after 200 to 400 procedures. (*Adapted from* Walsh CM, Ling SC, Walters TD, et al. Development of the gastrointestinal endoscopy competency assessment tool for pediatric colonoscopy (GiECATKIDS). J Pediatr Gastroenterol Nutr 2014;59(4):482; with permission.)

a mechanism since 2013 for members to gain MOC credit by examining their own endoscopy and colonoscopy documentation practices.[22] **Table 1** shows collective baseline responses from participants electing to participate in the first year of these MOC activities (NASPGHAN MOC Task Force Presentation at the Annual Meeting, 2014). These data not only reveal opportunities for improvements in processes of care, but also begin to provide benchmark data around key indicators, such as ileal intubation rates and typical procedural times. Ultimately, data collected through MOC activities may be useful for quality assurance across the field of pediatric gastroenterology.

PREPROCEDURE ELEMENTS OF QUALITY PEDIATRIC ENDOSCOPY

Indications for performing endoscopy in children can be diagnostic, as well as therapeutic. In either case, the indications for recommending and proceeding with a planned gastrointestinal procedure should be ideally made clear to both patients and other providers *before* it begins.[9] A number of studies in adults have shown higher diagnostic yield when endoscopic procedures are performed for appropriate reasons.[23–25] Another critical element of a high-quality preprocedure phase is evidence of patient assessment by the endoscopist.[13] One way to provide such evidence is to document a patient's physical status according to a classification system designed by the American Society of Anesthesiology (ASA), even if an anesthesiology-colleague has also made note of this in their procedural documentation.

Indeed, one of the most important preoperative assessments is relating patient risk factors for a given procedure to the proposed plan for sedation. The ASA has established suggestions for their nonanesthesiology colleagues to classify patients' physical status.[26,27] This classification system is commonly used as a metric of patient complexity, and serves as a common language among clinicians, as they discuss patients in terms of disease severity. However, the ASA is well known to suffer from

Table 1	
Example of baseline data collected from the providers enrolled in the North American Society for Pediatric Gastroenterology, Hepatology, and Nutrition endoscopy maintenance of certification (MOC) activity	
MOC Upper Endoscopy – Data Entry Period 1 (n = 81)	
1. Average compliance with procedural documentation requirements across 10 charts	84.2%
2. Average % of procedure reports shared with primary care or referring physician	63.8%
3. Average % documentation of discussion of biopsy results with patient/parent	90.4%
4. Average time from procedure to reporting of biopsy results	8.0 d
5. Average % upper endoscopies performed that resulted in change in clinical management	59.6%
MOC Colonoscopy – Data Entry Period 1 (n = 58)	
1. Average compliance with procedural documentation requirements across 10 charts	91.3%
2. Average total colonoscopy time (scope insertion through withdrawal)	35.7 min
3. Average total time to cecum	20.9 min
4. Average % successful terminal ileum intubation[a]	91.8%
5. Average % colonoscopies performed that resulted in change in clinical management	68.0%

[a] Record review restricted by protocol to cases with a priori intention to inspect the ileum.

interobserver agreement.[28] A brief preprocedural discussion with the anesthesiologist about patient ASA is a good way to make sure both anesthesiologist and endoscopist have the same considerations as they assess a patient. It also avoids discordant assessments of the same patient by 2 providers (the endoscopist and the anesthesiologist) treating the same patient during the same encounter, which could be used to signify inadequate coordination of care.

One caveat regarding ASA classification is that anesthesiologists may be inclined to label more children undergoing endoscopy as a higher ASA class when compared with ratings by endoscopists and pediatric endoscopy nurses. This may be because anesthesiologists routinely consider reflux, as well as patient age, in their decision-making. Another drawback to relying on ASA classification to document patient assessment is that the system is one of crude patient categories that cannot adequately capture complex clinical scenarios. For this reason, it may be very appropriate and useful to also document a patient's comorbidities.[13] Asthma, in particular, is a common pediatric comorbidity that could impact a patient receiving procedural sedation. Careful documentation of comorbidities does not only improve procedural outcomes, but also attests to the endoscopist's awareness of risks to a patient's safety and that they are in a position to take steps to mitigate them.

Despite its shortcomings, a patient's ASA class has been shown to be clearly associated with increased risk of adverse events in both adults and children.[29] In turn, ASA classifications may be useful in endoscopic risk stratification, leading to multisociety agreement that its documentation should be considered an important quality indicator for endoscopy.[13]

Informed consent is the final critical element of the preprocedure phase. The ASGE has defined informed consent as "voluntary agreement by a person with the capacity for decision making to make an informed choice about allowing an action proposed by another person."[30] By definition, obtaining informed consent in pediatrics almost always involves parents or legal guardians to provide consent. State laws should be used to determine the age at which pediatric patients can give legal consent or what exact capacity a patient requires for decision making.

There are few contraindications for performing endoscopy in children. New ASGE standards-of-practice for pediatric endoscopy state the only relative "absolute" contraindication may be when bowel perforation suspected, but even this is best recognized to be a relative risk.[31] Nevertheless, endoscopy in situations that may involve risk factors associated with concerns for patient safety during the procedure should involve a clearly documented risk-to-benefit discussion with the patient or the patient's family. These risk factors may include patient size, as very small premature neonates, in particular those weighing less than 2.0 kg, as well as obese children, may be at risk for respiratory compromise; patients with coagulopathies, which may increase their risks from biopsies; those with neutropenia, which may increase their risks of infection; and those with acute cardiac and/or pulmonary disease, who should also be assessed for risks of sedation-related events.[32–34]

To be of high quality, informed consent should include "professional disclosure," defined as what would be expected should a colleague in the same situation give either to another clinician or to a layperson.[35] Information within disclosure should include a patient's medical diagnosis and results, the proposed procedure and the reason, the benefits anticipated by performing the procedure, any risks the endoscopist has considered as he or she prepares for the procedure, as well as possible complications and/or adverse events that a reasonable patient should expect to know might be encountered during the procedure. Finally, patients should be advised as to any alternatives that might exist to doing the procedure, as well as their prognosis if the procedure is declined.

It is possible to directly relate each component of high-quality consent to specific procedures and their indications in children. For example, in the case of a diagnostic esophagogastroduodenoscopy with biopsies to evaluate esophagitis, the goals of the procedure are to obtain information by visualizing and sampling the mucosa of the upper gastrointestinal tract. Risks of the procedure are rare, but do include bleeding, perforation, and exposure to infectious disease. The alternative to not performing the procedure de facto would entail not gaining information unique to visualizing and/or sampling the mucosa.

COMPLICATIONS OF PEDIATRIC ENDOSCOPY

Although the safety of performing upper endoscopy in children has been well established, it is important to recognize that performing endoscopic procedures in children is inherently risky. In data from PEDS-CORI involving more than 10,000 endoscopies, the overall rate of complications was 2.3%, and mostly involved transient hypoxia from sedation (1.5%).[29] The risk of bleeding was second-most common at 0.3%.

Analysis of PEDS-CORI data also has suggested that characteristics of patients who are most at risk for complications during pediatric upper endoscopy include those who are younger, and those with higher ASA classes.[29] In addition, the presence of a trainee during a procedure may be more associated with adverse events. Presence of a trainee has also been shown to add time to procedures,[36,37] which to some extent should be viewed as a "necessary evil" of training the next generation of endoscopists. On the other hand, as procedural efficiency is increasingly rewarded, it may be important to document trainee presence to account for otherwise substandard metrics. Documentation of presence of a trainee during a procedure should be viewed as an element of high-quality endoscopy in gastrointestinal fellowship programs, as it allows both verification of procedural experience by the trainee, as well as clear evidence of their participation in the patient's medical record.

The ASGE has provided a lexicon for complications of endoscopy that is helpful for standardizing definitions.[38] It is fundamentally important to track complications, even though they may occur extremely infrequently. **Fig. 2** depicts an example of how the number of complications adjusted per 10,000 procedures, and analyzed at the provider level using a funnel plot of upper control limits for provider rates, can be used to identify endoscopists with special cause variation in their even rates. This approach rests on the assumption that if providers as a group are uniformly performing safe and competent gastrointestinal procedures, the rate of major complications during endoscopic procedures will be low and no special cause variation in complication rates across providers will be identified.

It also may be appropriate to risk stratify procedures so as to avoid misclassifying endoscopists with particular advanced expertise in procedures that may incur more risk, and/or those who are willing to take on the most difficult cases in a group. Our experience with adjusting procedures by ASA status (I/II vs III or greater), as well as to whether the procedures were diagnostic or therapeutic, has suggested these may be reasonable variables for risk adjustment. Further study is needed to better elucidate measures of complications, as well as best statistical approaches to understanding them appropriately.

INTRAPROCEDURAL ELEMENTS OF QUALITY

For both upper endoscopy and colonoscopy, high-quality procedures are reflected in documentation that attests to complete inspection, and that differentiates between examination by visualization only, and mucosal sampling. The implementation of

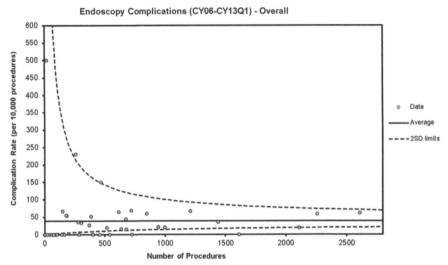

Fig. 2. Example of upper funnel methodology to identify providers (each orange dot represents one provider) with above expected, unadjusted, complication rates for pediatric endoscopy. N = 23,714. Complication Rate = 38.8/10,000 procedures. (*Data Courtesy of* JR Lightdale, MD, Worcester, MA.)

colorectal cancer (CRC) screening in adult medicine has guided development of most intraprocedural quality metrics in endoscopy. The most focus has been placed on cecal intubation rates, as well as adenoma detection rates and indications for procedures (ie, recommended intervals for postpolypectomy surveillance).[9] A multitude of studies have again found variation in care, as well as inconsistencies in documentation, to provide ample opportunities for CQI.[3,8,20,39]

At this time, thresholds for quality of CRC screening are generally considered to be a minimum cecal intubation rate of greater than 90%, a withdrawal time of at least 6 or better 9 minutes, and an adenoma detection rate of greater than 20%.[8] Furthermore, colonoscopy in adults should be completed with a complication rate lower than 1%, including polypectomy. To date, many quality improvement initiatives have focused on processes of care around bowel preparation and withdrawal rates that can help to ensure complete inspection during screening procedures.[40,41] The growing insight into factors that improve complete inspection and thereby CRC detection rates underscores a growing appreciation by adult colonoscopists into processes of care that can affect outcomes.

Colonoscopy in children is fundamental to the diagnosis and management of digestive disease in children, but is rarely performed to screen for CRC. As such, intraprocedural quality metrics for colonoscopy in children must be different from those in adults. Most indications for colonoscopy in children are lower gastrointestinal bleeding, abdominal pain, and diarrhea.[42] Colonoscopy is most commonly performed in infants and children when entertaining a diagnosis of inflammatory bowel disease,[43] but also may be used to identify common sources of rectal bleeding, including juvenile polyps.[42,44]

With respect to common indications, most pediatric colonoscopies require ileocecal intubation to screen for inflammatory bowel disease.[43] Thakkar and colleagues[10] recently proposed candidate quality metrics for pediatric colonoscopy to include ileal intubation, as well as procedure duration and bowel preparation quality. In a study of quality indicators for pediatric colonoscopy conducted through the PEDS-CORI network, they also reviewed preprocedural documentation of indications, as well as postprocedure unplanned events. In addition to wide variation in documentation, the investigators found approximately 30% of procedures to have no documentation of ileal inspection, and more than 50% to lack documentation of bowel preparation quality. A growing emphasis on improving processes of care, such as bowel preparation, while focusing on quality of documentation, is likely to improve diagnostic yield and help avoid need for repeat procedures.

Upper endoscopy is far more commonly performed in children as compared with colonoscopy, and may be specifically useful to evaluate for the possibility of common pediatric conditions, such as allergic, infectious, or peptic esophagitis; infectious or inflammatory gastritis; and celiac disease.[45] Again, complete inspection is key to diagnosis, and a typical upper gastrointestinal endoscopy should involve direct visualization of the esophagus, stomach, duodenal bulb, and the duodenum.

The preferred method of pediatric endoscope insertion when performing quality endoscopy, with or without endotracheal intubation, is direct visualization of structures in the pharynx, including the palate, epiglottis, arytenoids, and vocal cords. The esophagus should be partially distended to look for abnormalities and to also identify anatomic landmarks, such as the aortic notch and the gastroesophageal junction. The stomach should be considered as 3 areas: the fundus, corpus, and antrum. Most quality upper endoscopic procedures advance to the third part of the duodenum, past the major papilla.

According to new ASGE guidelines, biopsies should be obtained during endoscopic procedures if patients have an underlying immunocompromised state; if irregular or deep ulcerations of the mucosa are seen; or if there is proximal distribution of esophagitis, a mass lesion, or an irregular-appearing stricture.[46] Biopsies during colonoscopy should be obtained if there are irregularities of the mucosa. Generally speaking, obtaining biopsies should be considered a very safe practice, but inherently to involve increased risks, especially of bleeding or perforation.[47] Biopsies also should be recognized to add significant cost to endoscopic procedures. In turn, appropriate sampling may be key to ensuring endoscopic value.[48]

Regarding biopsies and pediatric endoscopy, the standard of care is to obtain them routinely, even in the absence of specific findings.[31] The resulting emphasis on obtaining nonfocal biopsies is based in large part on a consensus "risk-benefit calculation" that the downsides of performing repeat procedures in the pediatric population outweighs the downsides of obtaining biopsies from normal-appearing mucosa, on the off chance it might show disease. Evidence to support this practice has been limited, but impactful. For example, Khakoo and colleagues[49] examined the correlation between endoscopic and histologic findings in 167 children undergoing endoscopy for peptic symptoms, and found that only erosive disease was associated with high endoscopic-histologic correlation. In those patients with no findings endoscopically, 60% had evidence of gastritis on histology.

The likelihood that there may be pathologic findings if the mucosa appears normal to an endoscopist is considerably less during colonoscopy.[48] Nevertheless, it remains common practice during pediatric colonoscopy to obtain multiple nonfocal biopsies at multiple colonic segments, even if there is the appearance of normal colonic mucosa throughout. Recently, a few studies have suggested that current strategies of taking multiple biopsy specimens during pediatric colonoscopies add little to no benefit compared with strategies taking fewer biopsies, and may incur significant cost.[48,50] Future quality studies of pediatric colonoscopy are needed to evaluate biopsy strategies in pediatric colonoscopy in terms of diagnostic yield, patient safety, and procedural value.

Regardless, biopsy protocols during all pediatric procedures may benefit from standardization. For example, it is important to recognize that certain conditions common in children (eg, gastritis, celiac disease) may be patchy in distribution. One proposed method that has been shown consistently to increase diagnostic yield in the case of suspected gastritis is to use the Sydney system, which suggests 5 locations in the stomach[49,51] (**Fig. 3**).

Evidence-based guidelines may be critical to developing high-value biopsy protocols. In the case of celiac disease, the American College of Gastroenterology recommends 4 to 6 proximal small bowel biopsies, from parts 1 to 4 of the duodenum.[52] There has been growing evidence that diagnostic yield of pediatric celiac disease may be increased if the duodenal bulb is biopsied.[53] Eosinophilic esophagitis may be a patchy disease that also requires biopsies for diagnosis. There may be increased diagnostic yield if at least 5 biopsies are obtained from the distal, mid, and proximal esophagus.[54]

POSTPROCEDURAL ELEMENTS OF QUALITY

In the postprocedure period, there are several critical elements to ensuring high endoscopic quality. In particular, ensuring and documenting clear communication on the day of the procedure is important. In addition to communication of endoscopic findings, it is also important to convey that pathology has been sent and is pending. Documentation that the patient has been advised to await results of tissue sampling can attest to this communication.

Communication later of pathology findings is a fundamental responsibility associated with performing endoscopy in children.[55] As with all pathology, this is particularly true if the biopsies suggest disease or an unfavorable diagnosis; however, this responsibility is just as important when the biopsies do not show pathology. Either result is helpful for providing guidance regarding appropriate postprocedural follow-up. Failure to communicate pathology findings is often the result of poorly designed systems for ensuring communication practices.[56]

Role clarity is key, and it should be decided a priori in a practice as to who will communicate the findings. Candidates for this role include the providers themselves, a colleague who referred the patient for endoscopy, as well as nursing or administrative staff. It also should be determined ahead of time what form the communication will

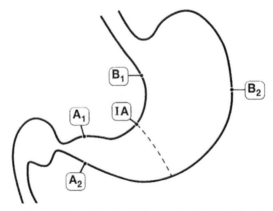

Fig. 3. The Sydney system for rigorously classifying each section of the stomach. (*From* Dixon MF, Genta RM, Yardley JH, et al. Classification and grading of gastritis. The updated Sydney System. International Workshop on the Histopathology of Gastritis, Houston 1994. Am J Surg Pathol 1996;20(10):1161–81; with permission.)

take, and the timing for notification. Finally, role clarity is also key in terms of documenting that communication about pathology results occurred, as well as follow-up plans that were made, in accordance.

Designing good systems for documenting communication of pathology findings requires a careful understanding of individual work-flow.[55] The ideal system for communicating results is meticulous, standardized, and sets clear expectations for everyone, including patients. For example, a practice may opt to provide a written handout during discharge from a procedural unit that gives a timeline for expecting notifications from the endoscopist regarding biopsies, who will call the patient, and how to reach the office if the communication appears to have broken down.

Clear documentation of communicating results should include information about how (eg, via phone call, letter, e-mail) and when patients were contacted, whether or not they appeared to understand the discussion, and what follow-up plan was recommended. It also may be appropriate to document the provider's impression of the patient's understanding and plan for next steps.

SUMMARY

In conclusion, gastrointestinal endoscopy is a fundamental tool for diagnosing gastrointestinal disease in children that is generally safe, but inherently risky. High-quality pediatric endoscopy should be recognized to involve technical, cognitive, and integrative skills. Quality of pediatric procedures should be reflected in documentation of key indicators, which are yet to be fully developed. Nevertheless, a plausible framework for CQI in pediatric endoscopy likely begins with standardization and consistency in documentation throughout all phases of a procedure.

Patient assessment preprocedure is critical and increasingly a nationally recognized quality metric. Likewise, a national emphasis on quality informed consent mandates that physicians explain the nature and purpose of the procedure, the probable risks and benefits, and any rare or unusual risks of which a reasonable person would want to be aware and any alternatives to performing the procedure or refusing care. Intraprocedural quality can be assured by allowing the indication for the procedure to a priori guide evidence-based strategies to ensure complete visualization of the anatomy and to obtain biopsies appropriately. Finally, postprocedural communication of results occurs both on the day of the procedure and subsequently, when pathology results are returned.

In short, ensuring quality in pediatric gastrointestinal procedures requires meticulous, carefully designed systems designed to capture key measures that endoscopists must be open to evaluating, at all stages of their careers.

REFERENCES

1. Bjorkman DJ, Popp JW Jr. Measuring the quality of endoscopy. Am J Gastroenterol 2006;101(4):864–5.
2. Chassin MR, Loeb JM, Schmaltz SP, et al. Accountability measures–using measurement to promote quality improvement. N Engl J Med 2010;363(7):683–8.
3. Hewett DG, Rex DK. Improving colonoscopy quality through health-care payment reform. Am J Gastroenterol 2010;105(9):1925–33.
4. Cotton PB, Hawes RH, Barkun A, et al. Excellence in endoscopy: toward practical metrics. Gastrointest Endosc 2006;63(2):286–91.
5. Brown RD, Goldstein JL. Quality assurance in the endoscopy unit: an emphasis on outcomes. Gastrointest Endosc Clin N Am 1999;9(4):595–607, vi.

6. Johanson JF, Schmitt CM, Deas TM Jr, et al. Quality and outcomes assessment in gastrointestinal endoscopy. Gastrointest Endosc 2000;52(6 Pt 1):827–30.
7. Institute of Medicine Committee on Quality of Health Care in America. To err is human: building a safer health system. In: Kohn L, Corrigan J, Donaldson M, editors. Washington, DC: National Academy Press; 2000. p. 287.
8. Pullens HJ, Siersema PD. Quality indicators for colonoscopy: current insights and caveats. World J Gastrointest Endosc 2014;6(12):571–83.
9. Rex DK, Petrini JL, Baron TH, et al. Quality indicators for colonoscopy. Am J Gastroenterol 2006;101(4):873–85.
10. Thakkar K, Holub JL, Gilger MA, et al. Quality indicators for pediatric colonoscopy: results from a multicenter consortium. Gastrointest Endosc 2015. [Epub ahead of print].
11. Aabakken L, Rembacken B, LeMoine O, et al. Minimal standard terminology for gastrointestinal endoscopy—MST 3.0. Endoscopy 2009;41(8):727–8.
12. Robertson DJ, Lawrence LB, Shaheen NJ, et al. Quality of colonoscopy reporting: a process of care study. Am J Gastroenterol 2002;97(10):2651–6.
13. Lieberman D, Nadel M, Smith RA, et al. Standardized colonoscopy reporting and data system: report of the quality assurance task group of the national colorectal cancer roundtable. Gastrointest Endosc 2007;65(6):757–66.
14. Lieberman DA, Faigel DO, Logan JR, et al. Assessment of the quality of colonoscopy reports: results from a multicenter consortium. Gastrointest Endosc 2009; 69(3 Pt 2):645–53.
15. Walsh CM, Ling SC, Khanna N, et al. Gastrointestinal endoscopy competency assessment tool: development of a procedure-specific assessment tool for colonoscopy. Gastrointest Endosc 2014;79(5):798–807.e5.
16. Leichtner AM, Gillis LA, Gupta S, et al. NASPGHAN guidelines for training in pediatric gastroenterology. J Pediatr Gastroenterol Nutr 2013;56(Suppl 1):S1–8.
17. Walsh CM, Ling SC, Walters TD, et al. Development of the gastrointestinal endoscopy competency assessment tool for pediatric colonoscopy (GiECATKIDS). J Pediatr Gastroenterol Nutr 2014;59(4):480–6.
18. Walsh CM, Ling SC, Mamula P, et al. The gastrointestinal endoscopy competency assessment tool for pediatric colonoscopy. J Pediatr Gastroenterol Nutr 2015; 60(4):474–80.
19. Rex DK, Bond JH, Winawer S, et al. Quality in the technical performance of colonoscopy and the continuous quality improvement process for colonoscopy: recommendations of the US Multi-Society Task Force on Colorectal Cancer. Am J Gastroenterol 2002;97(6):1296–308.
20. de Jonge V, Sint Nicolaas J, Cahen DL, et al. Quality evaluation of colonoscopy reporting and colonoscopy performance in daily clinical practice. Gastrointest Endosc 2012;75(1):98–106.
21. Available at: http://mocportfolioprogram.org/. Accessed August 30, 2015.
22. NASPGHAN. 2015. Available at: http://naspghan.org. Accessed August 30, 2015.
23. Balaguer F, Llach J, Castells A, et al. The European panel on the appropriateness of gastrointestinal endoscopy guidelines colonoscopy in an open-access endoscopy unit: a prospective study. Aliment Pharmacol Ther 2005;21(5):609–13.
24. Froehlich F, Repond C, Mullhaupt B, et al. Is the diagnostic yield of upper GI endoscopy improved by the use of explicit panel-based appropriateness criteria? Gastrointest Endosc 2000;52(3):333–41.
25. de Bosset V, Froehlich F, Rey JP, et al. Do explicit appropriateness criteria enhance the diagnostic yield of colonoscopy? Endoscopy 2002;34(5):360–8.

26. Practice guidelines for sedation and analgesia by non-anesthesiologists. Anesthesiology 2002;96(4):1004–17.
27. Anesthesiology ASo. ASA physical status classification system. 2014. Available at: http://www.asahq.org/resources/clinical-information/asa-physical-status-classification-system. Accessed April 19, 2015.
28. Mak PH, Campbell RC, Irwin MG. The ASA Physical Status Classification: interobserver consistency. American Society of Anesthesiologists. Anaesth Intensive Care 2002;30(5):633–40.
29. Thakkar K, El-Serag HB, Mattek N, et al. Complications of pediatric EGD: a 4-year experience in PEDS-CORI. Gastrointest Endosc 2007;65(2):213–21.
30. Committee ASoP, Chandrasekhara V, Eloubeidi MA, Bruining DH, et al. Open-access endoscopy. Gastrointest Endosc 2015;81(6):1326–9.
31. Committee ASoP, Lightdale JR, Acosta R, Shergill AK, et al. Modifications in endoscopic practice for pediatric patients. Gastrointest Endosc 2014;79(5):699–710.
32. Buderus S, Sonderkotter H, Fleischhack G, et al. Diagnostic and therapeutic endoscopy in children and adolescents with cancer. Pediatr Hematol Oncol 2012;29(5):450–60.
33. Seefelder C, Elango S, Rosbe KW, et al. Oesophageal perforation presenting as oesophageal atresia in a premature neonate following difficult intubation. Paediatr Anaesth 2001;11(1):112–8.
34. Long Y, Liu HH, Yu C, et al. Pre-existing diseases of patients increase susceptibility to hypoxemia during gastrointestinal endoscopy. PLoS One 2012;7(5):e37614.
35. Lofft AL. Informed consent for endoscopy. Gastrointest Endosc Clin N Am 1995;5(2):457–70.
36. Lightdale J, Valim C, Newburg A, et al. Efficiency of propofol sedation versus conscious sedation with midazolam and fentanyl in a pediatric endoscopy unit. Gastrointest Endosc 2005;61(5):AB92.
37. McCashland T, Brand R, Lyden E, et al. The time and financial impact of training fellows in endoscopy. CORI Research Project. Clinical Outcomes Research Initiative. Am J Gastroenterol 2000;95(11):3129–32.
38. Cotton PB, Eisen GM, Aabakken L, et al. A lexicon for endoscopic adverse events: report of an ASGE workshop. Gastrointest Endosc 2010;71(3):446–54.
39. Kaminski MF, Regula J, Kraszewska E, et al. Quality indicators for colonoscopy and the risk of interval cancer. N Engl J Med 2010;362(19):1795–803.
40. Lee TJ, Blanks RG, Rees CJ, et al. Longer mean colonoscopy withdrawal time is associated with increased adenoma detection: evidence from the Bowel Cancer Screening Programme in England. Endoscopy 2013;45(1):20–6.
41. Belderbos TD, Grobbee EJ, van Oijen MG, et al. Comparison of cecal intubation and adenoma detection between hospitals can provide incentives to improve quality of colonoscopy. Endoscopy 2015;47(8):703–9.
42. Thakkar K, Alsarraj A, Fong E, et al. Prevalence of colorectal polyps in pediatric colonoscopy. Dig Dis Sci 2012;57(4):1050–5.
43. Rufo PA, Denson LA, Sylvester FA, et al. Health supervision in the management of children and adolescents with IBD: NASPGHAN recommendations. J Pediatr Gastroenterol Nutr 2012;55(1):93–108.
44. Lee HJ, Lee JH, Lee JS, et al. Is colonoscopy necessary in children suspected of having colonic polyps? Gut Liver 2010;4(3):326–31.
45. Vandenplas Y, Rudolph CD, Di Lorenzo C, et al. Pediatric gastroesophageal reflux clinical practice guidelines: joint recommendations of the North American

Society for Pediatric Gastroenterology, Hepatology, and Nutrition (NASPGHAN) and the European Society for Pediatric Gastroenterology, Hepatology, and Nutrition (ESPGHAN). J Pediatr Gastroenterol Nutr 2009;49(4):498–547.

46. Committee ASoP, Sharaf RN, Shergill AK, Krinsky ML, et al. Endoscopic mucosal tissue sampling. Gastrointest Endosc 2013;78(2):216–24.

47. Yao MD, von Rosenvinge EC, Groden C, et al. Multiple endoscopic biopsies in research subjects: safety results from a National Institutes of Health series. Gastrointest Endosc 2009;69(4):906–10.

48. Badizadegan K, Thompson KM. Value of information in nonfocal colonic biopsies. J Pediatr Gastroenterol Nutr 2011;53(6):679–83.

49. Khakoo SI, Lobo AJ, Shepherd NA, et al. Histological assessment of the Sydney classification of endoscopic gastritis. Gut 1994;35(9):1172–5.

50. Manfredi MA, Jiang H, Borges LF, et al. Good agreement between endoscopic findings and biopsy reports supports limited tissue sampling during pediatric colonoscopy. J Pediatr Gastroenterol Nutr 2014;58(6):773–8.

51. Lash JG, Genta RM. Adherence to the Sydney System guidelines increases the detection of Helicobacter gastritis and intestinal metaplasia in 400738 sets of gastric biopsies. Aliment Pharmacol Ther 2013;38(4):424–31.

52. Rubio-Tapia A, Hill ID, Kelly CP, et al, American College of Gastroenterology. ACG clinical guidelines: diagnosis and management of celiac disease. Am J Gastroenterol 2013;108(5):656–76 [quiz: 677].

53. Weir DC, Glickman JN, Roiff T, et al. Variability of histopathological changes in childhood celiac disease. Am J Gastroenterol 2010;105(1):207–12.

54. Dellon ES, Gonsalves N, Hirano I, et al. ACG clinical guideline: evidenced based approach to the diagnosis and management of esophageal eosinophilia and eosinophilic esophagitis (EoE). Am J Gastroenterol 2013;108(5):679–92 [quiz: 693].

55. Coffin CM. Pediatric surgical pathology: pitfalls and strategies for error prevention. Arch Pathol Lab Med 2006;130(5):610–2.

56. Nakhleh RE. Quality in surgical pathology communication and reporting. Arch Pathol Lab Med 2011;135(11):1394–7.

Management of Upper Gastrointestinal Bleeding in Children: Variceal and Nonvariceal

 CrossMark

Richard A. Lirio, MD

KEYWORDS

- Upper gastrointestinal bleeding • Hematemesis • Coffee-ground emesis
- Nonvariceal bleeding • Variceal bleeding • Therapeutic endoscopy

KEY POINTS

- It is vital to obtain a detailed history to evaluate for the possible cause behind upper gastrointestinal (UGI) bleeding, paying close attention to comorbid conditions, medications, and exposures in addition to the severity, timing, duration, and volume of bleeding.
- Physical examination, laboratory evaluation, and trending vital signs are important in assessing for possible sources of UGI bleeding and can help differentiate between a medical (GI) or surgical case as well as the need for appropriate resuscitation.
- Acid suppression with proton-pump inhibitors is recommended to minimize bleeding and the risk of rebleeding, particularly in the intensive care setting.
- For nonvariceal bleeding, various endoscopic modalities, such as injection, cautery, and mechanical therapy, can be used to control bleeding.
- Endoscopic variceal ligation or banding is the modality of choice for esophageal varices and has been used with good success, but pediatric research and data are lacking.

INTRODUCTION

Upper gastrointestinal (UGI) bleeding can generally be defined as bleeding proximal to the ligament of Treitz, which leads to hematemesis.[1] More specifically, an UGI bleed is often characterized by vomiting bright red blood or coffee ground–like emesis. Melena, characterized by black, tarry stools, can also be a manifestation of UGI bleeding.

In the pediatric population, UGI bleeding has been noted to account for up to 20% of all GI bleeding in children.[1] In the critical care setting, a large prospective study

Disclosure statement: The author has no conflicts of interest to disclose and no funding resources to disclose.
Division of Pediatric Gastroenterology, Hepatology and Nutrition, Department of Pediatrics, UMass Memorial Children's Medical Center University Campus, University of Massachusetts Medical School, 55 Lake Avenue North, Worcester, MA 01655, USA
E-mail address: Richard.Lirio@umassmemorial.org

Gastrointest Endoscopy Clin N Am 26 (2016) 63–73
http://dx.doi.org/10.1016/j.giec.2015.09.003
1052-5157/16/$ – see front matter © 2016 Elsevier Inc. All rights reserved.

noted 6.4% of pediatric intensive care unit (PICU) admissions were secondary to UGI bleeding.[2] Further study of the risk factors for UGI bleeding in critical care settings, such as the PICU, have found that comorbid conditions (ie coagulopathy, pneumonia, multiple trauma, and so forth) increase the risk for pediatric UGI bleeds, particularly in patients not given prophylactic therapy.[3–5] Fortunately though, as noted by a recent study looking at emergency department data, most children presenting for care with UGI bleeds do not require hospitalization or intervention.[5]

CAUSE

Common and unusual causes of UGI bleeding depend on patient age, as noted in **Table 1**.[6–10] In addition, there may be geographic variability that can dictate the need for endoscopy (ie, prevalence of *Helicobacter pylori*). Outside of the United States, variceal bleeding may be more common in children, increasing their likelihood of requiring endoscopy and/or intervention to ensure hemostasis.[11] For example, schistosomiasis is a common infection in many parts of the developing world that can lead to periportal fibrosis, cirrhosis, and portal hypertension without overt hepatocellular injury. In areas where schistosomiasis is prevalent, such as sub-Saharan Africa and Southeast Asia, hepatic infestation and the possibility of variceal bleeding needs to be considered when presented with a patient with UGI bleeding. In these children, liver chemistries may return as normal and the singular presenting issue may strictly be the hematemesis.[11–13]

NEONATES

In the first few months of life, UGI bleeding is uncommon; however, it can still occur.[14,15] The most common cause of UGI bleeding in newborn infants is swallowed maternal blood from breastfeeding. An Apt test can be done to differentiate maternal blood from fetal blood by denaturing adult hemoglobin with sodium hydroxide (NaOH) causing a color change.[16,17]

Another consideration in this age group is vitamin K deficiency, particularly in babies born outside of the hospital setting and/or not receiving vitamin K prophylaxis at birth.[18] In severely ill newborns, stress gastritis and ulcers can also occur.[2–4] Coagulopathy

Table 1
Common and rare causes of pediatric UGI bleeding by age group

Neonates	Infants/Toddlers	Older Children/Adolescents
Swallowed maternal blood	Foreign bodies	Mallory-Weiss tears
Vitamin K deficiency	Mallory-Weiss tears	Ulcers/gastritis
Stress gastritis/ulcers	Ulcers/gastritis (NSAIDs, critically ill)	Esophagitis (ingestions, pill, and so forth)
Congenital anomalies (intestinal duplications, vascular anomalies)	Esophagitis (caustic ingestions)	Varices
Coagulopathy (infections, liver failure, hematologic issues, and so forth)	Varices	Rare: Dieulafoy, telangiectasia, AV malformation, parasites, and so forth
Milk protein intolerance (lower GI bleeding more common)	Rare: Dieulafoy, telangiectasia, AV malformation, parasites, and so forth	—

Abbreviations: AV, arteriovenous; NSAIDs, nonsteroidal antiinflammatory drugs.

from infections, hematologic issues, or liver disease can present with UGI bleeding in all age groups.[6] Intestinal duplications and vascular anomalies can present as acute UGI bleeds as well.[14,19] On rare occasions, milk protein intolerance may present with UGI bleeding; but lower GI bleeding/hematochezia would be the more common presentation.[20]

INFANTS/TODDLERS

Possible causes of UGI bleeding in the infant and toddler age range overlap with neonatal causes. Furthermore, in this more mobile and inquisitive population, foreign bodies must be considered more commonly as well as caustic ingestions. Also, Mallory-Weiss tears, or esophageal lacerations from chronic retching and/or vomiting, is another possible cause.[7] In addition, chronic use of medications, such as nonsteroidal antiinflammatory drugs (NSAIDs) used to treat febrile viral illnesses common in toddler populations, can lead to ulcers and gastritis with subsequent hematemesis.[8,9]

Rare causes of hematemesis in this age group can include *Helicobacter pylori*, Dieulafoy lesions, telangiectasias, hemangiomas, vascular malformations, duplications cysts, parasites, vasculitis, and gastric polyps.[14,15,19,21]

OLDER CHILDREN/ADOLESCENTS

In this age group, UGI bleeding causes are similar to that of adults. The most common considerations in otherwise healthy patients presenting with bright-red or coffee-ground emesis includes Mallory-Weiss tears, gastritis, esophagitis, peptic ulcers, and varices.[7,8,14,22,23] Coughs, which are usually thought of as a benign occurrence, can also lead to hematemesis secondary to a Mallory-Weiss tear. Unusual causes, though rare, still need to be considered in the differential, as it is with younger infants and children.

EVALUATION

Initial evaluation and assessment of patients presenting with UGI bleeding should focus on the achievement of hemodynamic stability (**Fig. 1**). Vital signs, such as heart rate, blood pressure, and capillary refill, should be continually monitored; the need for early fluid resuscitation should be assessed and initiated. This is particularly important in the pediatric population, which is more susceptible to hypovolemia. For severe, acute UGI bleeding in children, local pediatric gastroenterologists as well as GI surgeons should be consulted for help with the management and planning for interventions to effect hemostasis.[5,14]

While patients are being stabilized, a detailed history should be obtained to determine the initial presentation, time course, extent of bleeding, associated signs and symptoms, and other possible medical conditions, such as recent viral gastroenteritis or chronic illnesses.[5,14,22,23] Attention to the intake of breast milk or colored foods or drinks also needs to be considered. History regarding particular GI symptoms, such as poor feeding and irritability in neonates or dyspepsia, dysphagia, abdominal pain, or weight loss in older children, is important. Timing and presence of melena should also be determined.

Associated signs and symptoms, such as jaundice or easy bruising or recurrent and persistent epistaxis, should all be part of the history to help tease out the underlying cause of UGI bleeding, which could include liver diseases or hematologic diagnoses.[5,10,14] A thorough physical examination is also obviously vital.

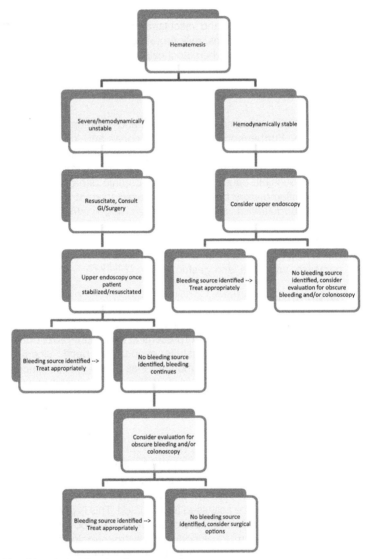

Fig. 1. Algorithm for evaluating hematemesis.

Obtaining a good medication history is also vital in assessing these patients. Certain medications, such as NSAIDs or corticosteroids, can predispose patients to ulcerations. Other medications, such as tetracycline, can lead to pill esophagitis.[9,23,24] And yet other medications can predispose patients to prolonged bleeding, such as anticoagulants. Additionally, medications, such as beta-adrenergic antagonists, may hide appropriate hypovolemic responses.[1]

To aid in assessing patients with UGI bleeding, laboratory evaluation should be done for more worrisome presentations. Testing should include a complete blood count, complete metabolic panel, and possibly coagulation studies as well. If the blood loss is significant enough, a type and cross-match blood sample should also be obtained in case of need for blood transfusion.[1,5,14]

Radiologic tests may be helpful in assessing UGI bleeding, particularly if a foreign body is suspected. For this, a plain radiograph should suffice. If liver disease is suspected, obtaining an abdominal ultrasound to rule out splenomegaly and portal hypertension can be a useful diagnostic tool. Generally speaking, an UGI series with contrast should not be performed in patients with acute UGI bleeding because this may delay or the hamper performance of subsequent procedures, such as endoscopy, angiography, or surgery.[14]

INTERVENTIONS

Lavage via nasogastric or orogastric tube has been described as a useful technique in assessing unexplained and significant UGI bleeding. Confirmation of a UGI bleed can be obtained by the return of bright red blood or coffee grounds on lavage; however, no therapeutic actions can be pursued with lavage. It is also important to note that in adult data, up to 15% of patients with active UGI bleeding can have a negative lavage.[25] In the past, ice water lavage was used with the hope of causing some vasoconstriction, leading to a slowing of UGI bleeding; however, this practice is no longer recommended and may actually be especially harmful, causing hypothermia, particularly in neonates and infants.

Acid suppression, although not well studied in the pediatric population, is recommended in pediatric UGI bleeds. Adult data support the role of acid suppression with a proton-pump inhibitor (PPI).[26] PPI usage in adults with active UGI bleeding has been shown to minimize the risk of rebleeding and decreases the length of the hospital stay. A meta-analysis found PPI therapy in adults resulted in reduced rates for rebleeding, surgery, and deaths when dealing with acute nonvariceal bleeding.[4,26,27] In a recent systematic review of critically ill pediatric patients, the use of PPIs showed some benefit in preventing UGI bleeding.[2]

Adjunctive therapy with somatostatin or octreotide can be used in active or difficult-to-control UGI bleeding. In adults, these medications are particularly effective in variceal bleeding but have also been helpful for nonvariceal bleeding.[25,28–30] No specific guidelines exist for the use of somatostatin or octreotide in the pediatric population; but for difficult-to-control bleeding, it is commonly given initially as a bolus of 1 µg/kg body weight to a maximum of 100 µg, then followed by a continuous intravenous (IV) infusion of up to 1 µg/kg/h.[14]

In adult UGI bleeding, prokinetics, such as erythromycin or metoclopramide, are used to try and clear the stomach of debris, food particles, blood, and clots, particularly in severe bleeding.[25,31] There are no data though to support the use of these agents in the pediatric population.

ENDOSCOPY

Endoscopy remains the intervention of choice in UGI bleeding because it can be diagnostic as well as therapeutic. Additionally, with endoscopy, a bleeding source can be identified and further risks for rebleeding can be assessed; however, its limitations do include the need for probable intubation and anesthesia. Another limiting factor to consider in neonates and infants is the fact that the smaller-diameter endoscopes cannot accommodate most of the therapeutic catheters and devices commonly used for hemostasis.[24,32–35]

Before performing endoscopy, informed consent should be obtained from the parent or responsible caretaker/guardian. Discussions regarding risks, such as possible anesthesia complications, aspiration, bleeding, infection, or perforation, should be undertaken before the procedure.[14,33]

Despite some limitations, however, endoscopy has been proven to be safe and effective in pediatric UGI bleeding.[24,32–35] Before performing endoscopy though, hemodynamic stability should be achieved as best as possible with resuscitation, transfusion, and correction of coagulopathy, if necessary. It is generally accepted that endoscopy for acute, severe, or persistent and uncontrolled UGI bleeding be performed within the first 24 to 48 hours of presentation. A recent retrospective review found it less common to find a UGI bleed in a patient undergoing upper endoscopy if done greater than 48 hours after a bleeding episode.[21]

As noted, endoscopy for UGI bleeding can be diagnostic and therapeutic. In terms of diagnosis, UGI bleeding can be classified into 2 subtypes, nonvariceal and variceal. Most acute UGI bleeding, particularly in the pediatric population, is nonvariceal.[14,22,23,33] Nonvariceal bleeding is commonly caused by Mallory-Weiss tears, peptic ulcers, and erosive esophagitis and less commonly Dieulafoy lesions, telangiectasias, or arteriovenous malformations.[19,21,23] Variceal hemorrhage in children is mostly associated with chronic liver disease and cirrhosis, leading to portal hypertension and eventually esophageal varices.[36]

NONVARICEAL BLEEDING

There are multiple therapeutic modalities that can be used to achieve hemostasis in nonvariceal UGI bleeds in children.[25,33] These modalities include injection, cautery, and mechanical therapy. These techniques are commonly used in adults with UGI bleeding but have also been found to be effective in pediatrics.[24,34,35]

The goal of injection is to achieve tamponade and eventual hemostasis in nonvariceal bleeding. Normal saline and diluted epinephrine are the most commonly used agents. Cautery techniques include heater probes, argon plasma coagulation, and electrocautery probes. Laser therapy can also be used but is not commonly available because of the high cost and lack of training.[25] Heater and electrocautery probes are used to apply tamponade to the bleeding area and combined with heat or electric current to coagulate blood vessels and stop bleeding.[25,33] Argon uses ionized gas to conduct electricity without tamponade, coagulating the bleeding area.[25]

Mechanical therapy includes the application of clips or band ligation to achieve tamponade of a bleeding site. These clips have been found to be effective in various types of UGI bleeding, including Mallory Weiss tears and Dieulafoy lesions. Endoscopic clips can be deployed through the endoscope and generally remain in place for a few days to weeks. There are limited pediatric-specific data available on the use of endoscopic clips; however, in adults, they have been shown to achieve effective hemostasis.[37] Theoretically, endoscopic clips minimize tissue injury via their mechanical tamponade.[38] The limiting factor for endoscopic clip usage is patients' size. Generally, endoscopic clips cannot be applied when using neonatal endoscopes.

VARICEAL BLEEDS

Compared with adult populations, variceal bleeding is less commonly seen in children. Some pediatric data does exist though, noting about 50% of children with cirrhosis have varices.[39,40] There are not much pediatric data on the actual incidence of variceal bleeding in children, although a recent prospective study noted there was 1 incident of portal hypertensive–associated bleeding per 200,000 Canadian children.[41]

Despite our lack of pediatric data on variceal bleeding, clinically, it is a serious event associated with severe risk and complications. A mortality rate of up to 19% within the first 35 days of variceal bleeding has been suggested by a North American study done in children with various liver diseases.[30]

Sclerosing agents, such as sodium morrhuate, ethanolamine, polidocanol, and sodium tetradecyl (with or without ethanol), can be used in conjunction with epinephrine to achieve hemostasis in esophageal variceal bleeding.[14–17,19] The eradication of varices using sclerosing agents in the pediatric population has been much better studied than the use of other hemostatic techniques in children. With the advent of band ligation though, sclerosing agents for bleeding esophageal varices are now less commonly used.[31,42]

Endoscopic variceal ligation or banding has become the therapy of choice for esophageal varices. Multiple adult studies have shown banding to be more effective at achieving lasting hemostasis with less risk for complications, such as rebleeding, ulcerations, stricture formation, and so forth, as compared with sclerotherapy.[31,42]

Before banding, patients should be resuscitated as best as possible and transfused as needed. As per the American Society for Gastrointestinal Endoscopy's (ASGE) adult guidelines on variceal bleeding eradication, intubation is strongly recommended in these patients secondary to a higher risk of aspiration. In addition, known variceal patients should be taken for endoscopy urgently or at least within the first 12 hours of presentation. It is also recommended that bleeding varices be reevaluated and banded to eradication.[31] Currently though, there is no well-defined interval between each endoscopy. Consensus guidelines in adults recommend repeat endoscopy every 1 to 2 weeks until eradication of the varices.[36] Once eradicated, surveillance endoscopy should be done every 3 to 6 months.[31,42]

As per the ASGE's guidelines for adults, nonselective beta-blockers can also be considered to minimize the risk of rebleeding as an adjunct to banding; however, there are no pediatric-specific data to support this. There are only limited data available to support the use of beta-blockers in children, with some concern for its use secondary to children's muted responses to hypovolemia while on beta-blockade.[42] That being said, there are no case reports of serious adverse effects of medications, such as propanolol, in portal hypertension and esophageal varices.

Adult patients with cirrhosis with acute UGI bleeding are generally given prophylactic antibiotics preferably before endoscopy to minimize the risk of infection because they are at an increased risk for mortality; however, as with most variceal bleeding in the pediatric setting, there is a lack of data regarding its use in children with cirrhosis.[42] It is, however, generally accepted clinical practice. In patients with recurrent variceal bleeding despite banding and/or sclerotherapy, transjugular intrahepatic portosystemic shunting should be considered.[31]

Unlike the adult population, there are no specific scoring systems to predict rebleeding for variceal bleeding in pediatrics. There is also not an adequate or validated test to assess for the possibility of variceal bleeding in children. Some noninvasive tests that look for splenomegaly, the ratio between platelet count and splenomegaly, and ultrasound elastography have been done to try and minimize the need for endoscopic evaluation but need further investigation before being put into clinical use.[43–45]

REBLEEDING

In adults, several endoscopic findings suggest a higher risk for rebleeding. We can generally extrapolate the use of these stigmata into the pediatric population. Endoscopic findings of active arterial bleeding (spurting) will most likely rebleed without endoscopic intervention.[4,25,26] As per the ASGE, up to about 50% of nonbleeding visible vessels will rebleed. Nonbleeding adherent clots can bleed up to 35% of the time. A point of contention and much debate arises in the management of adherent clots and whether or not to remove them, although it is generally acceptable to irrigate the clot and assess for possible intervention in order to decrease the risk of rebleeding.[25]

Flat pigmented lesions or clean-based ulcers generally have a much lower risk of rebleeding and most likely require little to no endoscopic intervention. Continued acid suppression for the entities at higher risk for rebleeding have been shown to decrease the rate of rebleeding and mortality and are generally recommended.[3,4,26,28]

OBSCURE BLEEDS

If upper endoscopy reveals no obvious sources of bleeding and there is persistent anemia or symptoms, such as melena, colonoscopy should be considered and is discussed in a separate article.[46] In patients with bleeding distal to the ligament of Treitz or even as distal as the right colon, presentation includes issues with melena and/or persistent anemia. If the upper and lower endoscopy on these patients proves to be negative, video capsule endoscopy or enteroscopy could be considered to evaluate the length of the small bowel for obscure sources of bleeding. Angiography is another consideration. In cases when endoscopy is unsuccessful in identifying the source of a large bleed, angiography can be helpful in diagnosing vascular anomalies. Nuclear red cell tags are another effective modality in diagnosing and identifying active, larger bleeds, particularly distal to the ligament of Treitz.[25]

SUMMARY AND RECOMMENDATIONS

When dealing with a UGI bleed, it is vital to obtain a detailed history to evaluate for possible causes, paying close attention to comorbid conditions, medications, and exposures in addition to the severity, timing, duration, and volume of bleeding. Physical examination and monitoring vital signs are also important in assessing for possible sources of UGI bleeding and can help differentiate between a medical (GI) or surgical case. Laboratory evaluation including complete blood count, comprehensive metabolic panel, coagulation studies, and/or type and crossmatch are an important tool in evaluating the severity and cause of the UGI bleeding. Appropriate resuscitation with IV fluids and/or blood products is important in achieving hemodynamic stability before any intervention.

Nasogastric lavage can be used to assess for the presence of blood or coffee-ground emesis in patients with hematemesis; however, it is no longer recommended using ice water lavage. Acid suppression with PPIs is recommended to minimize bleeding and the risk of rebleeding, particularly in the intensive care setting. Adjunct therapy with octreotide or somatostatin can also be considered for severe or difficult-to-control UGI bleeding.

Endoscopy remains the intervention of choice in UGI bleeding because it can be both diagnostic and therapeutic. For nonvariceal bleeding, various modalities, such as injection, cautery, and mechanical therapy, can be used to control bleeding. Endoscopic variceal ligation or banding is the modality of choice for esophageal varices and has been used with good success, but pediatric research and data are lacking. Beta-blockers can be considered as adjunct therapy to help eradicate esophageal varices; but again, there is lack of good pediatric data to support its use in children. Prophylactic antibiotics should be considered in cirrhotic children with acute UGI bleeding because they are at an increased risk for infection and mortality.

For obscure bleeding, other modalities, such as video capsule endoscopy, enteroscopy, angiography, and/or nuclear red cell tag, should be considered.

REFERENCES

1. Rodgers BM. Upper gastrointestinal hemorrhage. Pediatr Rev 1999;20:171.
2. Lacroix J, Nadeau D, Laberge S, et al. Frequency of upper gastrointestinal bleeding in a pediatric intensive care unit. Crit Care Med 1992;20:35.
3. Cochran EB, Phelps SJ, Tolley EA, et al. Prevalence of, and risk factors for, upper gastrointestinal tract bleeding in critically ill pediatric patients. Crit Care Med 1992;20:1519.
4. Lopez-Herce J, Dorao P, Elola P, et al. Frequency and prophylaxis of upper gastrointestinal hemorrhage in critically ill children: a prospective study comparing the efficacy of almagate, ranitidine, and sucralfate. The Gastrointestinal Hemorrhage Study Group. Crit Care Med 1992;20:1082.
5. Pant C, Olyaee M, Sferra TJ, et al. Emergency department visits for gastrointestinal bleeding in children: results from the Nationwide Emergency Department Sample 2006-2011. Curr Med Res Opin 2015;2:347–51.
6. Choe BH, Kim JY, Lee JH, et al. Upper gastrointestinal bleeding in children with haemophilia: a clinical significance of Helicobacter pylori infection. Haemophilia 2010;16:277–80.
7. Annunziata GM, Gunasekaran TS, Berman JH, et al. Cough-induced Mallory-Weiss tear in a child. Clin Pediatr (Phila) 1996;35:417.
8. Cannon RA, Lee G, Cox KL, et al. Gastrointestinal hemorrhage due to Mallory-Weiss syndrome in an infant. J Pediatr Gastroenterol Nutr 1985;4:323.
9. Kato S, Kobayashi M, Sato H, et al. Doxycycline-induced hemorrhagic esophagitis: a pediatric case. J Pediatr Gastroenterol Nutr 1988;7:762.
10. Armstrong KL, Fraser DK, Faoagali JL, et al. Gastrointestinal bleeding with influenza virus. Med J Aust 1991;154:180.
11. Mittal SK, Kalra KK, Aggarwal V, et al. Diagnostic upper GI endoscopy for hematemesis in children: experience from a pediatric gastroenterology centre in North India. Indian J Pediatr 1994;61:651.
12. Olveda DU, Olveda RM, Montes CJ, et al. Clinical management of advanced schistosomiasis: a case of portal vein thrombosis-induced splenomegaly requiring surgery. BMJ Case Rep 2014;2014. pii:bcr2014203897.
13. Okamoto K, Brown JD. Hepatosplenic schistosomiasis presenting as spontaneous hemoperitoneum in a Filipino immigrant. Am J Med Sci 2013;346:334–7.
14. Fox VL. Gastrointestinal bleeding in infancy and childhood. Gastroenterol Clin North Am 2000;29:37.
15. Smith TF, Welch TR, Allen JB, et al. Cutaneous mastocytosis with bleeding: probable heparin effect. Cutis 1987;39:241.
16. Bulstrode NW, Cuckow PM, Spitz LS, et al. Neonatal gastrointestinal pseudohaemorrhage. J R Coll Surg Edinb 1998;43:355.
17. Rosenthal P, Thompson J, Singh M, et al. Detection of occult blood in gastric juice. J Clin Gastroenterol 1984;6:119.
18. Burke CW. Vitamin K deficiency bleeding: overview and considerations. J Pediatr Health Care 2013;27(3):215–21.
19. Itani M, Alsaied T, Charafeddine L, et al. Dieulafoy's lesion in children. J Pediatr Gastroenterol Nutr 2010;51:672.

20. Yimyaem P, Chongsrisawat V, Vivatvakin B, et al. Gastrointestinal manifestations of cow's milk protein allergy during the first year of life. J Med Assoc Thai 2003; 86(2):116–23.
21. Cleveland K, Ahmad N, Bishop P, et al. Upper gastrointestinal bleeding in children: an 11 year retrospective endoscopic investigation. World J Pediatr 2012; 8:123–8.
22. Cox K. Upper gastrointestinal bleeding in children and adolescents. Pediatrics 1979;63:408.
23. Yaccha SK, Khanduri A, Sharma BC, et al. Gastrointestinal bleeding in children. J Gastroenterol Hepatol 1996;11:903.
24. Kato S, Nakagawa H, Harada Y, et al. A clinical study of upper gastrointestinal endoscopy in Japanese children. Acta Paediatr Jpn 1991;33:36.
25. Hwang JH, Fisher DA, Ben-Menachem T, et al. The role of endoscopy in the management of acute non-variceal upper GI bleeding – ASGE practice guidelines. Gastrointest Endosc 2012;75:1132.
26. Reveiz L, Guerrero-Lozano R, Camacho A, et al. Stress ulcer, gastritis, and gastrointestinal bleeding prophylaxis in critically ill pediatric patients: a systematic review. Pediatr Crit Care Med 2010;1:124–32.
27. Khuroo MS, Khuroo MS, Farahat KL, et al. Treatment with proton pump inhibitors in acute non-variceal upper gastrointestinal bleeding: a meta-analysis. J Gastroenterol Hepatol 2005;20:11–25.
28. Imperiale TF, Birgisson S. Somatostatin or octreotide compared with H2 antagonists and placebo in the management of acute nonvariceal upper gastrointestinal hemorrhage: a meta-analysis. Ann Intern Med 1997;127:1062.
29. Lam JC, Aters S, Tobias JD, et al. Initial experience with octreotide in the pediatric population. Am J Ther 2001;8:409.
30. Erogiu Y, Emerick KM, Whitingon PF, et al. Octreotide therapy for control of acute gastrointestinal bleeding in children. J Pediatr Gastroenterol Nutr 2004;38:41–7.
31. Hwang JH, Shergill AK, Acosta RD, et al. The role of endoscopy in the management of variceal hemorrhage – ASGE guidelines. Gastrointest Endosc 2014;80:221.
32. Zahavi I, Arnon R, Ovadia B, et al. Upper gastrointestinal endoscopy in the pediatric patient. Isr J Med Sci 1994;30:664.
33. Goenka AS, Dasilva MS, Cleghorn GJ, et al. Therapeutic upper gastrointestinal endoscopy in children: an audit of 443 procedures and literature review. J Gastroenterol Hepatol 1993;8:44.
34. Balsells F, Wyllie R, Kay M, et al. Use of conscious sedation for lower and upper gastrointestinal endoscopic examinations in children, adolescents, and young adults: a twelve-year review. Gastrointest Endosc 1997;45:375.
35. Chang MG, Wang TH, Hsu JY, et al. Endoscopic examination of the upper gastrointestinal tract in infancy. Gastrointest Endosc 1983;29:15.
36. Garcia-Tsao G, Sanyal AJ, Grace ND, et al. Prevention and management of gastroesophageal varices and variceal hemorrhage in cirrhosis – AASLD practice guidelines. Hepatology 2007;46:922.
37. Binmoeller KF, Thonke F, Soehendra N, et al. Endoscopic hemoclip treatment for gastrointestinal bleeding. Endoscopy 1993;25:167–70.
38. Yuan Y, Wang C, Hunt RH, et al. Endoscopic clipping for acute nonvariceal upper-GI bleeding: a meta-analysis and critical appraisal of randomized controlled trials. Gastrointest Endosc 2008;68:339–51.
39. Sokal EM, Van Hoorebeeck N, Van Obbergh L, et al. Upper gastro-intestinal tract bleeding in cirrhotic children candidates for liver transplantation. Eur J Pediatr 1992;151:326–8.

40. Stringer MD, Howard ER, Mowat AP, et al. Endoscopic sclerotherapy in the management of esophageal varices in 61 children with biliary atresia. J Pediatr Surg 1989;24:438–42.
41. Hussey S, Howard ER, Mowat AP, et al. Prospective study of major upper gastrointestinal hemorrhage in children [abstract]. Can J Gastroenterol 2008;22(Suppl A): 156A.
42. Ling SC, Walters T, McKiernan PJ, et al. Primary prophylaxis of variceal hemorrhage in children with portal hypertension: a framework for future research. J Pediatr Gastroenterol Nutr 2011;52:254–61.
43. Fagundes ED, Ferreira AR, Roquete ML, et al. Clinical and laboratory predictors of esophageal varices in children and adolescents with portal hypertension syndrome. J Pediatr Gastroenterol Nutr 2008;46:178–83.
44. Gana JC, Ferreira AR, Roquete ML, et al. Derivation of a clinical prediction rule for the noninvasive diagnosis of varices in children. J Pediatr Gastroenterol Nutr 2010;50:188–93.
45. Chang HK, Park YJ, Koh H, et al. Hepatic fibrosis scan for liver stiffness score measurement: a useful pre-endoscopic screening test for the detection of varices in postoperative patients with biliary atresia. J Pediatr Gastroenterol Nutr 2009; 49:323–8.
46. Sahn B, Bitton S. Lower gastrointestinal bleeding in children. Gastrointest Endosc Clin N Am 2015, in press.

Lower Gastrointestinal Bleeding in Children

Benjamin Sahn, MD, MS*, Samuel Bitton, MD

KEYWORDS

- Pediatric • Gastrointestinal bleeding • Hematochezia • Hemostasis • Resuscitation
- Colonoscopy

KEY POINTS

- Common causes of significant lower gastrointestinal bleeding (LGIB) in children are often different from those seen in adults.
- Endoscopy and colonoscopy are the mainstays of initial diagnostic testing in most children with LGIB.
- In the absence of an endoscopic diagnosis, other diagnostic modalities may be used, with varying degrees of diagnostic yield depending on the clinical scenario.
- The pediatric gastroenterologist is well served in becoming familiar with available hemostatic tools for small-diameter endoscopes, as well as developing comfort in performing at least 2 modes of therapeutic technique.

INTRODUCTION

Gastrointestinal (GI) bleeding in children, although uncommon, can be life threatening. Lower GI bleeding (LGIB) in pediatric patients occurs less commonly then upper GI bleeding (UGIB). However, its presentation often demands a similar degree of urgency. Causes of LGIB can run the gamut of severity from benign conditions such as anal fissures to an exsanguinating lesion, for example a vascular anomaly, and therefore deserves a careful yet expedient approach. This article reviews definitions and important causes of LGIB in children that typically require endoscopic knowledge and skill for diagnosis. We also discuss approaches to the management of LGIB from initial evaluation through definitive endoscopic therapies.

Disclosure: The authors have nothing to disclose.
Division of Pediatric Gastroenterology & Nutrition, Steven & Alexandra Cohen Children's Medical Center of New York, Hofstra North Shore-LIJ School of Medicine, North Shore – Long Island Jewish Health System, 1991 Marcus Avenue, Suite M 100, New Hyde Park, NY 11042, USA
* Corresponding author.
E-mail address: bsahn@nshs.edu

Gastrointest Endoscopy Clin N Am 26 (2016) 75–98
http://dx.doi.org/10.1016/j.giec.2015.08.007
1052-5157/16/$ – see front matter © 2016 Elsevier Inc. All rights reserved.

DEFINITIONS

LGIB can be acute or chronic, and assumed to be originating distal to the ligament of Treitz at the duodenojejunal junction, which marks the anatomic transition between the upper and lower GI tract. Acute LGIB is loosely characterized as active bleeding of less than 3 days' duration accompanied by anemia, hemodynamic compromise, altered consciousness, or the need for a blood transfusion.[1] In adults, at least 10% to 20% of GI bleeding is thought to occur from colonic and rectal sources, with diverticulitis considered the most common cause of clinically significant bleeding in adults.[1,2] In contrast, colonic diverticulitis is an extremely rare condition in children. The most common causes of LGIB in children include anal fissures, allergic colitis, enteric infections, and juvenile polyps.

Determining the source of either an upper or lower GI bleed is aided by accurate characterization of the appearance of stool during the bleeding event. In addition, it may be helpful to document the presence or absence of hematemesis, which is usually associated with bleeding proximal to the ligament of Treitz. Melena is stool that can be described as dark and sticky, like "tar," and usually represents the end-product of blood after traveling from the upper or middle digestive tract. Occasionally, bleeding from the proximal colon can appear melanotic. In contrast, hematochezia describes bright red blood per rectum, which often arises from the distal colon or rectum.

However, these stool patterns must be interpreted with caution, because profuse bleeding from the upper GI tract can appear as hematochezia, especially in younger patients with shorter intestinal transit times. Even in adult populations, up to 11% of patients with hematochezia were found to have an upper intestinal bleeding source.[3] This phenomenon is likely also because blood is a cathartic and any source of active bleeding can cause frequent loose melena or hematochezia. Furthermore, subjective variability in interpretation of stool color exists, although this can be minimized by using a standardized stool color card, which has been shown to aid in distinguishing upper (2 darker colors) from lower (2 brightest red colors) sources of GI bleed.[4]

EPIDEMIOLOGY

In the adult literature, UGIB is thought to occur at least 5 times as frequently as LGIB. In addition, the incidence of LGIB increases with age, reflecting its association with the onset of common conditions such as diverticulitis and angiodysplasia.[2] There is a paucity of data in the literature concerning the epidemiology of GI bleeding in childhood. A nationwide emergency department database analysis from 2006 to 2011 identified just fewer than 450,000 pediatric emergency department visits (ages birth to 19 years, with a median age of 9 years) to be associated generally with GI bleeding, of which UGIB accounted for 20% and LGIB for 30%.[5] Patients who were aged 15 to 19 years accounted for 40% of encounters, whereas patients aged 0 to 5 years comprised 38% of the total number of GI bleeding visits. This large dataset review also detected an increase in visits for GI bleeding during the study period from 82.18 per 100,000 children in 2006 to 93.93 per 100,000 in 2011. The greatest increase in encounters was seen in LGIB in patients 10 to 19 years old. Interestingly, 83% of children did not have other medical comorbidities. In multivariable logistic regression analysis, the investigators identified the following factors to be associated with increased risk of pediatric hospital admission for GI bleeding:

- Presence of ≥3 comorbid conditions (odds ratio [OR] 112.2)
- Presentation to a teaching hospital (OR 3.2)

- Occurrence of UGIB (OR 3.1)
- Age younger than 5 years (OR 1.3)

Mortality rates from LGIB in the adult literature are less than 5%,[6] and some reports are as low as 0.6%.[7] Recurrent bleeding occurs in 10% to 20% of LGIB, depending on the etiology and use of definitive therapy. The use of nonsteroidal anti-inflammatory drugs (NSAIDs) has been associated with an increased risk of rebleeding.[8]

CLINICAL PRESENTATION AND COURSE

Adult patients with LGIB may present with less hemodynamic instability than with UGIB, and demonstrate spontaneous resolution in up to 80% of cases.[1] However, this "truism" has not been replicated in studies of children. It is likely that children follow a similar course, as common causes of pediatric LGIB, such as milk protein colitis and juvenile polyps, are unlikely to cause prolonged and severe bleeding. Regardless of etiology, 3 parameters that may predict severe LGIB at time of initial presentation to an emergency department include initial hematocrit less than 35%, abnormal vital signs after the first hour, and gross blood on initial rectal examination.[9] In pediatrics, the age of the patient is one of the most important factors in narrowing the etiology of LGIB at presentation (**Table 1**). This article highlights some of the causes affecting the lower GI tract that are particularly amenable to endoscopy for diagnosis and therapy.

ETIOLOGY
Solitary Rectal Ulcer Syndrome

The prevalence of solitary rectal ulcer syndrome (SRUS) in children is unknown. Nevertheless, delay in diagnosis is common,[10] indicating SRUS may be more common than currently suspected. The condition usually presents with a constellation of symptoms that include rectal bleeding, mucous discharge, constipation with

Table 1
Differential diagnosis of lower gastrointestinal bleeding in children

Severity	Infant	Child	Adolescent

Often mild bleeding	Anal fissure
	Dietary protein allergy
	Vitamin K deficiency
	Lymphoid nodular
	  hyperplasia
		Anal fissure
		Infectious colitis
		Polyp: juvenile or
		  syndromic
		IBD
		SRUS
			Infectious colitis
			Anal fissure
			Hemorrhoids
			SRUS

Often moderate to
severe bleeding
	Necrotizing
	  enterocolitis
	Hirschsprung
	  enterocolitis
	Malrotation with
	  volvulus
	Duplication cyst
	Vascular malformation
		Meckel diverticulum
		Henoch-Schönlein
		  purpura
		Hemolytic uremic
		  syndrome
		Duplication cyst
		Vascular malformation
		Intussusception
		Typhlitis/neutropenic
		  colitis
		Dieulafoy lesion
			NSAID enteropathy
			IBD
			Vascular
			  malformation
			Meckel
			  diverticulum

Abbreviations: IBD, inflammatory bowel disease; NSAID, nonsteroidal anti-inflammatory drug; SRUS, solitary rectal ulcer syndrome.

Adapted from Neidich GA, Cole SR. Gastrointestinal bleeding. Pediatr Rev 2014;35(5):247; with permission.

prolonged straining, tenesmus, and lower abdominal and/or perianal pain.[11] Anemia is unusual in SRUS, unless the diagnosis is delayed.

SRUS results from asynchronous contraction of the pelvic floor and external anal sphincter muscles, leading to high intrarectal voiding pressures, which induces anterior rectal wall prolapse and ischemic changes.[12] If the process exists long enough, ulcer formation occurs. However identifying an ulcer on colonoscopy is not required for the diagnosis.

Endoscopic findings vary greatly, including nodularity, erythema, exudate, sessile or pedunculated polypoid lesions, frank ulceration, or may be normal.[10] The visualized lesion may be single or multiple, in any shape or size. Most often, SRUS is found on the anterior rectal wall within 5 to 10 cm of the anal verge. Obtaining multiple mucosal biopsies is essential even when minimal to no macroscopic findings are found, as histology is the gold standard for diagnosis. Histology of SRUS includes a thickened mucosal layer with smooth muscle bundles extending between the crypts, crypt architectural distortion, muscularis mucosae hyperplasia, and fibromuscular obliteration.

There are several methods of treatment depending on the severity with variable outcomes. Conservative management includes laxatives, steroid and mesalamine enemas, and defecation biofeedback therapy, the latter of particular importance in children who can cooperate with behavioral modification.[12] Endoscopic steroid injection and excisional surgery of the lesion have been used in cases resistant to conservative treatment. Endoscopic therapy with argon plasma coagulation (APC) has been used with some promise (**Fig. 1**). In a randomized controlled trial, 24 adult patients received biofeedback therapy, increased fiber intake, and laxatives, or the same regimen with several sessions of APC, with improved outcomes in those receiving APC therapy.[13] Further pediatric studies are needed to better determine the utility of APC in refractory cases of SRUS in children.

Polyps and Postpolypectomy Bleeding

Bleeding from polyps is described in pediatric patients of all ages, but is most commonly associated with juvenile polyps in children younger than 5 years. Juvenile polyps are hamartomatous lesions with little malignant potential. Other polyposis syndromes can present in childhood, including juvenile polyposis syndrome, PTEN hamartoma tumor syndromes (Cowden syndrome, Bannayan-Riley-Ruvalcaba syndrome), Peutz-Jeghers syndrome, familial adenomatous polyposis syndromes, and hereditary nonpolyposis colorectal cancer. Each GI polyposis syndrome must be monitored and surveyed according to available detailed guidelines.[14]

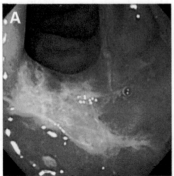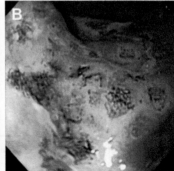

Fig. 1. (A) SRUS. (B) SRUS after successful treatment with argon plasma coagulation.

Colonoscopy is the most useful tool for diagnosis and treatment. A complete colonoscopy is necessary to thoroughly identify all polyps because they can be found proximal to the rectosigmoid colon in 35% of children with juvenile polyps.[15] Most polyps in children are pedunculated (**Fig. 2**) and amenable to polypectomy using a snare wire loop passed through the colonoscope working channel, coupled with electrocautery. A juvenile polyp is typically 1 to 3 cm or smaller, with a smooth or "chicken-skinned" red surface. Peutz-Jeghers syndrome polyps can be sessile or pedunculated with a lobulated surface. Tubular adenomas are typically pedunculated with smooth red surface, whereas villous adenomas are often sessile and broad based.

Each polyp type has distinct histologic characteristics, therefore polyp retrieval is important for pathologic analysis, especially to investigate its malignant potential. Intraprocedural bleeding after polypectomy can be controlled using hemostasis techniques, including clips, thermocoagulation, and detachable loop snares. In a study of 83 children with juvenile polyps, postpolypectomy bleeding occurred in 10%, and only 2 patients required endoscopic hemostasis for severe bleeding.[16]

Dieulafoy Lesion

A Dieulafoy lesion is a rare but potentially life-threatening cause of LGIB that can be found in children. It is a vascular abnormality that involves a large tortuous submucosal artery that reaches the mucosa without tapering its size. The theorized pathogenesis involves an ulcer that forms at the site of the exposed artery secondary to its pulsations on the surrounding tissue, and eventually the vessel ruptures into the lumen. Clinically, a Dieulafoy lesion presents with intermittent and painless gastrointestinal bleeding, which can be hematemesis, melena, or hematochezia depending on anatomic location.[17] Key elements to the diagnosis and management of a Dieulafoy lesion include the following:

- Most are found in the upper GI tract, with fewer than one-third of lesions found in the colon, with an absence of mucosal inflammation surrounding the artery.
- An actively spurting pulsatile arteriole from a mucosal defect with normal surrounding mucosa is characteristic. A dense clot with a narrow point of attachment to a mucosal defect may be found.
- A colonic Dieulafoy lesion may rupture due to stercoral ulceration over an abnormally dilated submucosal arterial vessel.

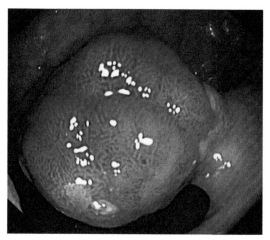

Fig. 2. Pedunculated polyp in a child with familial adenomatous polyposis.

- Endoscopy is the first-line diagnostic and therapeutic modality, with angiography reserved for endoscopic failure to localize or treat the lesion.
- Combination therapy with epinephrine injection followed by clip or band ligation has been shown to achieve permanent hemostasis in 95% of cases.

Angiodysplasias and Other Vascular Anomalies

The term angiodysplasia refers to a vascular ectasia manifesting as a thin-walled, dilated, punctate red vascular structure in the bowel mucosa or submucosa. It is most often found in the left colon or terminal ileum.[18] Therefore, detection necessitates a complete colonoscopy that reaches the terminal ileum, and enteroscopy should be considered for more proximal lesions.[19] Diagnosis of angiodysplasia can be made by cross-sectional imaging modalities, such as computed tomography angiography (CTA), or directly by colonoscopy. The preferred endoscopic treatment is by thermoablation or APC. Angiodysplasia often recurs despite treatment due to incomplete treatment or a newly developed lesion.[18]

Vascular malformations can present as nonisolated syndromic conditions at any age in childhood; each syndrome has a different endoscopic appearance in the bowel.

- Osler-Weber-Rendu syndrome: widespread or multiple capillary malformations similar to angiodysplasias[20] (also called hereditary hemorrhagic telangiectasias [HHT]).
- Klippel-Trénaunay syndrome: confluent bluish vascular discoloration from anus extending proximally.[21]
- Blue rubber bleb nevus syndrome (BRBNS) (**Fig. 3**): small, multifocal, well-circumscribed and demarcated venous malformations throughout the bowel.[22] This lesion is pathognomonic for BRBNS.

Management of vascular malformations includes therapeutic hemostasis to temporize significant acute or chronic bleeding, as well as surgical therapy. Medical therapy with sirolimus is now a promising treatment option for children with BRBNS,[23] in addition to endoscopic[24,25] and surgical[22] approaches. In adults with HHT, successful medical therapy has been reported with bevacizumab, a vascular endothelial growth factor inhibitor,[26] which may represent a future treatment option for children with this syndrome.

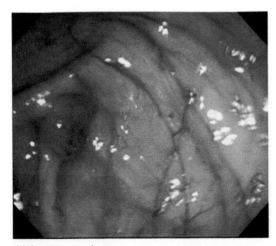

Fig. 3. Blue rubber bleb nevus syndrome.

Ileocolonic Ulceration

Infectious colitis

Infections with parasites, such as *Entamoeba histolytica*, and bacteria, such as *Clostridium difficile, Shigella, Salmonella, Escherichia coli*, and *Campylobacter*, can infect immune competent hosts, with varying degrees of colitis and ulceration detected macroscopically and microscopically. Treatment is typically supportive care or antimicrobial agents depending on pathogen and host comorbid conditions. In the immune-compromised patient, particular pathogens such as *Cryptosporidium* and *Cytomegalovirus* (CMV) should be considered; CMV is of particular importance in children with inflammatory bowel disease (IBD).

Endoscopic appearance of CMV infection can include diffuse colitis, only discrete ulcerations, or both (**Fig. 4**). CMV ulcers are often larger than 1 cm; can be round, oval, or irregular in shape; and with or without circumscribed boarders.[27] The diagnosis of CMV colitis can be made by endoscopic mucosal biopsy with routine hematoxylin and eosin staining, tissue CMV polymerase chain reaction, or viral culture. Treatment is with antiviral medications such as ganciclovir or foscarnet.

Inflammatory bowel disease

IBD often presents with LGIB and has a distinct mucosal pattern. Colonoscopic appearance in Crohn disease is characterized by variable degree of aphthous ulceration and sometimes luminal narrowing,[28] whereas ulcerative colitis is characterized by diffuse erythema, loss of vascular markings, friability, erosions, ulcers, and spontaneous bleeding.[29] In the setting of acute severe ulcerative colitis, complete colonoscopy may incur increased risk of excess bleeding, as well as perforation. At the least, flexible sigmoidoscopy in the setting of acute severe colitis can contribute to diagnostic clarification and to evaluate for infection, such as CMV.[30] Endoscopic hemostasis is rarely necessary for bleeding secondary to IBD colitis; rather, anti-inflammatory therapy to heal the mucosa is critical to resolution of ongoing bleeding.

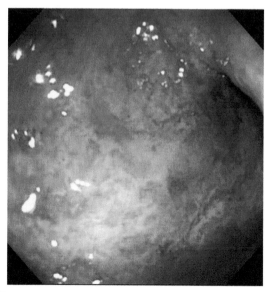

Fig. 4. CMV colitis.

Anastomotic ulceration

Postoperative anastomotic ulcers (AUs) are a complication after bowel resection and reanastomosis, and occur more in children than adults. Bleeding from these ulcers can be occult or life threatening, and should be suspected in any patient with history of previous bowel surgery. In a multicenter study of 11 children over 22 years, congenital bowel malformations and necrotizing enterocolitis were the most common initial underlying reason for bowel resection, and there was a median delay of nearly 4 years from onset of symptoms to diagnosis of AU.[31]

Endoscopic features of AU include round 1-cm to 3-cm ulcers surrounded by normal mucosa at the proximal or distal side of the anastomosis. If therapeutic endoscopy is performed, rebleeding risk within 30 days may be less with hemoclips compared with injection and thermocoagulation.[32] Some patients will require surgical resection of the AU.

Graft-versus-host disease

Gastrointestinal graft-versus-host disease (GVHD) can develop 3 or more weeks after hematopoietic stem cell transplantation. When present, rectal bleeding can be life threatening, and is often accompanied by diarrhea, abdominal pain, nausea, and vomiting. Sometimes a fleshy material can be excreted from the rectum in severe cases, recognized as a "colon cast."[33] In children with significant diarrhea with or without LGIB, sigmoidoscopy with biopsy alone (avoiding upper endoscopy) is usually sufficient for diagnosis. Endoscopic appearance can be normal, or have nonspecific findings of erythema, edema, erosions, and ulceration.[34]

Because the diagnosis of GVHD relies on obtaining biopsies, attention must be paid to correcting coagulopathy and thrombocytopenia before the procedure as needed. Medical therapy of the underlying GVHD is preferred when possible, although at times a focal bleeding lesion requires endoscopic therapy. A therapeutic procedure in the setting of GVHD should be performed by an experienced endoscopist and used with caution given potentially higher risks of bleeding or perforation.

Heterotopic gastric mucosa

Heterotopic gastric mucosa (HGM) in the rectum is a rare etiology of LGIB, due to hydrochloric acid secretion leading to ulceration of surrounding rectal mucosa. Unlike Meckel diverticulum, the rectal bleeding from heterotopic rectal gastric mucosa can be painful. Scintigraphy should identify HGM in the rectum and elsewhere if present. Surgical excision is often required, but endoscopic treatment has been attempted.[35]

Stercoral ulcer

Stercoral ulcer is thought to develop secondary to impacted feces causing pressure necrosis of the bowel wall with a significant risk of perforation. Although it usually occurs in elderly patients with a history of chronic constipation, it also has been described on rare occasion in children, especially when vascular perfusion is compromised.[36] Clinical presentation involves significant lower abdominal pain with hematochezia. The rectosigmoid colon with relatively poor blood supply and harder stool consistency is the typical location. Endoscopically, an irregular ulcer that conforms to the contours of the impacted stool can be found. Endoscopic hemostasis using thermocoagulation and injection therapy has been successful, with surgery reserved for uncontrollable bleeding.[37]

Severe Upper Gastrointestinal Bleeding

Extensive bleeding proximal to the ligament of Treitz can cause melena or hematochezia without hematemesis. Life-threatening etiologies of UGIB that may present with LGIB that should be considered in every child include esophageal variceal bleeding and aortoesophageal fistula secondary to button battery ingestion. A more detailed description of the differential diagnosis and management of UGIB can be found elsewhere (discussed by Lirio (Management of Upper Gastrointestinal Bleeding in Children: Variceal and Nonvariceal) elsewhere in this issue).

EVALUATION AND RESUSCITATION

The initial evaluation and resuscitation of a child with LGIB occurs simultaneously at presentation. A targeted history and physical examination (**Box 1**) attempt to identify the cause of bleeding and location within the GI tract, whereas evaluation of hemodynamic status and initial laboratory tests further guide the clinician to the severity of the bleed. Clinically based scoring systems to evaluate the severity of bleed and need for endoscopic intervention in LGIB have not been developed as rigorously as in UGIB.[38,39]

As a first time bleeding episode in childhood may herald the presentation of a congenital or genetic condition, family history of IBD, polyposis syndromes, liver

---

Box 1
Key elements of evaluation and resuscitation

Targeted history

Hematochezia versus melena

Fatigue, dyspnea, orthostatic changes, syncope

Previous gastrointestinal bleeding, recent polypectomy, or other procedures

Comorbidities: liver disease, inflammatory bowel disease, bleeding diathesis, previous intestinal surgery

Medications: antithrombotics, nonsteroidal anti-inflammatory drugs, aspirin

Foreign body ingestion

Vital signs

Tachycardia

Hypotension

Physical Examination

Head, ears, eyes, nose, and throat: sclera icterus, lip pigmentation, petechiae, trauma

Cardiovascular: murmur, capillary refill, extremity perfusion

Abdominal: tenderness, distension, ascites, hepatosplenomegaly

Rectal: gross blood, fissures, fistulae

Skin: vascular malformations/hemangiomas, jaundice, pallor

Laboratory evaluation

Complete blood count

Prothrombin time/international normalized ratio, partial thromboplastin time

Complete metabolic panel

Blood type and cross match

Resuscitation measures

Crystalloid

Blood products

Vasoactive medications

diseases, and bleeding diatheses should be inquired. For toddler and adolescent-age patients, accidental or intentional ingestions of foreign bodies or medications belonging to family members living in the same household may be useful information to investigate. Commonly ingested substances that may color the stool red (fruit punch, beets, candies) or black (licorice, blueberries, spinach, iron) and lead to false report of LGIB may be inquired in the very well-appearing child with no identifiable abnormality.

Once an endoscopic evaluation is determined likely, nasogastric tube (NGT) placement to obtain a gastric aspirate should be considered, particularly in those with hemodynamic instability who may have severe UGIB presenting with blood per rectum.[40] This practice is a debated one without clear evidence to standardize its use. Cuellar and colleagues[41] evaluated 62 adult patients accounting for 73 GI bleeding episodes and found an NGT aspirate appearance had a sensitivity and specificity of 79% and 55%, respectively, for determination of active UGIB, leading the investigators to conclude this practice is not supported. There are no studies evaluating the relationship between the volume of saline infused into the stomach to clear an initial bloody aspirate, and the likelihood of needing endoscopic intervention. Ultimately, a case-by-case approach for using NGT aspirate to guide therapy is needed that also accounts for the age and developmental status of the patient, as some children will become intensely agitated with this maneuver, making resuscitation more difficult.

DIAGNOSTIC ASSESSMENT

Following the initial evaluation and resuscitation, one must determine if an endoscopic procedure or imaging study will be performed to further localize the bleeding source. Various algorithms for adult patients have been previously published.[1,40,42] In children, there are multiple suitable approaches as well. In the pediatric patient with moderate to severe bleeding suspected to be from a lower intestinal source (eg, no hematemesis, stigmata of portal hypertension), the authors' approach is often to consider the presence or absence of pain in the decision process (**Fig. 5**).

Additionally, as blood and stool pass per rectum, it is often prudent to collect samples for infectious testing, particularly in the setting of fever or overt diarrhea. Results of tests for *Clostridium difficile* and a culture for pathogenic bacteria will have delay of hours to days and directly affect treatment.

Endoscopy

The initial diagnostic tests for identification of the bleeding source is typically esophagogastroduodenoscopy (EGD) and colonoscopy given the therapeutic potential; the decision of which to perform first will depend on the degree of suspicion for an upper GI source based on history and/or positive aspirate for blood from NGT lavage.

Colonoscopy has a diagnostic yield between 48% and 90% in the setting of LGIB.[2] Performing only sigmoidoscopy may obviate the need for complete bowel preparation, but has a much lower diagnostic yield of 9%,[2] making this a less-appealing initial approach if a complete colonoscopy is feasible. If an EGD and colonoscopy (after bowel preparation) fail to identify the bleeding source, a small bowel source of bleeding should be sought. The utility of a repeat colonoscopy to evaluate for a missed lesion is likely very low.[43]

Technetium-99 Pertechnetate Disodium Scintigraphy (Meckel Scan)

Hemorrhage from a Meckel diverticulum with HGM should be considered early in the course of diagnostic evaluation of children. Depending on the timing between initial

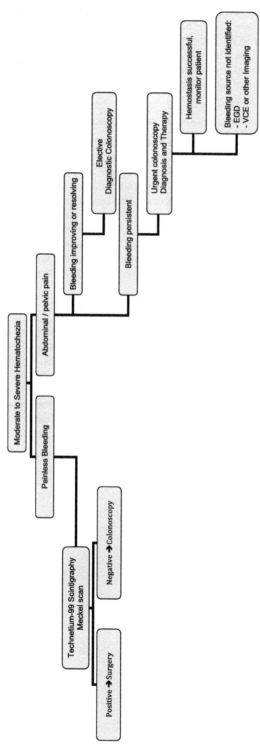

Fig. 5. Diagnostic algorithm when lower GI source of bleeding suspected.

presentation and feasibility to complete a bowel preparation, a Meckel scan could be considered before colonoscopy, particularly in young children with painless bleeding. The test can identify HGM throughout the bowel, such as in a duplication cyst. An important limitation of scintigraphy is the sensitivity of 60% and negative predictive value of 76%,[44] although the sensitivity may increase to 87% with use of ranitidine before the scan.[45] Even with premedication, a negative Meckel scan does not rule out the possibility of HGM.

Technetium-99–Labeled Red Blood Cell Scan (Nuclear Bleeding Scan)

A nuclear bleeding scan may noninvasively identify the bleeding location within the GI tract. It requires a brisk bleeding rate greater than 0.1 mL/min,[46] and therefore is not appropriate for occult obscure GI bleeding. Images are obtained frequently in the first few hours (dynamic phase) and again every few hours up to 24 hours after injection of the tagged red blood cells (delayed phase). The bleeding scan may become positive only in up to 73% of patients in the delayed phases,[47] highlighting the utility to complete both phases. However, in a study of 23 scans performed in children, the bleeding scan had an overall sensitivity of 39% and only the scans positive in the first 2 hours highly correlated with correctly identifying the location of the lesion.[48] A bleeding scan is often used as a second-line test if other methods of investigation fail to localize the bleeding site.

Angiography: Mesenteric and Radiologic

Direct mesenteric angiography also requires a brisk bleeding rate of 0.5 mL/min or more.[49] The specificity is 100%; however, the sensitivity is variable depending on multiple factors, including the skill of the interventional radiologist. A sensitivity of 30% to 47% was found in one study that included 44 adults with acute bleeding.[50] The therapeutic potential is only for arterial sources of bleeding, which can be directly accessed for embolization. Additional therapeutic benefits include preoperative coil placement in or near the bleeding location for easier identification at time of surgery (**Fig. 6**).[51] There are major potential risks of mesenteric angiography, including femoral

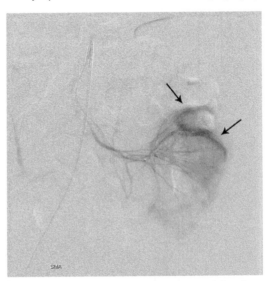

Fig. 6. Superior mesenteric artery angiography identifying a jejunal arteriovenous malformation (*arrows*). (*Courtesy of* Anne Marie Cahill, MD, Philadelphia, PA.)

artery thrombosis and bowel ischemia, which limit its use as a first-line diagnostic modality.

CTA and magnetic resonance angiography (MRA) are appealing alternatives to mesenteric angiography given diminished invasiveness and risk of adverse events. In the setting of brisk bleeding, CTA has been reported to have a sensitivity and specificity of 70% to 90% and 99% to 100%, respectively.[52,53] However, with obscure gastrointestinal bleeding (OGIB), the sensitivity may be closer to 55%.[54] CTA offers faster examination times, which will allow some children to complete the study without sedation who would require it for MRA. However, advantages of MRA include lack of ionizing radiation, better contrast resolution, and ability to perform dynamic contrast enhancement and diffusion studies, which makes MRA the preferred test if IBD or polyposis is the suspected cause of bleeding.[55]

Video Capsule Endoscopy

In the pediatric population, OGIB is the second most common indication for use of video capsule endoscopy (VCE), with a diagnostic yield of 38.4% in this setting.[56] In children younger than 8 years, OGIB is the most common indication for VCE, with positive diagnostic findings in 53% of patients, including identification of polyps, vascular anomalies, Meckel diverticulum, intestinal duplications, and AUs.[57] The primary complication related to use of VCE is capsule retention; therefore, it should not be used as an initial study if there is suspicion for bowel obstruction, stricture, fistula, or tumor. The children with highest risk for capsule retention are those with known IBD.[58]

Small Bowel Enteroscopy

The use of small bowel enteroscopy in children with GI bleeding is typically reserved for patients with OGIB who previously had a VCE or CTA to localize the lesion. Procedural options include push, single or double balloon, and spiral enteroscopy. Push enteroscopy refers to per-oral passage of a colonoscope or enteroscope into the jejunum without any assisting advancement device. Spiral enteroscopy uses a specialized overtube and a pediatric colonoscope,[59] which has not been studied in detail in children. There is a growing experience with balloon enteroscopy in children, which allows evaluation of the entire small bowel, particularly when both antegrade (transoral) and retrograde (transanal) approaches are used together. In pediatric patients, the diagnostic yield of double balloon enteroscopy for OGIB is 50% to 77%.[19,60,61] Oliva and colleagues[62] evaluated an algorithm in 22 children using single-balloon enteroscopy when a positive or suspicious finding was found on VCE, with a combined diagnostic yield of 95% in this approach. A study in adults with OGIB found the most cost-effective approach is to use double-balloon enteroscopy as the initial diagnostic test[63]; however, this approach has yet to be widely adopted in management of pediatric patients.

PREENDOSCOPY PREPARATION AND CONSIDERATIONS

Before attempting endoscopic hemostasis, a comprehensive management plan must be developed that accounts for numerous preprocedure considerations. Hemodynamic resuscitation is paramount before endoscopic intervention for gastrointestinal bleeding.[64] While the initial evaluation and resuscitation are ongoing, the pediatric endoscopist should consider the potential venues to perform a therapeutic procedure and the support staff available to complete a procedure effectively. Within each medical center, a dedicated procedure suite, operating room, intensive care unit, or emergency department may be considered appropriate or not, depending on availability of anesthesia resources, personnel, and certain specialized endoscopic equipment.

Although simpler therapeutic GI procedures can be performed under gastroenterologist-administered moderate sedation,[65] the major trend in pediatric endoscopy is to use anesthesiologist-administered deep sedation or general anesthesia.[66] Given the differences in how children respond to anesthesia compared with adults,[67] and the possibility of complex comorbid medical conditions, a pediatric-trained anesthesiologist may be preferred or essential to safely completing a therapeutic endoscopy.

At least one other team member should be knowledgeable in the procedure and tools used in achieving hemostasis before beginning an endoscopic procedure. In situations in which the pediatric endoscopist is not expert with therapeutic modalities, it is appropriate to consult with adult gastroenterology colleagues who may provide technical support and guidance. Lack of appropriate procedure space, pediatric size endoscopes and devices, support staff, anesthesia resources, or technical endoscopic skill available are grounds to consider transporting a pediatric patient to another venue with pediatric expertise. No patient with GI bleeding should undergo diagnostic or therapeutic endoscopy in the setting of significant cardiopulmonary instability, bowel perforation, or peritonitis.

Once it is determined a procedure will be undertaken, one should obtain informed consent from the patient or appropriate caregiver with communication of potential benefits, risks, and alternatives to endoscopic intervention.[68] It is also important to identify the surgical or interventional radiology staff who may be able to assist in the event of uncontrolled bleeding or other complication, and to determine the need for preprocedure antibiotic prophylaxis, such as in patients with cirrhosis.[69]

A number of bowel preparations are currently used in children.[70] In the setting of acute bleeding, a preparation with a polyethylene glycol–based solution given by mouth or NGT is often preferred, with a readiness to begin the procedure as close to the time of preparation completion as allowable.[71] An unprepared colonoscopy can be completed successfully on emergent basis,[72,73] however preparation is preferable.

ENDOSCOPIC HEMOSTASIS

Multiple therapeutic options exist for endoscopic hemostasis. Regardless of the modality chosen, there are principles that consistently give the endoscopist the best chance to achieve a successful result and minimize adverse events:

- Use the largest endoscope feasible for patient size and weight, including a therapeutic scope with dual working channels when available. Ensure the available hemostatic devices are compatible with the size of working channel (**Table 2**). Specifications for each endoscope model are available elsewhere.[74]
- The endoscopist should use the modalities he or she is most experienced with that are appropriate for the particular lesion encountered.
- Prepare 2 modalities (injection, thermal, mechanical) before beginning the procedure.
- Prepare a jet irrigation pump coupled to the endoscope, controlled by foot pedal to provide uninterrupted irrigation. Depending on irrigation pump and size of colonoscope, an adaptor may be needed to insert the tip of tubing through a working channel. An alternative is 60-mL syringes with water or saline manually pushed into the working channel.

Table 2
Endoscopes and hemostatic devices in pediatric colonoscopy

Patient Weight	Endoscope	Working Channel/Outer Diameter Range, mm	Hemostatic Accessory
<5 kg	Ultrathin gastroscope	2.0/4.9–5.9	Injection needle 23 or 25 G APC 5-Fr probe Polypectomy snare <30 mm Bipolar 5-Fr probe
5–15 kg	Standard gastroscope	2.8/8–11.6	Injection needle 19–22 G Bipolar 7-Fr probe APC 7-Fr probe Through-the-scope clips
>15 kg[a]	Pediatric or adult colonoscope	3.2–3.8 mm[b]/11.5–13.2	Injection needle 19–22 G Bipolar 7–10 Fr[c] APC 7–10 Fr[c] Through-the-scope clips
Older child	Dual-channel therapeutic colonoscope	2.8–3.2 mm, 3.7–3.8 mm/11.5–13.7	Injection needle 19–22 G Bipolar 7–10 Fr[c] APC 7–10 Fr[c] Through-the-scope clips

Abbreviation: APC, argon plasma coagulation.
[a] Endoscope choice individualized, gastroscope may still be preferred at lower limits of this weight range.
[b] Pentax (Montvale, NJ) EC 2990Li colonoscope, 2.8-mm working channel.
[c] 10-Fr probes require >3.4-mm channel.

- Establish clear communication between endoscopist and assistant for each step of the therapeutic sequence (eg, instructing to "expose," "retract," or "deploy" a device may use more specific language than the terms "out," "in," or "go").

Injection Therapy

Epinephrine, sclerosants, tissue adhesives, and ethanol are available agents for injection therapy. Although sclerosants and tissue adhesives can be used in the small bowel and colon, their primary role is in esophageal variceal, and gastric ulcer or variceal bleeding, respectively. A single injectable agent should be used in any one session, as combining multiple agents together is associated with increased complications.[75] The endoscope should be close to the bleeding vessel to limit the distance needed to extend the needle sheath. Kinking of the needle may be more likely if extended long distances and with plastic compared with metal sheaths.

Injection therapy is a high-yield modality in gaining immediate control of a spurting artery and before washing away an adherent blood clot overlying the bleeding site. In both of these instances, injection followed by a thermal or mechanical hemostatic modality in combination is superior to using injection therapy alone. A meta-analysis of 20 studies including 2472 adult patients identified that dual therapy significantly decreases rebleeding and emergency surgery risks compared with injection monotherapy.[76]

Epinephrine

Epinephrine has multiple mechanisms of action, including immediate volume tamponade followed by vasoconstriction and platelet aggregation. A safe and effective epinephrine concentration of 1:10,000[77] for gastric and intestinal bleeding is prepared with a mixture of 1 mL epinephrine 1:1000 + 9 mL normal saline. A more dilute concentration of 1:100,000 should be considered in the esophagus due to bypassing of first-pass metabolism,[78] or in some patients with severe cardiac disease. There are no studies identifying the ideal injection volume in children. Typically, aliquots of 0.5 to 2 mL are used per injection, in 4 injection quadrants 2 to 3 mm from an ulcer base or bleeding vessel,[79] with a maximum injection volume of 10 mL. There are caveats to these standards. Injections into 4 quadrants are advantageous because the path of the underlying feeding vessel is unknown; however, fewer injections may be elected to avoid changing the orientation of the target to a less direct access for a second modality. Larger injection volumes up to 20 mL have been shown to be safe and decrease rebleeding risk in adults.[80] However, it is unknown if these data can be extrapolated to pediatric patients. In general, larger volumes per injection are used for actively spurting vessel and smaller volumes (ie, $\leq$0.5 mL) may be considered for thinner-walled areas (eg, right colon) where systemic absorption and perforation risk may be greater. Other important risks of injection therapy include bowel ischemia and bleeding.

Ethanol
Ethanol achieves hemostasis through its mucosal dehydrating effects. Its use has had variable success in studies of adult patients,[79] and is not well studied in children. Caution should be taken if using ethanol, as the volume of each injection is less than epinephrine and may be more difficult to control.[81]

Thermal Devices

Thermal energy leads to tissue edema, coagulation, and blood vessel contraction. Coaptation coagulation is used with contact probes, and refers to the combined mechanism of direct pressure tamponade by the probe onto the vessel followed by delivery of thermal energy to destruct the vessel wall.[82] Use of monopolar devices, such as hot biopsy forceps, have fallen out of favor, as the depth of thermal energy is less controlled, and a grounding pad on the patient is required. Most endoscopists prefer bipolar and heater probes (HPs), given the ease of use, availability, and safety, including the lack of need for a grounding pad because the entire circuit is closed at the tip of the device. In clinical practice, many pediatric endoscopists prefer bipolar probes compared with HPs due to a wider clinical experience.

Heater probe
HPs are teflon-coated cylinders containing a heating coil. A predetermined amount of heat energy (joules) is delivered with each pulse to the probe tip and transferred to the tissue to induce coagulation. There is no electrocautery. The increased resistance that occurs with tissue desiccation does not limit depth of injury with an HP, thus deeper coagulation and perforation risk is greater with HP compared with bipolar probes.

Multipolar/Bipolar probe
Multipolar/bipolar electrocoagulation (MPEC) probes deliver an electrical current through tissue not yet desiccated. The endoscopist uses a foot pedal to deliver the electrical current. The power output (watts) is adjusted on the electrosurgical unit by the endoscopist. The power selected, number of applications (times pressing on the foot pedal), and duration of each application determines the amount of energy delivered to the tissue, and may differ depending on type and location of the lesion and endoscopist preference.[83] A power setting of 15 to 20 W is appropriate for most lesions encountered in any GI tract location,[84] although some prefer to use a lower setting range of 12 to 15 W for lesions in the small bowel and colon.[78] The coaptation

force applied by the probe contributes to the depth of energy delivered. Technique in treatment of gastric lesions is often with firm pressure and application times up to 10 seconds, whereas it is safer in the small bowel and colon to apply light pressure and 3 to 4 seconds of electrocautery pulse time owing to thinner walls of the bowel. These generalities must be adapted in each situation, as a fibrotic ulcer in the colon may require greater current than angiodysplasia in the same location. Unique probes include a 5-French bipolar probe available for use through the 2-mm channel of a pediatric endoscope (ConMed Endoscopic Technologies, Chelmsford, MA) and the Injector Gold Probe that has an integrated 25-G injection needle (Boston Scientific, Natick, MA) for the ability to apply dual modalities with a single device.

Argon plasma coagulation

APC is a noncontact electrocoagulation device that delivers monopolar current to the tissue target through ionized argon plasma gas.[85] Grounding pads on the patient are required. The energy delivered is controlled by the endoscopist through adjustments of the gas flow rate and power settings on the electrosurgical generator, application time through a foot pedal to discharge the gas, and probe distance from the tissue. A gas flow rate of 1 L per minute and power of 30 to 50 W for most lesions can be used, with lower power settings within this range in the right colon, while delivering pulses for 1-second to 2-second intervals.[71] As the tissue desiccates and coagulum forms at the surface, the gas begins to conduct to adjacent intact tissue, which limits depth of injury. However, APC can still generate deeper bowel wall injury compared with contact modalities like bipolar electrocautery depending on the amount of power used.[86]

A major difference between available APC probes is the direction gas can fire from the probe tip. A probe may fire directly forward, to the side, or circumferentially (ERBE, Marietta, GA), forward and to the side (Canady, Hampton, VA) or only directly forward (ConMed Endoscopic Technologies, Chelmsford, MA). More firing directions offers the endoscopist more options when approaching a lesion perpendicular or tangential. Regardless of angle, the probe should be maintained 1 to 3 mm from the target, which requires fine control of the endoscope tip, and represents a pitfall for many endoscopists using this modality. If the probe is too far, inert gas is infused into the bowel lumen, which can be combustible, and should be suctioned out readily. If tissue contact is made while firing the gas, injury depth can increase, and coagulum accumulates on the probe tip, which must be frequently removed and cleaned.

APC has a wide range of applications. It has been reported to be effective in children with multiple upper GI tract lesions.[87] In adults, use in the rectum is well described to treat radiation proctitis[88] and SRUS.[13] APC has become one of the therapeutic modalities of choice for angiodysplasias and other vascular malformations,[89,90] and has been used in BRBNS in children.[91] However, other modalities should be considered for larger caliber vessels in the stomach (eg, gastric Dieulafoy lesion), as the depth of electrocautery may not be satisfactory for obliteration.[78] In comparison with other hemostatic modalities, APC has been shown to be safe and produce similar therapeutic results.[92,93]

Clips

Clips provide mechanical tamponade without inducing tissue injury. Multiple clips can be placed in a sequential fashion (**Fig. 7**) to tamponade either side of a vessel after first securing the direct point of bleeding.[81] Nomenclature in the literature for this accessory includes endoclip, hemoclip, and through-the-scope (TTS) clip. Three manufacturers of TTS clips are available; all have particular specifications, are single use, and

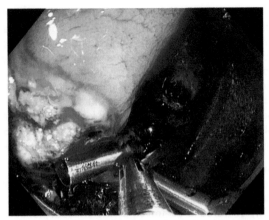

Fig. 7. Multiple hemoclips placed in colon after endoscopic mucosal resection. (*Courtesy of* Michael Kochman, MD, FACP, Philadelphia, PA.)

require a minimum of a 2.8-mm working channel. The QuickClip2 (Olympus America, Center Valley, PA) is rotatable once exposed from the sheath, and the Resolution clip (Boston Scientific) can be reopened after initial closure before final deployment. The TriClip (Cook Medical, Bloomington, IN) is a 3-pronged clip compared with the others with 2 prongs.

In pediatric patients, TTS clips may be useful for immediate or delayed postpolypectomy bleeding, as well as sustained bleeding after mucosal biopsy. They also may be useful when encountering a bleeding vessel within an ulcer base. Patients with thrombocytopenia and coagulopathy or on anticoagulation medications may have a favorable result with use of clips because preventing additional tissue injury minimizes bleeding risk. Clips are also favored in the thinner-walled right colon and cecum. Monotherapy[94–96] and combination therapy[97,98] have demonstrated equally good results. Clips compared with epinephrine injection and/or thermocoagulation in the colon have demonstrated no difference in 30-day rebleeding rates.[99]

Regardless of the particular clip being used or the type of bleeding lesion, success or failure of this device is often determined by the knowledge and precision of its use by both the endoscopist and assistant. Before clip exposure through the sheath, the endoscopist is best advised to approach the bleeding vessel tangentially or directly with minimal endoscope tip angulation and to suck excess air from the lumen to soften the wall. The assistant must be familiar with the uses of both sliding fixtures on the handle: one for exposing and retracting the clip in the sheath and the other for controlling the remaining steps from opening through deployment. Once the clip is exposed beyond the sheath and jaws are opened, the endoscopist will work in a coordinated fashion with the assistant to maximize tissue amount and apposition, followed by jaw closure and deployment.

Emerging Technologies for Hemostasis in Pediatric Lower Gastrointestinal Bleeding

Hemospray

Hemospray (Cook Medical, Winston Salem, NC) is a powder delivered via a through-the-scope catheter and a carbon dioxide pressurized system. The powder absorbs moisture at the site of bleeding and concentrates clotting factors, forming a mechanical plug on the bleeding vessel.[100] Active bleeding is required, thus it cannot be used for a nonbleeding visible vessel. Most of the current published experience with

Hemospray in GI endoscopy has been in the treatment of UGIB,[101] although experience treating colonic bleeding is growing.[102–104] This modality has not been studied in children with LGIB to date.

Over-the-scope clip

The over-the-scope clip (OTSC) (Ovesco Endoscopy AG, Tubingen, Germany) is a clip preloaded to the endoscope with the jaws open. Compared with TTS clips, the OTSC has higher compression force and capacity to capture larger volumes of tissue, making it effective for both hemostasis and perforation closure.[105] A pitfall of this device in treating an active-bleeding lesion is the need to withdraw the scope after the bleeding site is identified to load the OTSC, and then advance the scope again. This device has been used in children[106] to close gastrocutaneous fistula and for hemostasis in adults,[107] but has not been studied in children to date for control of LGIB.

SUMMARY

Children presenting to medical attention with LGIB may have underlying conditions that range from completely benign to immediately life threatening. Awareness of the most likely etiologies based on the patient's age and associated symptoms will guide the diagnostic evaluation and expedite therapy. The resuscitation, preprocedure preparation, and technical understanding of available therapeutic modalities are integral in achieving optimal outcomes.

REFERENCES

1. Barnert J, Messmann H. Management of lower gastrointestinal tract bleeding. Best Pract Res Clin Gastroenterol 2008;22:295–312.
2. Zuckerman GR, Prakash C. Acute lower intestinal bleeding: part I: clinical presentation and diagnosis. Gastrointest Endosc 1998;48:606–17.
3. Jensen DM, Machicado GA. Diagnosis and treatment of severe hematochezia. The role of urgent colonoscopy after purge. Gastroenterology 1988;95:1569–74.
4. Zuckerman GR, Trellis DR, Sherman TM, et al. An objective measure of stool color for differentiating upper from lower gastrointestinal bleeding. Dig Dis Sci 1995;40:1614–21.
5. Pant C, Olyaee M, Sferra TJ, et al. Emergency department visits for gastrointestinal bleeding in children: results from the Nationwide Emergency Department Sample 2006-2011. Curr Med Res Opin 2015;31:347–51.
6. Peura DA, Lanza FL, Gostout CJ, et al. The American College of Gastroenterology bleeding registry: preliminary findings. Am J Gastroenterol 1997;92:924–8.
7. Kollef MH, O'Brien JD, Zuckerman GR, et al. BLEED: a classification tool to predict outcomes in patients with acute upper and lower gastrointestinal hemorrhage. Crit Care Med 1997;25:1125–32.
8. Foutch PG. Diverticular bleeding: are nonsteroidal anti-inflammatory drugs risk factors for hemorrhage and can colonoscopy predict outcome for patients? Am J Gastroenterol 1995;90:1779–84.
9. Velayos FS, Williamson A, Sousa KH, et al. Early predictors of severe lower gastrointestinal bleeding and adverse outcomes: a prospective study. Clin Gastroenterol Hepatol 2004;2:485–90.
10. Perito ER, Mileti E, Dalal DH, et al. Solitary rectal ulcer syndrome in children and adolescents. J Pediatr Gastroenterol Nutr 2012;54:266–70.
11. Urganci N, Kalyoncu D, Eken KG. Solitary rectal ulcer syndrome in children: a report of six cases. Gut Liver 2013;7:752–5.

12. Blackburn C, McDermott M, Bourke B. Clinical presentation of and outcome for solitary rectal ulcer syndrome in children. J Pediatr Gastroenterol Nutr 2012;54: 263–5.

13. Somani SK, Ghosh A, Avasthi G, et al. Healing of a bleeding solitary rectal ulcer with multiple sessions of argon plasma. Gastrointest Endosc 2010;71:578–82.

14. Burt RW, Cannon JA, David DS, et al. Colorectal cancer screening. J Natl Compr Canc Netw 2013;11:1538–75.

15. Lehmann CU, Elitsur Y. Juvenile polyps and their distribution in pediatric patients with gastrointestinal bleeding. W V Med J 1996;92:133–5.

16. Lee BG, Shin SH, Lee YA, et al. Juvenile polyp and colonoscopic polypectomy in childhood. Pediatr Gastroenterol Hepatol Nutr 2012;15:250–5.

17. Jeon HK, Kim GH. Endoscopic management of Dieulafoy's lesion. Clin Endosc 2015;48:112–20.

18. Chuang FJ, Lin JS, Yeung CY, et al. Intestinal angiodysplasia: an uncommon cause of gastrointestinal bleeding in children. Pediatr Neonatol 2011;52: 214–8.

19. Urs AN, Martinelli M, Rao P, et al. Diagnostic and therapeutic utility of double-balloon enteroscopy in children. J Pediatr Gastroenterol Nutr 2014;58:204–12.

20. Regula J, Wronska E, Pachlewski J. Vascular lesions of the gastrointestinal tract. Best Pract Res Clin Gastroenterol 2008;22:313–28.

21. Thosani N, Ghouri Y, Shah S, et al. Life-threatening gastrointestinal bleeding in Klippel-Trenaunay syndrome. Endoscopy 2013;45(Suppl 2 UCTN):E206.

22. Fishman SJ, Smithers CJ, Folkman J, et al. Blue rubber bleb nevus syndrome: surgical eradication of gastrointestinal bleeding. Ann Surg 2005;241(3):523–8.

23. Yuksekkaya H, Ozbek O, Keser M, et al. Blue rubber bleb nevus syndrome: successful treatment with sirolimus. Pediatrics 2012;129:e1080–4.

24. Mavrogenis G, Coumaros D, Tzilves D, et al. Cyanoacrylate glue in the management of blue rubber bleb nevus syndrome. Endoscopy 2011;43(Suppl 2 UCTN): E291–2.

25. Suksamanapun N, Trakarnsanga A, Akaraviputh T. Blue rubber bleb nevus syndrome. Endoscopy 2011;43(Suppl 2 UCTN):E411–2.

26. Epperla N, Hocking W. Blessing for the bleeder: bevacizumab in hereditary hemorrhagic telangiectasia. Clin Med Res 2015;13:32–5.

27. Kim CH, Bahng S, Kang KJ, et al. Cytomegalovirus colitis in patients without inflammatory bowel disease: a single center study. Scand J Gastroenterol 2010; 45:1295–301.

28. Sipponen T, Nuutinen H, Turunen U, et al. Endoscopic evaluation of Crohn's disease activity: comparison of the CDEIS and the SES-CD. Inflamm Bowel Dis 2010;16:2131–6.

29. Travis SP, Schnell D, Krzeski P, et al. Developing an instrument to assess the endoscopic severity of ulcerative colitis: the Ulcerative Colitis Endoscopic Index of Severity (UCEIS). Gut 2012;61:535–42.

30. Turner D, Travis SP, Griffiths AM, et al. Consensus for managing acute severe ulcerative colitis in children: a systematic review and joint statement from ECCO, ESPGHAN, and the Porto IBD Working Group of ESPGHAN. Am J Gastroenterol 2011;106:574–88.

31. Charbit-Henrion F, Chardot C, Ruemmele F, et al. Anastomotic ulcerations after intestinal resection in infancy. J Pediatr Gastroenterol Nutr 2014;59:531–6.

32. Lee YC, Wang HP, Yang CS, et al. Endoscopic hemostasis of a bleeding marginal ulcer: hemoclipping or dual therapy with epinephrine injection and heater probe thermocoagulation. J Gastroenterol Hepatol 2002;17:1220–5.

33. Al Ashgar H, Peedikayil M, Chaudhri N, et al. Defecation of a "colon cast" as a rare presentation of acute graft-versus-host disease. Ann Saudi Med 2009;29:231–3.
34. Sultan M, Ramprasad J, Jensen MK, et al. Endoscopic diagnosis of pediatric acute gastrointestinal graft-versus-host disease. J Pediatr Gastroenterol Nutr 2012;55:417–20.
35. Cheli M, Alberti D, Vavassori D, et al. Heterotopic rectal gastric mucosa: a rare cause of lower gastrointestinal bleeding in children. Case report and review of pediatric literature. Eur J Pediatr Surg 2007;17:50–4.
36. Al Omran Y, Al Hindi S, Alarayedh S, et al. Stercoral perforation in a child: a rare complication of NSAID use. BMJ Case Rep 2014;2014.
37. Huang CC, Wang IF, Chiu HH. Lower gastrointestinal bleeding caused by stercoral ulcer. CMAJ 2011;183:E134.
38. Blatchford O, Murray WR, Blatchford M. A risk score to predict need for treatment for upper-gastrointestinal haemorrhage. Lancet 2000;356:1318–21.
39. Rockall TA, Logan RF, Devlin HB, et al. Risk assessment after acute upper gastrointestinal haemorrhage. Gut 1996;38:316–21.
40. ASGE Standards of Practice Committee, Pasha SF, Shergill A, et al. The role of endoscopy in the patient with lower GI bleeding. Gastrointest Endosc 2014;79:875–85.
41. Cuellar RE, Gavaler JS, Alexander JA, et al. Gastrointestinal tract hemorrhage. The value of a nasogastric aspirate. Arch Intern Med 1990;150:1381–4.
42. Green BT, Rockey DC, Portwood G, et al. Urgent colonoscopy for evaluation and management of acute lower gastrointestinal hemorrhage: a randomized controlled trial. Am J Gastroenterol 2005;100:2395–402.
43. Gilbert D, O'Malley S, Selby W. Are repeat upper gastrointestinal endoscopy and colonoscopy necessary within six months of capsule endoscopy in patients with obscure gastrointestinal bleeding? J Gastroenterol Hepatol 2008;23:1806–9.
44. Dolezal J, Vizda J. Experiences with detection of the ectopic gastric mucosa by means of Tc-99m pertechnetate disodium scintigraphy in children with lower gastrointestinal bleeding. Eur J Pediatr Surg 2008;18:258–60.
45. Rerksuppaphol S, Hutson JM, Oliver MR. Ranitidine-enhanced 99m technetium pertechnetate imaging in children improves the sensitivity of identifying heterotopic gastric mucosa in Meckel's diverticulum. Pediatr Surg Int 2004;20:323–5.
46. Concha R, Amaro R, Barkin JS. Obscure gastrointestinal bleeding: diagnostic and therapeutic approach. J Clin Gastroenterol 2007;41:242–51.
47. Zettinig G, Staudenherz A, Leitha T. The importance of delayed images in gastrointestinal bleeding scintigraphy. Nucl Med Commun 2002;23:803–8.
48. Lee J, Lai MW, Chen CC, et al. Red blood cell scintigraphy in children with acute massive gastrointestinal bleeding. Pediatr Int 2008;50:199–203.
49. Zuckerman DA, Bocchini TP, Birnbaum EH. Massive hemorrhage in the lower gastrointestinal tract in adults: diagnostic imaging and intervention. AJR Am J Roentgenol 1993;161:703–11.
50. Fiorito JJ, Brandt LJ, Kozicky O, et al. The diagnostic yield of superior mesenteric angiography: correlation with the pattern of gastrointestinal bleeding. Am J Gastroenterol 1989;84:878–81.
51. Sahn B, Blinman TA, Cahill AM, et al. Vascular malformation as a cause of occult gastrointestinal bleeding. J Pediatr Gastroenterol Nutr 2015;60:e28.
52. Junquera F, Quiroga S, Saperas E, et al. Accuracy of helical computed tomographic angiography for the diagnosis of colonic angiodysplasia. Gastroenterology 2000;119:293–9.

53. Yoon W, Jeong YY, Shin SS, et al. Acute massive gastrointestinal bleeding: detection and localization with arterial phase multi-detector row helical CT. Radiology 2006;239:160–7.
54. Lee SS, Oh TS, Kim HJ, et al. Obscure gastrointestinal bleeding: diagnostic performance of multidetector CT enterography. Radiology 2011;259:739–48.
55. Rondonotti E, Marmo R, Petracchini M, et al. The American Society for Gastrointestinal Endoscopy (ASGE) diagnostic algorithm for obscure gastrointestinal bleeding: eight burning questions from everyday clinical practice. Dig Liver Dis 2013;45:179–85.
56. Cohen SA. The potential applications of capsule endoscopy in pediatric patients compared with adult patients. Gastroenterol Hepatol 2013;9:92–7.
57. Fritscher-Ravens A, Scherbakov P, Bufler P, et al. The feasibility of wireless capsule endoscopy in detecting small intestinal pathology in children under the age of 8 years: a multicentre European study. Gut 2009;58:1467–72.
58. Atay O, Mahajan L, Kay M, et al. Risk of capsule endoscope retention in pediatric patients: a large single-center experience and review of the literature. J Pediatr Gastroenterol Nutr 2009;49:196–201.
59. Akerman PA, Agrawal D, Chen W, et al. Spiral enteroscopy: a novel method of enteroscopy by using the Endo-Ease Discovery SB overtube and a pediatric colonoscope. Gastrointest Endosc 2009;69:327–32.
60. Nishimura N, Yamamoto H, Yano T, et al. Safety and efficacy of double-balloon enteroscopy in pediatric patients. Gastrointest Endosc 2010;71:287–94.
61. Liu W, Xu C, Zhong J. The diagnostic value of double-balloon enteroscopy in children with small bowel disease: report of 31 cases. Can J Gastroenterol 2009;23:635–8.
62. Oliva S, Pennazio M, Cohen SA, et al. Capsule endoscopy followed by single balloon enteroscopy in children with obscure gastrointestinal bleeding: a combined approach. Dig Liver Dis 2015;47:125–30.
63. Somsouk M, Gralnek IM, Inadomi JM. Management of obscure occult gastrointestinal bleeding: a cost-minimization analysis. Clin Gastroenterol Hepatol 2008; 6:661–70.
64. Jairath V, Barkun AN. The overall approach to the management of upper gastrointestinal bleeding. Gastrointest Endosc Clin N Am 2011;21:657–70.
65. Standards of Practice Committee of the American Society for Gastrointestinal Endoscopy, Lichtenstein DR, Jagannath S, et al. Sedation and anesthesia in GI endoscopy. Gastrointest Endosc 2008;68:815–26.
66. ASGE Standards of Practice Committee, Lightdale JR, Acosta R, et al. Modifications in endoscopic practice for pediatric patients. Gastrointest Endosc 2014; 79:699–710.
67. Schwarz SM, Lightdale JR, Liacouras CA. Sedation and anesthesia in pediatric endoscopy: one size does not fit all. J Pediatr Gastroenterol Nutr 2007;44: 295–7.
68. Standards of Practice Committee, Zuckerman MJ, Shen B, et al. Informed consent for GI endoscopy. Gastrointest Endosc 2007;66:213–8.
69. Chavez-Tapia NC, Barrientos-Gutierrez T, Tellez-Avila F, et al. Meta-analysis: antibiotic prophylaxis for cirrhotic patients with upper gastrointestinal bleeding—an updated Cochrane review. Aliment Pharmacol Ther 2011;34: 509–18.
70. Pall H, Zacur GM, Kramer RE, et al. Bowel preparation for pediatric colonoscopy: report of the NASPGHAN endoscopy and procedures committee. J Pediatr Gastroenterol Nutr 2014;59:409–16.

71. Wong Kee Song LM, Baron TH. Endoscopic management of acute lower gastrointestinal bleeding. Am J Gastroenterol 2008;103:1881–7.
72. Rossini FP, Ferrari A, Spandre M, et al. Emergency colonoscopy. World J Surg 1989;13:190–2.
73. Chaudhry V, Hyser MJ, Gracias VH, et al. Colonoscopy: the initial test for acute lower gastrointestinal bleeding. Am Surg 1998;64:723–8.
74. ASGE Technology Committee, Varadarajulu S, Banerjee S, et al. GI endoscopes. Gastrointest Endosc 2011;74:1–6.e6.
75. Loperfido S, Patelli G, La Torre L. Extensive necrosis of gastric mucosa following injection therapy of bleeding peptic ulcer. Endoscopy 1990;22:285–6.
76. Marmo R, Rotondano G, Piscopo R, et al. Dual therapy versus monotherapy in the endoscopic treatment of high-risk bleeding ulcers: a meta-analysis of controlled trials. Am J Gastroenterol 2007;102:279–89 [quiz: 469].
77. Randall GM, Jensen DM, Hirabayashi K, et al. Controlled study of different sclerosing agents for coagulation of canine gut arteries. Gastroenterology 1989;96:1274–81.
78. Prabhu NC, Song LM. Achieving hemostasis and the risks associated with therapy. Gastrointest Endosc Clin N Am 2015;25:123–45.
79. Park WG, Yeh RW, Triadafilopoulos G. Injection therapies for nonvariceal bleeding disorders of the GI tract. Gastrointest Endosc 2007;66:343–54.
80. Lin HJ, Hsieh YH, Tseng GY, et al. A prospective, randomized trial of large-versus small-volume endoscopic injection of epinephrine for peptic ulcer bleeding. Gastrointest Endosc 2002;55:615–9.
81. Kay MH, Wyllie R. Therapeutic endoscopy for nonvariceal gastrointestinal bleeding. J Pediatr Gastroenterol Nutr 2007;45:157–71.
82. Harrison JD, Morris DL. Does bipolar electrocoagulation time affect vessel weld strength? Gut 1991;32:188–90.
83. Laine L. Determination of the optimal technique for bipolar electrocoagulation treatment. An experimental evaluation of the BICAP and Gold probes. Gastroenterology 1991;100:107–12.
84. Morris ML, Tucker RD, Baron TH, et al. Electrosurgery in gastrointestinal endoscopy: principles to practice. Am J Gastroenterol 2009;104:1563–74.
85. Asge Technology C, Conway JD, Adler DG, et al. Endoscopic hemostatic devices. Gastrointest Endosc 2009;69:987–96.
86. Garrido T, Baba ER, Wodak S, et al. Histology assessment of bipolar coagulation and argon plasma coagulation on digestive tract. World J Gastrointest Endosc 2014;6:304–11.
87. Khan K, Schwarzenberg SJ, Sharp H, et al. Argon plasma coagulation: clinical experience in pediatric patients. Gastrointest Endosc 2003;57:110–2.
88. Sarin A, Safar B. Management of radiation proctitis. Gastroenterol Clin North Am 2013;42:913–25.
89. Kwan V, Bourke MJ, Williams SJ, et al. Argon plasma coagulation in the management of symptomatic gastrointestinal vascular lesions: experience in 100 consecutive patients with long-term follow-up. Am J Gastroenterol 2006;101:58–63.
90. Sami SS, Al-Araji SA, Ragunath K. Review article: gastrointestinal angiodysplasia—pathogenesis, diagnosis and management. Aliment Pharmacol Ther 2014;39:15–34.
91. Agnese M, Cipolletta L, Bianco MA, et al. Blue rubber bleb nevus syndrome. Acta Paediatr 2010;99:632–5.

92. Cipolletta L, Bianco MA, Rotondano G, et al. Prospective comparison of argon plasma coagulator and heater probe in the endoscopic treatment of major peptic ulcer bleeding. Gastrointest Endosc 1998;48:191–5.

93. Havanond C, Havanond P. Argon plasma coagulation therapy for acute non-variceal upper gastrointestinal bleeding. Cochrane Database Syst Rev 2005;(2):CD003791.

94. Yuan Y, Wang C, Hunt RH. Endoscopic clipping for acute nonvariceal upper-GI bleeding: a meta-analysis and critical appraisal of randomized controlled trials. Gastrointest Endosc 2008;68:339–51.

95. Sung JJ, Tsoi KK, Lai LH, et al. Endoscopic clipping versus injection and thermo-coagulation in the treatment of non-variceal upper gastrointestinal bleeding: a meta-analysis. Gut 2007;56:1364–73.

96. Saltzman JR, Strate LL, Di Sena V, et al. Prospective trial of endoscopic clips versus combination therapy in upper GI bleeding (PROTECCT–UGI bleeding). Am J Gastroenterol 2005;100:1503–8.

97. Park CH, Joo YE, Kim HS, et al. A prospective, randomized trial comparing mechanical methods of hemostasis plus epinephrine injection to epinephrine injection alone for bleeding peptic ulcer. Gastrointest Endosc 2004;60:173–9.

98. Lo CC, Hsu PI, Lo GH, et al. Comparison of hemostatic efficacy for epinephrine injection alone and injection combined with hemoclip therapy in treating high-risk bleeding ulcers. Gastrointest Endosc 2006;63:767–73.

99. Kumar A, Artifon E, Chu A, et al. Effectiveness of endoclips for the treatment of stigmata of recent hemorrhage in the colon of patients with acute lower gastrointestinal tract bleeding. Dig Dis Sci 2011;56:2978–86.

100. Holster IL, van Beusekom HM, Kuipers EJ, et al. Effects of a hemostatic powder hemospray on coagulation and clot formation. Endoscopy 2015;47(7):638–45.

101. Tjwa ET, Holster IL, Kuipers EJ. Endoscopic management of nonvariceal, non-ulcer upper gastrointestinal bleeding. Gastroenterol Clin North Am 2014;43:707–19.

102. Holster IL, Brullet E, Kuipers EJ, et al. Hemospray treatment is effective for lower gastrointestinal bleeding. Endoscopy 2014;46:75–8.

103. Kratt T, Lange J, Konigsrainer A, et al. Successful Hemospray treatment for recurrent diclofenac-induced severe diffuse lower gastrointestinal bleeding avoiding the need for colectomy. Endoscopy 2014;46(Suppl 1 UCTN):E173–4.

104. Curcio G, Granata A, Traina M. Hemospray for multifocal bleeding following ultra-low rectal endoscopic submucosal dissection. Dig Endosc 2014;26:606–7.

105. ASGE Technology Committee, Wong Kee Song LM, Banerjee S, et al. Emerging technologies for endoscopic hemostasis. Gastrointest Endosc 2012;75:933–7.

106. Wright R, Abrajano C, Koppolu R, et al. Initial results of endoscopic gastrocutaneous fistula closure in children using an over-the-scope clip. J Laparoendosc Adv Surg Tech A 2015;25:69–72.

107. Manta R, Galloro G, Mangiavillano B, et al. Over-the-scope clip (OTSC) represents an effective endoscopic treatment for acute GI bleeding after failure of conventional techniques. Surg Endosc 2013;27:3162–4.

Button Battery Ingestion in Children

A Paradigm for Management of Severe Pediatric Foreign Body Ingestions

Kristina Leinwand, DO, David E. Brumbaugh, MD,
Robert E. Kramer, MD, FASGE*

KEYWORDS

- Button battery ingestion • Aortoesophageal fistula • Gastrointestinal hemorrhage
- Pediatric • Foreign body ingestion • Caustic ingestion • Esophageal stricture • MRI

KEY POINTS

- Button battery ingestions are the most dangerous form of foreign body ingestion commonly encountered in pediatrics.
- A multidisciplinary approach is needed to most effectively manage these patients, including emergency medicine, anesthesia, pediatric gastroenterology, pediatric surgery/cardiothoracic surgery, otolaryngology, interventional cardiology, and radiology.
- Even after removal of the battery from the esophagus, there may be ongoing evolution of the injury for up to several weeks thereafter, placing patients at risk for a catastrophic aortoesophageal fistula or other severe sequelae.
- Endoscopic intervention for asymptomatic gastric button batteries remains controversial but may be considered in high-risk patients in order to evaluate for esophageal injury.
- Surveillance of esophageal injury with MRI may be used to stratify the risk of severe hemorrhage and guide management decisions.

INTRODUCTION

Management of foreign body ingestion (FBI) can be one of the most challenging issues in pediatric endoscopy. The myriad variations in size, type, and timing of foreign object ingested, compounded by patient factors, such as age, underlying medical issues, and clinical presentation, make each case inherently unique. Button battery (BB)

Disclosure: The authors have no significant financial relationships to disclose related to the content of this article.
Department of Pediatrics, Digestive Health Institute, Children's Hospital Colorado, University of Colorado, 13123 E 16th Ave, B290, Aurora, CO 80045, USA
* Corresponding author.
E-mail address: Robert.Kramer@childrenscolorado.org

Gastrointest Endoscopy Clin N Am 26 (2016) 99–118
http://dx.doi.org/10.1016/j.giec.2015.08.003
giendo.theclinics.com

ingestions (BBIs) epitomize the challenge of pediatric FBI, as the outcome can range from harmless to death. As the authors' center has personally experienced, when death occurs as a consequence of BBIs in an otherwise healthy child, it is one of the most tragic occurrences that a physician may encounter in a career.

US surveillance data have demonstrated a clear increase in morbidity and mortality due to BBI in the last 2 decades,[1,2] fueling public health and advocacy efforts to broadcast the danger of BBs for small children. The urgency to endoscopically remove esophageal batteries is now well appreciated, but further consensus on management has been difficult to develop.[3–5] From the clinical standpoint, there are 2 specific areas of management where there is considerable controversy and/or ambiguity. First is the postremoval management of children with moderate/severe esophageal injury. Clinicians must first appreciate the spectrum of esophageal and para-esophageal complications associated with BBI in children and the specific management dilemmas encountered. The risk for delayed occurrence of aortoenteric fistula (AEF) days or weeks following BB removal[3] further challenges our decision making, specifically around patient disposition after battery removal.

The second controversial area in the management of BBI surrounds the management of asymptomatic patients with batteries beyond the esophagus (eg, intragastric, duodenal, and so forth). Recent expert opinion-based guidelines from the Endoscopy Committee of the North American Society for Pediatric Gastroenterology, Hepatology, and Nutrition (NASPGHAN) recommended consideration of endoscopic assessment and removal in certain cases of BBI whereby the battery lies beyond the esophagus.[5] This recommendation contradicts previous guidelines from the National Battery Ingestion Hotline (NBIH) and the National Capital Poison Center, which had suggested only conservative initial management in asymptomatic children with postesophageal BB.[1,6] In this article, the authors review their single-center experience with BBI with the primary aim of presenting data that may help better inform and support management decisions.

BACKGROUND

Ingestion of batteries has long been recognized as a potential health hazard for children.[7,8] Voluntary reporting data, as collected through the NBIH and National Poison Data System since the 1980s, has revealed several important trends in the epidemiology of BBI.[9] Although the rate of battery ingestion (per million population) has remained stable in children over the past 30 years,[1] data from the National Electronic Injury Surveillance System has shown the absolute number of emergency department (ED) visits for battery-related injury has more than doubled from 1990 to 2009.[2]

More concerning, the rate of significant complications and death resulting from BBI has increased almost 7-fold.[1] This emergence of greater BBI-associated morbidity and mortality appeared in the mid 1990s and temporally corresponds to a change in battery production toward larger-diameter, higher-voltage lithium cells. The composition of swallowed batteries has subsequently trended toward larger-diameter lithium batteries, as these are now ubiquitous in the household environment.

More than 90% of serious outcomes from BBI in children between 2000 and 2009 were due to greater than 20-mm diameter lithium cells.[1] Because of its size, the 20- to 25-mm diameter lithium BB is more likely to become impacted in the pediatric esophagus compared with the traditional, previously standard, less than 15-mm alkaline BB. Serious outcomes are most common in small children less than 5 years of age.[9] Small children are more likely to mouth objects in the environment, and the smaller diameter of the esophagus in young children predisposes to foreign body impaction. More than 50% of serious outcomes due to BBI occur after unwitnessed ingestions, in which case there is likely a delay in recognition and diagnosis.[9]

Lithium cells are typically 3.0 V, as compared with the 1.5 V of traditional alkaline BBs. The increased voltage is a major factor in the type and degree of injury transmitted by these newer-age batteries as, per Ohm's law, higher voltage drives an increase in current.

Animal studies have been helpful in understanding the pathophysiology of BBI-caused injury[10] to be caustic rather than thermal. When a BB becomes entrapped in the digestive tract, mucosa bridges the positive and negative terminals of the battery, thus completing a circuit and allowing current to flow. Electrical current from the battery results in generation of hydroxide radicals in the esophageal tissue. The presence of hydroxide radicals rapidly raises the pH of the tissue leading to caustic injury and associated coagulative necrosis. Depending on the site of battery impaction, necrosis weakens the esophageal wall over a short period of time and may extend through to adjacent tissue, such as the trachea or great vessels. The process of coagulative necrosis has been demonstrated to start within 15 minutes of contact.[10] Even with batteries that have been ingested after use (and presumably without significant residual capacitance), significant injury may still be possible.[6] This reality provides further evidence of the power of the newer lithium cells, which have a much longer storage life than traditional alkaline cells.

Most deaths reported due to BBI involve the development of AEF with resulting catastrophic hemorrhage. Data from the National Capital Poison Center indicate that among the 41 reported fatalities, 19 (46.3%) were confirmed to be due to AEF, with another 12 (29.2%) reported as either merely "aortovascular" or unknown.[11] Most concerning have been reports of this catastrophic lesion occurring more than 2 weeks after BB removal.[3] AEF secondary to BBI has proven to be extremely difficult to manage even when properly recognized. Short- and long-term fatality rates in adult AEF have been reported at 46.8% and 70.3%, respectively.[12] There have been a few reported cases of survival in children after AEF from other causes,[13,14] but only one after AEF associated with BBI.[15] These reports, however, stress the importance of prompt recognition and intervention to maximize the potential for patient survival after BBI.

With the recognition of the increased risk associated with newer-age lithium BBs, public education and advocacy efforts have been launched, resulting in much greater awareness within the medical and parental communities.[16,17] Partnerships with industry have led to increased resources to deal with these hazards and, it is hoped, will result in decreased incidence of severe events (BatteryControlled.com). Furthermore, toy manufacturers have largely answered the call to secure the battery compartments in their products, and battery manufacturers have changed packaging to make the batteries more childproof. Most recently, new technology is being developed that would potentially make batteries incapable of transmitting a charge unless firmly seated within a battery compartment, rendering them safe within the human digestive tract.[18] For those who work in the clinical setting, however, the increased awareness has resulted in a parallel increase in calls and referrals following BBI. Given the complexity and potential severity each of these cases represents, pediatric departments and EDs have been challenged to develop appropriate clinical care pathways to rapidly assess and manage them.

CASE DESCRIPTIONS

The following 13 cases describe the most significant and severe esophageal BBIs that have occurred in the authors' institution over a 6-year period, from 2009 to 2015. With each case there have been important lessons to be learned that have subsequently impacted the authors' institutional approach to managing these patients in the future. These points are highlighted after each vignette, and the impact on clinical care is summarized in the discussion section. Additional data on the timing of BB removal in relationship to the distance from the authors' institution are presented in **Table 1**.

BUTTON BATTERY INGESTION CASE SERIES
Case 1

A 2-year-old previously healthy boy presented to the ED after a witnessed BBI. He had one episode of emesis after the ingestion and was drooling on arrival to the ED. Approximately 2 hours after ingestion, a radiologic foreign body series confirmed a retained BB at the proximal esophagus; he was transferred 20 miles to Children's Hospital Colorado (CHCO). Endoscopic removal was attempted in the procedure center by the gastroenterology team approximately 2.5 hours after arrival. Attempts at removal with flexible endoscopy were unsuccessful because of the dense adhesion of the battery to the esophageal mucosa, despite a total BB exposure time of only 6 hours. The BB was successfully removed by pediatric surgery using rigid esophagoscopy, but a nasogastric tube was unable to be placed because of esophageal edema. The patient was extubated after the procedure and transferred to the inpatient medical floor, where he remained ordered to take nothing by mouth. At 48 hours after removal, a Gastrografin esophagram demonstrated focal perforation of the upper esophagus into the retropharyngeal soft tissues at the level of C4. At 72 hours after removal, a nasogastric tube was placed by interventional radiology and he received enteral nutrition. He was discharged home on hospital day 6 with nasogastric tube feedings. Repeat esophagram 16 days after initial ingestion showed overall improvement but persistence of the esophageal perforation, which ultimately resolved on repeat esophagram 23 days after ingestion. Two days later, the nasogastric tube was removed; he tolerated a regular diet well without further complications. He was subsequently lost to follow-up 1 month after the ingestion, and it is unknown if he ever developed an esophageal stricture.

Lessons Learned

A BB can fuse to the mucosa rapidly, leading to difficult removal that may require rigid esophagoscopy.

Case 2

A 16-month-old previously healthy girl presented to her local ED with 1 day of irritability and approximately 2 ounces of bright red hematemesis. Within 2 hours of initial presentation, an abdominal radiograph was obtained that showed a round, radiopaque foreign body in the abdomen, possibly the transverse colon, suspicious for a BB. She was transferred 20 miles to CHCO ED, where a repeat abdominal radiograph showed an intra-abdominal foreign body consistent with a disc battery; but it was still unclear if it was located in the stomach or colon.

A computed tomography (CT) abdomen without contrast was then used to further delineate the location of the foreign body, which was shown to be in the central portion of the gastric body with a moderate amount of surrounding ingested material. The patient's vital signs were stable, and she was well appearing without any further hematemesis. In line with the guidelines for gastric BBs, she was scheduled to go to the operating room (OR) for foreign body removal the following morning, which was 7 hours later.

Table 1
Single-center case series of serious BBIs

Case	Times: Ingestion to Diagnosis, Center to Intervention, Total BB Exposure	Anatomic Location	Distance to Removal Center	Timing to Significant Outcome	CHCO Hospital Duration
1	2 h, 2.5 h, 6 h	Proximal esophagus	20 miles	Contained esophageal perforation at 2 d	6 d
2	2 h, 9 h, 15 h	Stomach	20 miles	Death by exsanguination ~15 h after ingestion	9 h
3	3 h, 3 h, 8 h	Distal esophagus	25 miles	Readmission at 18 d with death by exsanguination	5 d; 15 h
4	2 h, 1 h, 2.5 h	Proximal esophagus	20 miles	Ulceration visualized 6 h after ingestion	15 d
5	1 h, 1 h, 2.5 h	Proximal esophagus	20 miles	Contained esophageal perforation at 4 d	12 d
6	Unknown, 4 h, unknown	Unknown; ? esophagus	10 miles	Death by exsanguination ~6 h after admission	6 h
7	2 d, 1.5 h, 2 d	Proximal esophagus	175 miles	Ulceration visualized 2 d after ingestion	8 d
8	1 h, 1.5 h, 2.5 h	Distal esophagus	10 miles	Ulceration visualized at 2.5 h after ingestion	5 d
9	24 h, <2.5 h, 27 h	Proximal esophagus	30 miles	Contained esophageal perforation at 4 d	24 d
10	>2 d, 2 h, >2 d	Midesophagus	70 miles	Ulceration; esophageal stricture at 4 wk	7 d
11	3 h, <3 h, 6 h	Proximal esophagus	15 miles	Sinus tract in proximity to R carotid artery at 2 d	15 d
12	3 d, unknown, 3 d	Proximal esophagus	10 miles	Ulceration; esophageal stricture at 12 wk	7 d
13	3 h, unknown, 7.5 h	Proximal esophagus	190 miles	Tracheoesophageal fistula at 7 d	29 d

Abbreviations: CHCO, Childhren's Hospital Colorado; R, right.

While in the OR preoperative area of the authors' referral center, within 9 hours of initial presentation to the outside hospital, the patient developed further hematemesis and was taken to the OR for resuscitation because of rapid clinical decompensation. She was intubated and resuscitated with albumin and blood infusions. She suffered 3 episodes of cardiac arrest. During resuscitation, the patient was noted to have many hemorrhages from her mouth and nose despite a large nasogastric tube in place. The procedure was converted to open laparotomy, which revealed a markedly distended stomach with a large clot encasing a 20-mm BB in the fundus. Compression of the abdominal aorta was attempted without achieving control of bleeding; after ongoing resuscitation attempts, she remained asystolic and was pronounced dead in the OR just 15 hours after the initial presentation to our facility.

Autopsy revealed 2 linear midesophageal mucosal erosions, focal collection of blood in the paraesophageal soft tissue adjacent to the erosions, as well as accumulation of blood within the adventitia of the aorta and in the soft tissue of the distal trachea. There were no erosions or ulcerations within the stomach. Cause of death was identified as hypovolemic shock due to ulceration of the midesophagus and hemorrhage from large arterial source due to battery ingestion.

Lessons Learned

Identification of a gastric foreign body does not preclude esophageal injury, especially in unwitnessed ingestions when the total time of BB exposure is unknown. BBs can transiently lodge in the esophagus and cause severe erosion and ongoing injury. Even after passage of the battery to the stomach, necrosis of the esophagus and surrounding tissues is an ongoing process that can lead to fistulization and associated severe outcomes.

Case 3

A 2-year-old previously healthy girl presented to the ED with chest pain, coughing, and vomiting. A chest radiograph 3 hours after presentation showed a round radiopaque 25-mm foreign body in the distal esophagus concerning for BBI, and she was transferred 25 miles to the CHCO ED for further management. Flexible endoscopy was successful in removal of the BB from the distal esophagus, where the underlying tissue was ulcerated and friable (**Fig. 1**). She was extubated to room air, and repeat complete blood count and chest radiograph in the postanesthesia care unit revealed stable blood counts and no evidence of pneumomediastinum. She was admitted to the inpatient medical floor, where she remained ordered to take nothing by mouth. One day after admission, the esophagram revealed mucosal irregularity and mild narrowing of the distal esophagus in the region of removed BB but no evidence of esophageal perforation/leak. At 48 hours after removal, she was started on a clear-liquid diet, was advanced to a mechanical soft diet at hospital day 4, and was discharged home on hospital day 5.

Thirteen days after discharge (18 days following BB removal), the patient presented to the ED with a history of abdominal pain and diarrhea for 5 days as well as new-onset hematemesis and hematochezia and was admitted to the ICU. Repeat esophagram revealed mucosal irregularity of the distal esophagus without clear stricture or evidence of perforation. In the ICU, she developed hematemesis and shock. Emergent bedside endoscopy revealed an intact lower esophageal ulceration and copious blood and a large clot in the gastric fundus. Endoscopic attempts at hemostasis, including Blakemore tube inflation and epinephrine injections, were unsuccessful; despite 4 hours of aggressive attempts at stabilization and resuscitation, cardiorespiratory support was withdrawn.

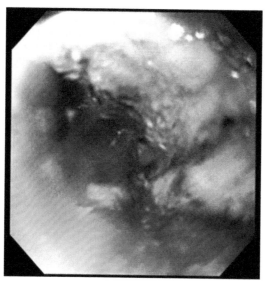

Fig. 1. Severe esophageal injury at site of BB removal, with necrosis and eschar.

Lessons Learned

Despite a reassuring esophagram and clinical stability 5 days after ingestion, devastating hemorrhage from esophageal erosion secondary to BBI can unexpectedly occur weeks out from the initial ingestion. Because of the high arterial pressure from AEF, Blakemore tubes may not be able to control or stabilize bleeding.

Case 4

A 6-year-old previously healthy girl presented to the ED after witnessed BBI. She complained of throat pain and intermittent nonbloody emesis; 2 hours after arrival to the ED, a chest radiograph revealed a BB at the proximal esophagus. She was transferred 20 miles to the CHCO ED, where emergent endoscopic removal of a 20-mm BB by the surgery team was performed. There was extensive proximal esophageal erosion and ulceration despite just 6 total hours of BB exposure. She was extubated after the procedure and transferred to the pediatric ICU (PICU) where she remained ordered to take nothing by mouth on total parenteral nutrition (TPN). Five days after ingestion, MRI of the chest with magnetic resonance angiography showed significant inflammation of the anterior esophageal wall, sparing the posterior wall, without disruption of surrounding vasculature. This study was thought to be reassuring, as no immediate major vessels seemed to be threatened by the location of necrotic injury. On hospital day 7, an esophagram showed mucosal ulceration and probable edema or stricture without visible fistula or evidence of perforation. With these imaging studies, the patient was determined to be at a decreased risk of hemorrhage and perforation. In turn, she was advanced to an oral soft diet and was discharged home on hospital day 15. It was unknown if there were further complications, such as stricture, as she was subsequently lost to follow-up.

Lessons Learned

As mucosal injury occurs with even short exposure to BBs, every effort should be made to expedite removal when possible. MRI is a useful tool for post–battery-ingestion evaluation of the extension of injury beyond the esophagus and may help guide treatment decisions.

Case 5

A 6-year-old boy with a history of repaired tracheoesophageal fistula presented to the ED after witnessed BBI. He was clinically stable, and a chest radiograph demonstrated the BB to be retained in the proximal esophagus. Shortly after presentation (within 1–2 hours), the patient developed hematemesis and vomited up the BB, which was noted to be corroded, and had an adherent blood clot; he was immediately transferred 20 miles to the CHCO ED. Within 1 hour of transfer, endoscopy was performed in the CHCO OR with findings of noncircumferential proximal esophageal ulceration and eschar formation, without bleeding. The BB exposure time at endoscopy was estimated to be 2.5 hours. The patient was extubated and admitted to the general medical floor and was advanced to a soft diet 1 day after admission. Four days later, he developed dysphagia and pain with eating; MRI of the chest revealed a focal fluid collection with a beak directed to the esophagus concerning for contained esophageal perforation. He was made to take nothing by mouth on TPN and placed on intravenous (IV) antibiotics. Seven days later, a repeat MRI showed a persistent esophageal fluid collection with improvement of the proximal esophageal mucosal inflammation. An esophagram demonstrated no extravasation of fluid. On hospital day 8, he was advanced to a soft diet and was discharged home on hospital day 12. A repeat esophagram 1 month after discharge did not demonstrate a leak or stricture; on the follow-up visit 2 years after the initial ingestion, he was tolerating a regular diet without any dysphagia or complications.

Lessons Learned

A total BB exposure time of just 2.5 hours was associated with contained esophageal perforation, giving credence to the growing concern for potential morbidity associated with any BB exposure to the esophageal mucosa. As with other type of esophageal foreign bodies, children with a history of tracheo-esophageal fistula (TEF) have an increased risk of impaction.

Case 6

An 18-month-old previously healthy girl presented to the ED after 24 hours of hematemesis and mild abdominal pain. She was noted on vital signs to be hypotensive and tachycardic, and her laboratory test results revealed normocytic anemia. The patient received IV fluid resuscitation with subsequent normalization of vital signs and was transferred to the PICU for monitoring. In addition, chest and abdominal radiographs were obtained and read as normal, without a visualized foreign body. A nasogastric tube was placed, which showed a small amount of bright red blood in the tube. Consultation with the gastrointestinal (GI) service led to a plan for endoscopy after stabilization and transfusion of packed red blood cells.

Approximately 4 hours after admission to the ICU, the patient developed gasping respirations and clinical decompensation requiring intubation and was noted to have substantial esophageal bleeding. Gastroenterology and surgery coordinated an emergent bedside endoscopy with active resuscitation including chest compressions. On endoscopic intubation of the esophagus, a moderate amount of red blood was flushed away and the visualized esophageal mucosa was not determined to show lesions. The stomach was noted to have a large clot present that could not be suctioned or flushed, without signs of active bleeding. After 2 hours of aggressive resuscitation attempts and just 6 hours after initial presentation, the patient was pronounced dead. Autopsy revealed erosions in the midesophagus extending into the aorta, consistent with injury from a BB, though no battery was identified at any site.

Lessons Learned

Although this case could not be completely confirmed to be secondary to BBI, the opinion of the pathologist and the clinicians involved support this as the most likely underlying cause of death. This case again highlights that the absence of a battery within the esophagus at the time of presentation does not preclude significant injury at some point prior. In otherwise healthy toddlers with acute onset of severe hematemesis, a high index of suspicion for battery ingestion should be maintained.

Case 7

A 2-year-old previously healthy boy presented to his pediatrician's office with 1 day of fever, sore throat, and nonbloody emesis. He was initially treated with azithromycin; but after he developed food refusal the following day, a chest radiograph was obtained that showed a BB in the proximal esophagus. The patient was transferred 175 miles to the CHCO ED and had endoscopic removal in the OR 1.5 hours after transfer. Before removal, surgery and cardiothoracic surgery were called and placed on standby as an additional precautionary measure because of the prolonged time of BB exposure. Flexible esophagosocopy by gastroenterology and rigid esophagoscopy by otolaryngology were initially unsuccessful in removal. Otolaryngology then used a Miller laryngoscope and alligator forceps and successfully removed the battery. Subsequently, there was concern for circumferential necrotic ulceration where the BB had been impacted, and a nasogastric tube was placed. The patient was extubated to room air and transferred to the medical inpatient floor where he remained ordered to take nothing by mouth.

The following day, a CT angiogram of the neck showed no evidence of soft tissue or vessel injury, and an esophagram showed no evidence of perforation. The patient's diet was advanced to clears by mouth and nasogastric feeds on hospital day 2. A repeat esophagram on hospital day 7 showed extensive mucosal irregularity in the proximal esophagus, extending 3.5 cm, which represented mucosal ulceration. On hospital day 8, repeat CT angiogram again did not show evidence of injury to large vessels. The patient was discharged home on hospital day 8 on a combination of nasogastric feeds and a limited amount of a soft mechanical diet. He was quickly weaned from nasogastric tube feeds; at the follow-up visit 4 months after discharge, he had no difficulties with oral intake.

Lessons Learned

Coordination between gastroenterology and otolaryngology and precautionary measures with surgery and cardiothoracic surgery on standby allowed for a well-controlled environment with prompt removal of the BB in this clinical scenario that was at high risk for morbidity/mortality because of 48 hours of esophageal BB exposure. In this case, neither flexible nor rigid esophagoscopy was able to remove the battery; but a laryngoscope with alligator forceps was effective.

Case 8

A 4-year-old previously healthy boy presented to a local urgent care with abdominal pain and chest pain and a self-report of swallowing a magnet. Within 1 hour of ingestion, chest and abdominal radiographs confirmed a retained BB in the distal esophagus; he was transferred 10 miles to a CHCO satellite campus where he vomited up a 19-mm BB. Endoscopy approximately 2.5 hours after the initial diagnosis demonstrated 2 small linear erosions of the distal esophagus with surrounding dusky mucosa concerning for necrosis. He was transferred to the CHCO main campus PICU for monitoring. One day after removal, a CT angiogram of the neck showed no large vessel injury; on hospital day 4, an MRI of the chest showed no evidence of aortoeso-phageal fistula. He was started on an oral soft mechanical diet, which he tolerated well, and discharged home on hospital day 5. Three weeks later, a follow-up esoph-agoscopy showed healing ulcers without stricture formation. The patient was lost to follow-up after this procedure.

Lessons Learned

CT angiography and MRI can be used concurrently to help estimate the risk of injury beyond the esophagus and to guide treatment decisions, including discharge planning from the ICU as well as when to initiate feeding.

Case 9

An 11-month-old previously healthy boy presented to his pediatrician with 24 hours of cough, increased oral secretions, refusal to eat, and fever. A chest radiograph showed a retained proximal esophageal BB, and he was transferred 30 miles to a local ED for further management. Removal of the BB with esophagoscopy by otolaryngology in the local ED within 3 hours after initial diagnosis was difficult but successful. After battery removal, laryngoscopy was noted to reveal circumferential ulceration in the proximal esophagus.

The patient was then transferred to the CHCO PICU and ordered to take nothing by mouth on IV fluids. On hospital day 2, an esophagram showed significant esophageal wall irregularity and deep mucosal ulceration along the posterior lateral wall, without evidence of perforation or fistulous tract formation. On hospital day 3, endoscopy demonstrated severe edema, exudates, and necrosis of the proximal esophagus. A nasojejunal tube was placed. Rigid bronchoscopy and laryngoscopy showed vocal cord paralysis but with normal trachea.

An MRI of the chest with angiogram on hospital day 4 showed extensive perieso-phageal inflammatory changes tracking between the esophagus and trachea, with a localized perforation along the left cervical esophagus, as well as loculated pockets of fluid extending into the mediastinum between the proximal right innominate artery and the left common carotid artery without disruption of the vessels. On hospital day 5, nasojejunal feedings were started and tolerated well. Repeat endoscopy 2 days before discharge showed healing ulcers without stricture formation. However, because of the anticipated prolonged duration of tube feedings due to aspiration from vocal cord pa-ralysis, a gastrostomy tube was placed simultaneously.

Repeat esophagram was normal before discharge, and he went home on hospital day 24 with gastrostomy tube feeds and an oral pureed diet. In the follow-up visit 3 months after discharge, he continued on oral purees and gastrostomy tube feeds because of persistent aspiration from vocal cord paralysis, without evidence of stric-ture formation on repeat esophagram.

Lessons Learned

Morbidity and mortality associated with BBI is not strictly limited to vascular injury and bleeding events but also includes vocal cord paralysis and perforation.

Case 10

A 15-month-old previously healthy girl presented to the pediatrician's office with a barking cough for 1 week and 2 days of decreased oral intake and fever. She had pro-gressive coughing and sputtering with eating, and the follow-up visit with a chest radiograph showed a midesophageal BB. She was transferred 70 miles to the

CHCO ED, where she was taken to the hybrid OR within the cardiac catheterization laboratory, with endoscopic removal by gastroenterology performed within 2 hours of transfer in the presence of interventional cardiology and cardiothoracic surgery. Because of the high risk and concern for AEF formation because of the long duration of battery impaction in this case, arteriogram of the aorta was performed before removal and showed the BB to be approximately 3 to 4 mm from the aortic arch. This distance was thought to be reasonably safe to allow endoscopic removal without surgical intervention. On endoscopic removal of the BB, there were 2 large ulcerations of the midesophagus with friability and edema.

The patient was extubated after the procedure and transferred to the PICU, where she was made to take nothing by mouth and started on TPN. Her hospital course was complicated by left leg hypoperfusion secondary to focal occlusive thrombus in the proximal left superficial femoral artery from the cardiac catheterization, which was treated with continuous heparin for 4 days and then stopped because of the risk of esophageal ulceration bleed. On hospital day 3, an MRI of the chest with angiogram showed circumferential periesophageal wall thickening extending 6.8 cm and separated by 4 mm from the descending thoracic aorta at the level of the aortic arch, with the esophageal lumen separated from the proximal descending thoracic aorta by 1 cm. The lack of progression of injury on MRI was assessed to be reassuring; on hospital day 4, she was started on a soft mechanical diet, which she tolerated well up to discharge on hospital day 7.

Approximately 4 weeks after ingestion, an esophagram showed a focal stricture of the patient's upper esophagus, requiring esophageal dilation and localized injection of steroid at the stricture site. She has not been reevaluated since her procedure and is now considered lost to follow-up.

Lessons Learned

Endoscopic removal in the cardiac catheterization laboratory OR with fluoroscopic guidance and arteriogram of the aorta allowed direct visualization of the BB and proximity to the aorta, which improved preparedness for potential complications to the multidisciplinary team involved in the procedure. The use of arteriography, however, does carry the risk of thrombus formation, which must be weighed against the benefit of identifying proximity of injury to the aorta.

Case 11

A 4-year-old previously healthy girl presented to a local ED with drooling and self-reported, unwitnessed FBI. Chest radiograph 3 hours after presentation confirmed a proximal esophageal BB; she was taken to the OR for removal by otolaryngology approximately 6 hours after presentation to the ED, with mild edema and irritation of the proximal esophagus on removal of the battery. The patient was subsequently transferred to the CHCO medical inpatient floor, where she remained ordered to take nothing by mouth. One day after admission, an esophagram demonstrated mild cervical esophageal edema/irregularity without stricture; she was started on a clear-liquid diet. Because of pain and difficulty swallowing on hospital day 3, she had a repeat endoscopy that showed severe ulceration of the proximal esophagus and had an MRI of the chest with angiogram that demonstrated formation of a sinus tract from the right lateral wall of the esophagus, in close proximity to her right carotid artery. She was immediately made to take nothing by mouth, transferred to the PICU, and started on TPN.

A repeat esophagram on hospital day 7 showed no perforation, and a repeat MRI of the chest with angiogram on hospital day 9 showed no evidence of arterial or venous irregularity at the site of prior sinus tract formation. She was started on a soft mechanical diet on hospital day 11, which was tolerated well without complication; she was discharged home on a regular diet on hospital day 15. One month after discharge, the patient was assessed to be doing well without dysphagia, with no stricture noted on repeat esophagram.

Lessons Learned

Despite minimal findings of edema and ulceration on initial esophagoscopy at removal of the BB, esophageal necrosis and surrounding inflammation progresses despite no further exposure, making timing of associated morbidity from BB exposure somewhat unpredictable. Although there was no clinical vascular complication in this case, MRI helped to evaluate the risk and take appropriate precautionary measures until subsequent imaging showed resolution of potential danger to vascular structures.

Case 12

A previously healthy 20-month-old girl presented to her local ED with 2 days of drooling, congestion, fever, vomiting, retching, and dysphagia. In the ED, she had labored breathing and refusal to move her neck; a CT of her neck showed a retained proximal esophageal BB. A 25-mm BB was removed in the OR by otolaryngology; surrounding mucosa showed erythema, ulceration, and necrosis. A nasogastric tube was placed, and the patient was transferred to the CHCO PICU. On hospital day 2, an MRI of the chest showed inflammatory changes, with wall thickening noted to be most extensive in the posterior esophageal wall, with no evidence of approximation between the esophagus and large vessels. On hospital day 3, the patient underwent a repeat esophagoscopy that demonstrated severe ulceration without evidence of stricture or fistula; she started a limited clear-liquid diet and nasogastric tube feedings. She was discharged home on hospital day 7 on a regular diet. The patient subsequently complained of dysphagia and blood tinged spit-up at the follow-up 1 month later, and endoscopy showed a mild esophageal stricture that was dilated. She has had no further dysphagia since esophageal dilation and remains clinically well 10 months after discharge.

Lessons Learned

Stricturing of the esophagus can be a common complication after BB exposure but does not often present before 4 weeks after initial ingestion.

Case 13

A 20-month-old boy developed drooling, watery eyes, neck pain, and neck extension and was taken to a local ED because of suspected FBI. A chest radiograph 3 hours after the onset of symptoms demonstrated a retained proximal esophageal BB, and he was transferred 187 miles to CHCO for removal. Endoscopic removal of the battery was performed 7.5 hours after diagnosis and demonstrated circumferential necrosis. A nasogastric tube was placed, and the patient was transferred from the OR to the CHCO PICU with continued mechanical ventilation via endotracheal intubation for further management. MRI of the neck/chest with angiography on hospital day 1 showed esophageal wall thickening and paraesophageal inflammation most pronounced at the level of the aortic arch, with a paraesophageal fluid collection just above the aortic arch without compromise of the surrounding vasculature. An esophagram showed no evidence of perforation, and he was extubated after repeat endoscopy showed healing ulceration on hospital day 5. Four days later, he developed biphasic stridor and fever and was urgently intubated. Subsequently he was found to have vocal cord paralysis, with bronchoscopy demonstrating an 11-mm tracheal erosion with communication to the mediastinum and the tip of the endotracheal tube terminating in the esophagus. Because of persistent fevers and concern for mediastinitis that was unresponsive to intravenous antibiotics, the patient underwent diversion of the proximal esophagus to a spit fistula and temporary closure of the distal esophagus as well as gastrostomy tube placement for nutritional support.

During the patient's prolonged hospitalization, he underwent microlaryngoscopy with bronchoscopy 5 times, with the final bronchoscopy before discharge showing persistent tracheoesophageal fistula and left vocal cord paralysis. The patient was discharged home on hospital day 29 with gastrostomy tube feeds and a pureed oral diet. One month after discharge, he was readmitted for 24 hours because of a spit fistula stricture that was dilated.

The patient was scheduled for repeat endoscopy approximately 3 months after initial ingestion that showed marked improvement and a well-healed tracheoesophageal fistula. In turn, he underwent a takedown of cervical esophagostomy with cervical esophageal anastomosis followed by a 14-day hospitalization for recovery. Repeat esophagram has demonstrated anastomotic cervical esophageal leak; but because of financial stressors, the patient has not returned for recommended evaluation, including repeat esophagram, esophagoscopy with possible dilation, bronchoscopy for vocal cord assessment, and swallow evaluation.

Lessons Learned

Respiratory symptoms after battery removal should prompt emergent evaluation for vocal cord and tracheal complications, including tracheoesophageal fistula.

Summary Data

Although these data do not encompass the numerous calls the authors' institution receives on a regular basis regarding more benign cases of BBI (beyond the esophagus and estimated to be at low risk for esophageal injury), it does illustrate the spectrum of severe morbidity and mortality that occur when there is significant esophageal injury. In this series of 13 severe cases, 4 (30.8%) resulted in esophageal perforation, 3 (23.1%) developed an esophageal stricture, and 2 (15.4%) required gastrostomy placement. Mortality in this series of patients with severe esophageal injury from BBI was 23.1%. For survivors, the average hospital stay was 12.1 days.

DISCUSSION
Initial Presentation and Assessment

Successful management of BBIs demands a multidisciplinary approach and coordinated care across the ED, anesthesia, pediatric gastroenterology, pediatric surgery, otolaryngology, cardiothoracic surgery, and radiology physicians. First contact may occur by phone from a referring institution or from direct presentation in the ED. In general, any child presenting to the ED with symptoms consistent with a foreign body should have both anteroposterior and lateral films of the chest and airway to help differentiate the ubiquitous coin ingestions from BB.[19] Careful examination of these films for the halo sign, as well as the step-off between the positive and negative nodes of BBs, should be performed. If a BB is found, orientation of the slightly smaller negative pole (anode) should be noted, as this is the direction of most serious injury.

Once the diagnosis of an esophageal BBI is confirmed, rapid assessment of the risk level must be performed in order to mobilize the appropriate resources. This initial assessment should minimally include the age of the patient, size of the battery, timing of ingestion, and current location of the battery, whenever possible. These factors encompass the most important risk factors for predicting severe injury. As illustrated in the cases discussed earlier and from the national data,[11] esophageal impaction at the level of the aortic arch, age less than 5 years, battery size of 20 mm or greater, and prolonged time of impaction are all factors that should prompt the greatest level of concern. Similarly, a child who has recently undergone endoscopic removal of a battery and then presents with any degree of hematemesis or coffee-ground emesis should be considered as an impending AEF and treated accordingly.

Recommended indications for endoscopic intervention in cases of BBI beyond the esophagus in asymptomatic patients are variable across published guildelines.[1,5,6] Based on most of the national data, which shows postesophageal batteries have not been associated with significant morbidity and mortality, guidelines from the NBIH[1] and the Button Battery Taskforce[6] currently advocate abdominal radiographs and observation in asymptomatic patients. In higher-risk patients (<6 years of age and BB $\geq$15 mm), the radiograph is in 4 days and 10 to 14 days in low-risk patients. These guidelines do advocate for endoscopic removal in high-risk asymptomatic patients if the battery is still in the stomach after 4 days.

However, more recent recommendations[5] by the Endoscopy Committee of the NASPGHAN call for consideration of endoscopic intervention even in cases of asymptomatic postesophageal BBI in high-risk patients (aged <5 years, BB $\geq$20 mm). The rationale for this more conservative guideline is not primarily due to concerns regarding the risk of gastric injury, though this has been reported.[20] It is instead based on concerns for unrecognized esophageal injury before passage into the stomach, as noted in 2 of the fatalities cited earlier (case 2 and case 6). The role of endoscopy is, therefore, primarily diagnostic, rather than the therapeutic removal of the battery itself. In this fashion, one may consider radiographic studies (CT, esophagram) as alternative methods to assess for unrecognized esophageal injury. Nevertheless, these have the disadvantage of not allowing for removal of the battery and may be less sensitive than endoscopy. (MRI is contraindicated with a metallic foreign body present.)

In addition to mobilizing all the necessary personnel, critical management decisions include whether endoscopic intervention is needed as well as what is the most appropriate site for the procedure. Location of endoscopic intervention may vary by case and by institution, depending on what resources are available and the timing of presentation. At the authors' institution, with the highest-risk cases, they have found that the cardiac catheterization laboratory (case 10) has offered the best combination of imaging capability and ability to convert to an open surgical case. In cases whereby there is less suspicion for direct aortic involvement but still concerns about hemorrhage or the ability to remove the battery with a flexible endoscope, the general OR may be the most appropriate choice. In lower-risk cases, whereby the battery has already passed into the stomach or beyond, but the endoscopic assessment of any subsequent esophageal injury is desired, a well-equipped endoscopic procedure unit may be used.

In addition to determining the appropriate venue for endoscopic removal, timing of removal and a corresponding anesthesia/sedation plan are needed. In the case of an esophageal BBI, there is an obvious premium on removal as urgently as possible. With the potential for long-term injury in as short as 15 minutes after impaction,[10] the sooner removal is achieved the better. In the authors' institution, triage guidelines for surgical and endoscopic procedures have been created that characterize BB removal at the highest priority level. With this designation, the authors' institutional goal is to have patients in the OR within 60 minutes of entry into the facility.

Achieving this level of response requires rapid and efficient communication between all of the medical and surgical subspecialists appropriate for the case. Principal among these is anesthesiology. With the emphasis on rapid preparation for surgical/endoscopic intervention, usual nothing-by-mouth guidelines are circumvented, by definition. As with all FBI cases, the airway must be secured and protected, especially with the potential for a full stomach. Therefore, rapid sequence intubation will likely be needed.

ENDOSCOPIC REMOVAL

After the decision of where to perform the removal and the assembly of the appropriate personnel for the procedure, the specifics of the removal itself should be determined. As illustrated in case 10, in high-risk cases whereby esophageal impaction has been prolonged and injury to vascular structures is suspected, localization of the battery in relation to the aorta and other large vessels through angiography may be performed immediately before endoscopic removal. Although this may further delay actual removal by up to 30 minutes, in cases whereby there has already been prolonged exposure of the tissue, this additional delay may be negligible compared with the value of determining proximity to the aorta.

In terms of actual endoscopic removal, use of the smallest gastroscope available that still has a 2.8-mm biopsy channel is advised to allow the use of the full complement of foreign body retrieval devices. In the authors' institution, this is the Olympus GIF-160 (Olympus America, Center Valley, PA, USA), with an outer diameter of 8.6 mm. Although newer endoscopes have better optics and field of view, the narrower diameter may provide some additional measure of safety in preventing perforation, as most of these patients with BBI are younger than 4 years of age. In larger patients, the additional 0.5 to 1.0 mm in diameter may be negligible in terms of increased risk.

Once the battery is visualized within the esophageal lumen, the depth (in centimeters) and orientation of the impaction should be noted as best as possible. Examination of the surrounding tissue for eschar formation and fusion to the surface of the battery may help indicate how difficult removal will be. Although gastric batteries may be effectively removed with nets, these may be difficult to pass between the battery and esophageal mucosa and are typically not helpful when the battery is adherent to the esophagus. Within the esophagus, grasping devices are usually most successful. In the authors' institution, the use of the Raptor forceps (BX00711177, US Endoscopy, Mentor, OH, USA) has been effective in most cases. The combination of alligator and rat tooth jaws helps provide a firm grip in the crevice between the positive and negative poles of the battery. Nevertheless, the authors' experience has also dictated that, in some instances, as in case 1, the battery is so densely adherent to the mucosa that flexible endoscopy tools are not able to generate enough traction for removal necessitating the use of rigid esophagoscopy.

Alternatively, a case report has been published on the use of a modified magnet endoscope to capture esophageal BBs that were not retrievable with conventional devices.[21] In this report, a magnet head tube (Cook Co, Bloomfield, IL, USA) was attached to an infant endoscope, with a 0.5-cm step-off between the tip of the endoscope and the end of the magnet tube. With a battery firmly fused to the mucosa, however, the authors suspect it would still be unlikely that a magnet would provide sufficient traction.

POSTREMOVAL EVALUATION

After battery removal, the scope should be reinserted into the esophagus and another careful examination of the mucosa performed to better assess the severity and location of any injury as well as to determine the most likely complications (**Fig. 2**). Trauma

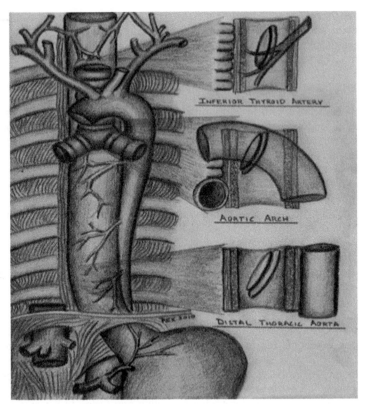

Fig. 2. Sites of esophageal button battery impaction and related risk of injury.

to the anterior aspect of the esophagus prompts greater concern for vascular and tracheal injury, whereas posteriorly oriented inflammation has been associated with the development of spondylodiscitis.[22] Anterior injury in the proximal esophagus should prompt concern for thyroid artery involvement or tracheoesophageal fistula as well as vocal cord injury (case 9). Location in the midesophagus should evoke the greatest concern for AEF. Although injury in the distal esophagus is perhaps reassuring against atrioesophageal complications, one of the 3 fatalities in this series (case 3) did show erosion at this level; caustic burns anywhere in the esophagus have the potential to result in perforation and stricture formation. Circumferential involvement in particular should increase concerns about long-term complications of stricture or stenosis, as seen in cases 10, 12, and 13.

After reexamination of the esophagus, passage of the endoscope into the stomach and proximal duodenum to exclude additional foreign bodies is prudent, presuming that this is not hampered by esophageal trauma and/or edema.

POSTREMOVAL MANAGEMENT

Postendoscopy management is perhaps the most difficult and controversial aspect of the care of these patients. The level of care necessary depends highly on the location, duration, and difficulty of removal of the BBI. In more than half of the cases (63.6%) in the authors' institution when removal was performed, patients were admitted to the

PICU for monitoring, with a trend toward a lower threshold in more recent years. Patients are generally taking nothing by mouth for a variable amount of time (range 1–29 days), depending on the degree of injury and the risk of complications. As in 5 of the cases described earlier, a nasogastric tube may be placed to initiate enteral nutrition.

The role of repeat endoscopy in the management of these patients is also ripe for debate. Although others have cited the value of a second-look endoscopy 2 to 4 days after ingestion to help determine the timing of feeding introduction,[23] based on what we now appreciate to be the pathophysiology of injury in these cases, such timing for a second look may lead to false reassurance about continued risks for complications. In the authors' series, a repeat endoscopy was performed before patient discharge in 5 patients (38.5%).

Over time, the authors' center has come to favor MRI for evaluation after removal in order to assess the proximity of submucosal and extraesophageal injury to the aorta and other important structures (**Fig. 3**). In cases whereby the extent of injury has been beyond 3 mm from the aorta, it has been thought to be safe to reinitiate feeds (case 10). Although most of these patients will still require anesthesia to perform MRI, the value of this modality over endoscopy is the less invasive nature as well as the ability to follow the evolution of unseen injury over time and determine when inflammation is receding away from the vascular structures. The authors have found this information to be invaluable in making management decisions, such as when to start oral feeds, transfer from the PICU, and discharge home. With the potential for catastrophic complications several weeks after removal, this modality seems the most promising for stratifying risk.

Esophagram is another useful noninvasive study for assessing injury, primarily for the purpose of detecting perforation and/or stricture formation. It is obviously prudent to use water-soluble contrast in these cases whereby the perforation risk is relatively

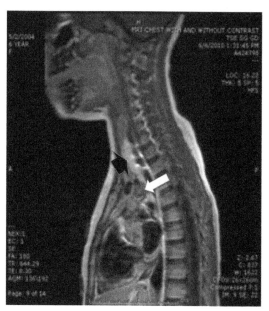

Fig. 3. T1 MRI with contrast 5 days after BB removal showing persistent inflammation anterior to esophagus (*black arrow*) above aortic arch (*white arrow*).

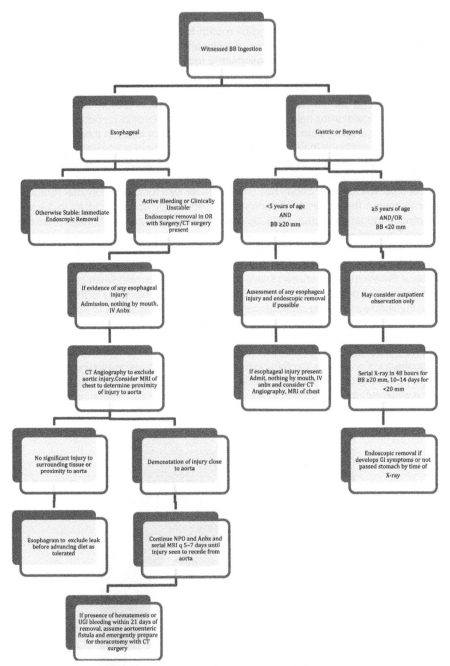

Fig. 4. Suggested algorithm for management of BBIs in children. Anbx, antibiotics; UGI, upper gastrointestinal. (*Adapted from* Kramer RE, Lerner DG, Lin T, et al. Management of ingested foreign bodies in children: a clinical report of the NASPGHAN Endoscopy Committee. J Pediatr Gastroenterol Nutr 2015;60(4):564; with permission.)

high. In the authors' institution, an initial esophagram is typically performed 1 to 7 days after battery removal, with a repeat study 7 to 14 days later.

Discharge criteria for patients with injury after BBI have generally been either tolerance of oral feeds or stable tube feeds (nasogastric or via gastrostomy), along with reassuring indications that their injury is not involving any vascular structures. However, even with these criteria met, there may be fatality (as in the authors' case 3), which can occur many days after discharge and more than 2 weeks after successful battery removal. The details of case 3 highlight the danger of ongoing injury and the importance of continued vigilance necessary to manage these patients. Factors such as the reliability of the family to return for follow-up visits as well as the distance patients live from the responsible medical providers need to be carefully considered before discharge. Exhaustive discharge instructions need to be provided that outline the signs and symptoms of upper GI bleeding. Use of acid blockade to minimize the impact of acid reflux on the esophageal injury has not been studied but would seem well justified. Minor sentinel bleeding has been noted in the authors' patients (cases 2, 3, and 6) and others before impending AEF hemorrhage and should prompt immediate referral and emergent activation of the cardiothoracic team. At some point during patient care, cases should be reported to the National Battery Ingestion Hotline (US phone number: [202] 625–3333).

Follow-up care for patients after BBI is essential to assess for midterm complications (ie, bleeding) and long-term sequelae (ie, stricture formation). In most cases of significant esophageal injury (and especially those with circumferential injury), a repeat esophagram 4 weeks after removal is prudent to assess for stricture. If this is normal and patients are asymptomatic, no additional surveillance is necessary unless feeding issues develop. In the event of a stricture, endoscopic dilation should be considered promptly (as illustrated by case 10), as 4 weeks should represent sufficient healing time to minimize perforation risk. Respiratory issues should prompt evaluation for tracheal erosion/injury. See **Fig. 4** for an algorithm summarizing the suggested management of BBI in children.

SUMMARY

Although the existence of national data on BBIs provides much-needed information on the epidemiology of these serious injuries, there are no prospective studies available to guide management decisions. As a result, treatment recommendations are primarily based on expert opinion from related clinical experience. The single-center experience of the serious esophageal BBI cases presented in this article is the largest published outside of the compiled national data and offers important lessons for the management of future cases. Additional study is needed to better define the role of acid blockade, endoscopy, and MRI in the postremoval management of these cases and determine optimal timing for initiation of enteral feeding. Advocacy efforts are ongoing and vital in order to minimize the occurrence of these potentially fatal injuries.

REFERENCES

1. Litovitz T, Whitaker N, Clark L, et al. Emerging battery-ingestion hazard: clinical implications. Pediatrics 2010;125(6):1168–77.
2. Sharpe SJ, Rochette LM, Smith GA. Pediatric battery-related emergency department visits in the United States, 1990–2009. Pediatrics 2012;129(6):1111–7.
3. Brumbaugh DE, Colson SB, Sandoval JA, et al. Management of button battery-induced hemorrhage in children. J Pediatr Gastroenterol Nutr 2011;52(5):585–9.

4. Russell RT, Griffin RL, Weinstein E, et al. Esophageal button battery ingestions: decreasing time to operative intervention by level I trauma activation. J Pediatr Surg 2014;49(9):1360–2.

5. Kramer RE, Lerner DG, Lin T, et al. Management of ingested foreign bodies in children: a clinical report of the NASPGHAN Endoscopy Committee. J Pediatr Gastroenterol Nutr 2015;60(4):562–74.

6. Jatana KR, Litovitz T, Reilly JS, et al. Pediatric button battery injuries: 2013 task force update. Int J Pediatr Otorhinolaryngol 2013;77(9):1392–9.

7. Dinary G, Rosenbach Y, Zahavi I, et al. Hazards of button battery ingestion by children. Harefuah 1983;105(11):361–2 [in Hebrew].

8. Litovitz TL. Button battery ingestions. A review of 56 cases. JAMA 1983;249(18): 2495–500.

9. Litovitz T, Whitaker N, Clark L. Preventing battery ingestions: an analysis of 8648 cases. Pediatrics 2010;125(6):1178–83.

10. Tanaka J, Yamashita M, Kajigaya H. Esophageal electrochemical burns due to button type lithium batteries in dogs. Vet Hum Toxicol 1998;40(4):193–6.

11. Center NCP. Fatal button battery ingestions: 41 reported cases. 2015; Case data on BBI fatalities to date. Available at: http://www.poison.org. Accessed June 15, 2015.

12. Akashi H, Kawamoto S, Saiki Y, et al. Therapeutic strategy for treating aortoeso-phageal fistulas. Gen Thorac Cardiovasc Surg 2014;62(10):573–80.

13. Hill SJ, Zarroug AE, Ricketts RR, et al. Bedside placement of an aortic occlusion balloon to control a ruptured aorto-esophageal fistula in a small child. Ann Vasc Surg 2010;24(6):822.e8–9.

14. Sigalet DL, Laberge JM, DiLorenzo M, et al. Aortoesophageal fistula: congenital and acquired causes. J Pediatr Surg 1994;29(9):1212–4.

15. Spiers A, Jamil S, Whan E, et al. Survival of patient after aorto-oesophageal fistula following button battery ingestion. ANZ J Surg 2012;82(3):186–7.

16. Button Battery Task Force: the hazards of button batteries. Available at: http://www. aap.org/en-us/advocacy-and-policy/aap-health-initiatives/Pages/Button-Battery. aspx. Accessed June 15, 2015.

17. Coin lithium battery safety. Available at: http://www.energizer.com/responsibility/coin-lithium-battery-safety. Accessed June 15, 2015.

18. Laulicht B, Traverso G, Deshpande V, et al. Simple battery armor to protect against gastrointestinal injury from accidental ingestion. Proc Natl Acad Sci U S A 2014;111(46):16490–5.

19. Thabet MH, Basha WM, Askar S. Button battery foreign bodies in children: hazards, management, and recommendations. Biomed Res Int 2013;2013:846091.

20. Honda S, Shinkai M, Usui Y, et al. Severe gastric damage caused by button battery ingestion in a 3-month-old infant. J Pediatr Surg 2010;45(9):e23–6.

21. Soong WJ, Yuh YS. Ingested button battery retrieved by a modified magnet endoscope. J Chin Med Assoc 2007;70(3):132–5.

22. Tan A, Wolfram S, Birmingham M, et al. Neck pain and stiffness in a toddler with history of button battery ingestion. J Emerg Med 2011;41(2):157–60.

23. Ruhl DS, Cable BB, Rieth KK. Emergent treatment of button batteries in the esophagus: evolution of management and need for close second-look esophago-scopy. Ann Otol Rhinol Laryngol 2014;123(3):206–13.

Pediatric Considerations in Endoscopic Retrograde Cholangiopancreatography

David M. Troendle, MD*, Bradley A. Barth, MD, MPH

KEYWORDS

- Endoscopic retrograde cholangiopancreatography (ERCP) • Pediatrics • Equipment
- Indications • Adverse events

KEY POINTS

- The utilization of endoscopic retrograde cholangiopancreatography (ERCP) in the pediatric population is rapidly expanding.
- Technical and clinical outcomes following pediatric ERCP seem to mirror those seen in adult patients when performed for similar indications.
- Well-designed pediatric studies are needed to clarify appropriate indications and patient selection algorithms, identify pediatric-specific risk factors for adverse events, and develop pediatric specific risk mitigation strategies.

OVERVIEW

Endoscopic retrograde cholangiopancreatography (ERCP) is an advanced endoscopic technique used in the diagnosis and treatment of biliary and pancreatic diseases in patients of all ages. To date, the relative infrequency with which this procedure has been performed in children has resulted in a paucity of pediatric-specific data about ERCP. In turn, it has historically been necessary to adapt patient selection algorithms and risk mitigation strategies for children undergoing ERCP from studies involving adult patients. More recently, with increasing use of ERCP in children, has come a better understanding of appropriate indications as well as expected technical and clinical outcomes specific to this population. Recent reports, although limited by retrospective single-center design, suggest that additional well-designed pediatric studies are feasible and warranted. In particular, it is becoming clearer that there are indications for ERCP that may be unique to the pediatric population, whereas other studies have shown the historic practice of adapting adult-based practices to children may be inappropriate in certain instances. With these recent developments in mind, this article serves to update the reader on the current role of ERCP in

Division of Pediatric Gastroenterology, University of Texas Southwestern Medical Center, 5323 Harry Hines Boulevard, Dallas, TX 75390-8548, USA
* Corresponding author. 5323 Harry Hines Boulevard, Dallas, TX 75390-8548.
E-mail address: david.troendle@utsouthwestern.edu

Gastrointest Endoscopy Clin N Am 26 (2016) 119–136
http://dx.doi.org/10.1016/j.giec.2015.08.004
1052-5157/16/$ – see front matter © 2016 Elsevier Inc. All rights reserved.

the management of biliary and pancreatic disease with a focus on pediatric indications, patient preparation, equipment, as well as technical and clinic outcomes following the procedure when it is performed in children.

INDICATIONS

ERCP is a technically demanding procedure in patients of all ages that is associated with a relatively high rate of adverse events (AE) as compared with standard upper and lower endoscopy. Thus, significant efforts have been made to emphasize careful patient selection to limit procedural exposure to those who are most likely to benefit. Recording an indication from a published list of appropriate indications, such as that presented by the American Society for Gastrointestinal Endoscopy (ASGE)[1] in **Box 1**,

---

Box 1
List of approved indications for endoscopic retrograde cholangiopancreatography

- The jaundiced patient suspected of having biliary obstruction (appropriate therapeutic maneuvers should be performed during the procedure)
- The patient without jaundice whose clinical and biochemical or imaging data suggest pancreatic duct or biliary tract disease
- Evaluation of signs or symptoms suggesting pancreatic malignancy when results of direct imaging (eg, endoscopic ultrasound, ultrasound, computed tomography, MRI) are equivocal or normal
- Evaluation of pancreatitis of unknown cause
- Preoperative evaluation of the patient with chronic pancreatitis or pseudocyst
- Evaluation of the sphincter of Oddi by manometry
- Empirical biliary sphincterotomy without sphincter of Oddi manometry is not recommended in patients with suspected type III sphincter of Oddi dysfunction
- Endoscopic sphincterotomy
  - Choledocholithiasis
  - Papillary stenosis or sphincter of Oddi dysfunction
  - To facilitate placement of biliary stents or dilation of biliary strictures
  - Sump syndrome
  - Choledochocele involving the major papilla
  - Ampullary carcinoma in patients who are not candidates for surgery
  - Facilitate access to the pancreatic duct
- Stent placement across benign or malignant strictures, fistulae, postoperative bile leak, or in high-risk patients with large unremovable common duct stones
- Dilation of ductal strictures
- Balloon dilation of the papilla
- Nasobiliary drain placement
- Pancreatic pseudocyst drainage in appropriate cases
- Tissue sampling from pancreatic or bile ducts
- Ampullectomy of adenomatous neoplasms of the major papilla
- Therapy for disorders of the biliary and pancreatic ducts
- Facilitation of cholangioscopy or pancreatoscopy

From Early DS, Ben-Menachem T, Decker GA, et al. Appropriate use of GI endoscopy. Gastrointest Endosc 2012;75(6):1130; with permission.

has been recommended as a critical preprocedural quality indicator that should be monitored and reported.[2] Such lists were generated primarily with adult patients in mind, with a goal of emphasizing the utilization of less invasive diagnostic modalities in lieu of diagnostic ERCP when possible, as well as limiting exposure to ERCP in settings where it has been shown to be ineffective by well-designed studies. As pediatric-specific studies are produced and additional experience is gained with alternative diagnostic modalities in children, pediatric-specific indications will likely reflect a similar evidence-basis and rationale.

The evolution of ERCP in the pediatric population has mirrored the adult experience closely. Early studies (those before 2004) have been summarized previously[3,4] and were primarily focused on demonstrating the feasibility and diagnostic utility of pediatric ERCP. More recent publications emphasize its utilization as a primarily therapeutic modality and highlight applications of ERCP unique to the pediatric population (**Table 1**).[5–22] Based on these primarily single-center experiences, the most common clinical scenarios in which ERCP is undertaken in the pediatric population are pancreaticobiliary and include the following:

Biliary scenarios (**Fig. 1**)

- Management of choledocholithiasis
- Management of biliary strictures, typically benign and seen after liver transplantation or in the setting of primary sclerosing cholangitis
- Management of bile leak, typically encountered after cholecystectomy
- Preoperative evaluation of choledochol cyst and management of acute obstruction when present
- Preoperative evaluation of pancreaticobiliary maljunction
- Investigation of neonatal cholestasis
- Investigation of biliary pathologic abnormality of unclear cause when results of less invasive imaging modalities are equivocal or unavailable

Pancreatic scenarios (**Fig. 2**)

- Management of chronic pancreatitis, with the goal of improving pancreatic drainage (removal of stones, dilation/stenting of strictures)
- Management of pancreatic divisum with minor papillotomy
- Investigation of recurrent acute pancreatitis of unclear cause
- Management of pancreatic duct leak, typically encountered in setting of abdominal trauma
- Management of pancreatic pseudocyst via transpapillary approach
- Investigation of pancreatic ductal pathologic abnormality of unclear cause when results of less invasive imaging modalities are equivocal or unavailable

A recent review of a large US pediatric inpatient database demonstrated an overall increase in ERCP utilization by 26% from 2000 to 2009.[23] During this time period, there was a decrease in utilization of diagnostic ERCP by 43% and an increase in the utilization of therapeutic ERCP by 69%. Although it is true that ERCP is being used more and more as a therapeutic modality in most patient populations, diagnostic ERCP may be of unique benefit in carefully chosen pediatric populations. Although not routinely recommended as part of the workup of neonatal cholestasis,[24] small case series initially suggested that under select circumstances ERCP may be beneficial.[25–27] It may be particularly useful in the setting of cholestasis of unclear cause where laparotomy is being contemplated to rule out biliary atresia (BA). In one relatively large study of neonates referred for laparotomy to rule out BA, prelaparotomy ERCP was able to obviate surgery in 25% of 140 patients.[8] The sensitivity and specificity for ERCP for

Table 1
Pediatric endoscopic retrograde cholangiopancreatography series since 2004

Author (Year)	Procedures (N)	Mean Age (Range)	Success (%)	Therapeutic (%)	Unique Aspects
Varadarajulu et al,[5] 2004	163	9.3 y (1 mo–17 y)	98	67	Similar technical outcomes between children and adults when performed for similar indications
Rocca et al,[6] 2005	48	10 y (1 mo–17 y)	97	84	ERCP largely a therapeutic modality
Cheng et al,[7] 2005	329	12.3 y (2 mo–17 y)	98	71	17% of procedures performed for chronic pain of suspected pancreatic or biliary origin; rates of PEP much higher in this cohort
Petersen et al,[8] 2009	140	60 d (15–174 d)	87	0	ERCP prevented laparotomy in 25% of patients with suspected BA
Iqbal et al,[9] 2009	343	NR	NR	43	• Therapeutic procedures are risk factors for PEP • Stenting in CP patients is risk factor for PEP
Vegting et al,[10] 2009	99	7 y (3 d–16.9 y)	71	61	• 51% of patients <1 y of age • ERCP prevented laparotomy in 12% of patients with suspected BA
Jang et al,[11] 2010	245	8 y (1 mo–16 y)	98	78	25% of procedures performed for choledochal cyst
Keil et al,[12] 2010	104	7 wk (3–25 wk)	91	0	Highlights utility of diagnostic ERCP in the workup of neonatal cholestasis
Otto et al,[13] 2011	231	11.4 y (62 d–21 y)	NR	69	64% of ERCPs performed for AP, ARP, and CP
Shteyer et al,[14] 2012	27	55 d (33 d–89 d)	81	0	Highlights utility of diagnostic ERCP in the workup of neonatal cholestasis
Troendle et al,[15] 2013	65	15.2 y (1 mo–18.4 y)	100	100	Evaluated ERCP for choledocholithiasis when performed by a pediatric gastroenterologist

Study	N	Age			Notes
Halvorson et al,[16] 2013	70	12 y (6 y–17 y)	99	94	Pediatric ERCP performed by adult gastroenterologist
Enestvedt et al,[18] 2013	429	14.9 y (3 mo–21 y)	95	64	• Highlights increasing utilization of ERCP over time • High rate of cholangitis in patients with PSC (50%)
Agarwal et al,[17] 2014	221	13.8 y (5 y–18 y)	NR	71	Highlights therapeutic utility in pediatric patients with ARP and CP, particularly when coupled with ESWL
Saito et al,[19] 2014	235	4 y (8 d–20 y)	96	3.4	Diagnostic utility in setting of BA and CC
Giefer et al,[20] 2015	425	13.6 (72 d–18 y)	95	81	• Identification of PEP risk factors (PD injection, PS) • Any pancreatic stenting increased rates of PEP
Troendle et al,[21] 2015	432	12.7 y (1 mo–19 y)	NR	86	• Identification of PEP risk factors (PD injection, PS) • Prophylactic pancreatic stenting increased rates of PEP in high-risk patients
Hiramatsu et al,[22] 2015	63	3.9 y (4 mo–13 y)	100	0	Superior role of ERCP compared with MRCP in preoperative examination of children with pancreaticobiliary malunion

Abbreviations: AP, acute pancreatitis; ARP, acute recurrent pancreatitis; CC, choledochal cyst; CP, chronic pancreatitis; ESWL, extracorporeal shock wave lithotripsy; MRCP, magnetic resonance cholangiopancreatography; NR, not specifically reported; PD, pancreatic duct; PS, pancreatic sphincterotomy; PSC, primary sclerosing cholangitis.

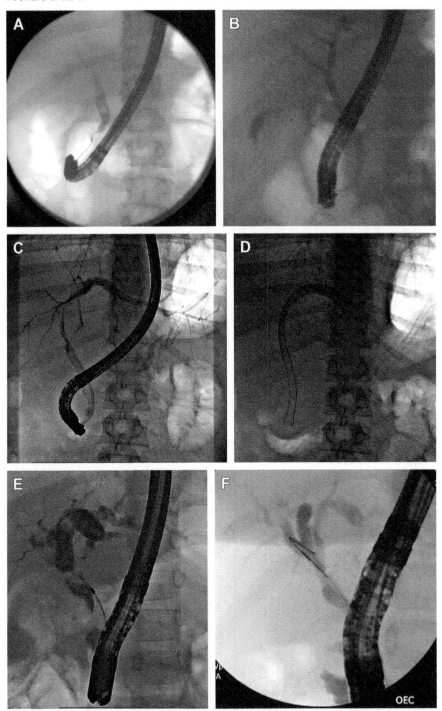

Fig. 1. Examples of pediatric biliary ERCP. (*A*) Choledocholithiasis before removal. (*B*) Bile leak after cholecystectomy. Malignant hilar biliary obstruction (*C*) before and (*D*) after placement of overlapping uncovered metal biliary stents resulting in improved drainage of left system. Benign hilar biliary stricture with significant upstream dilation (*E*) before and (*F*) after serial stenting.

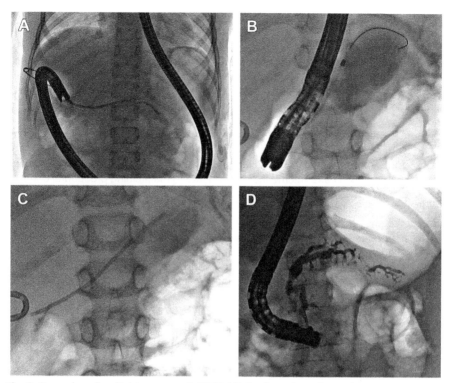

Fig. 2. Examples of pediatric pancreatic ERCP. (*A*) Confirmation of complete pancreatic divi-sum before minor papillotomy with duodenoscope in the long position. Communicating pancreatic pseudocyst (*B*) before and (*C*) after transpapillary drainage with plastic stent showing intraduodenal drainage of contrast. (*D*) Features of chronic pancreatitis.

diagnosing BA in this series were 92% and 73%, respectively. Smaller studies have demonstrated similar utility of ERCP in this setting, where ERCP has been shown to obviate laparotomy in 19% to 42% of cases.[12,14,28] Although procedural failure rates ranged from 6% to 18%, the negative predictive value approached 100%, suggesting it may be useful in avoiding diagnostic laparotomy in cholestatic neonates. Further work is needed to clarify the role of diagnostic ERCP in this clinical scenario, wherein timely diagnosis of biliary atresia is critically important to optimize clinical outcomes.

TECHNICAL CONSIDERATIONS

There are several specific technical considerations to planning and performing ERCP in children. In particular, it is important to identify and develop an ideal, pediatric-safe operating environment, and to prepare the patient for the procedure in line with age-appropriate guidelines. Patient monitoring during ERCP must take into account pediatric-specific data and use appropriately sized equipment, while ensuring safety during sedation for the procedure is paramount.

Operating Environment

Once an appropriate indication for ERCP has been established, efforts must be made to identify the most appropriate clinical environment for performing the procedure. The ideal environment will be one in which an appropriately trained, high-volume endoscopist, with significant pediatric experience, performs the procedure while surrounded by support staff familiar with the unique aspects of pediatric care. When ERCP was initially introduced as a feasible technique in children, it was almost exclusively performed by high-volume adult-trained endoscopists in the setting of an adult facility where the equipment was located.

More recently, pediatric-trained endoscopists have reported performing the procedure in the confines of tertiary pediatric facilities with comparable technical success and AE rates.[15,29] Although ERCP is performed less commonly in children when compared with adults, its utilization is increasing rapidly,[18,23] leading many larger pediatric facilities to provide access to the procedure at their center.[30] It is critical that endoscopists performing ERCP in children be appropriately trained in the procedure and have an ongoing case volume that is adequate to maintaining procedural competency. Although the ASGE has recommended that 180 ERCPs be performed before competency be assessed,[31] a recent meta-analysis evaluating initial ERCP training and competency suggests that this threshold may be inadequate,[32] and that further research is needed in this arena. Although the optimal ongoing procedural volume remains unknown, it has been suggested that greater than 50 cases per year are necessary to remain competent, because studies have suggested that ongoing case volume less than this threshold may be an independent risk factor for AE in adult patients.[33,34]

Patient Preparation

As emphasized in a recent ASGE consensus document on endoscopic practice in pediatric patients,[35] there are at least several general considerations that should be taken into account as children and their families are prepared for the procedure:

- Psychological preparation and age-appropriate preprocedural education for both patients and their families
- Obtaining written informed consent from the legal guardian as well as assent from older pediatric patients
- Observation of standard age-appropriate pre-endoscopy dietary restrictions: typically 2 hours for clear liquids, 4 hours for breast milk, and 6 hours for non-human milk and solids
- Consideration of early procedure times for younger patients, who are at risk for dehydration with prolonged fasting
- Attention to ambient temperature throughout all phases of the procedure. Small infants are at risk for developing hypothermia with prolonged procedure times as can occur with ERCP; thus, ready access to warmers as well as the ability to control the temperature of the procedure room is important for these patients.

Furthermore, if the procedure is to be performed by an offsite endoscopist, as occurs at many institutions, mechanisms need to be in place to allow for seamless communication between endoscopist and the physicians caring for the patient before and after the procedure.

Sedation

Best sedation practices for pediatric endoscopic procedures remain controversial. Although pediatric ERCP has been described as safely being performed with either endoscopist-administered moderate sedation or anesthesiologist-administered general anesthesia (GA), there are insufficient outcome data to firmly recommend one form of sedation over another. Although some have described exclusive use of moderate sedation, even for prolonged procedures of high-difficulty grade without apparent ill effect,[17] at least one large pediatric case series has described a need to prematurely discontinue ERCPs or to convert to GA in 7.1% of cases in which such endoscopist-administered procedural sedation was attempted.[20] Ultimately, the decision on the type of sedation to be used will depend on the comfort level of the endoscopist and the ERCP team as well as the resources that are available to them.

Even experienced proceduralists attempting to provide moderate sedation for pediatric patients undergoing ERCP should be aware that the soft-walled trachea of smaller children may be compressed by the relatively large duodenoscopes currently available. This knowledge is particularly pertinent for children near 10 to 15 kg (22–33 lbs), in which it may be appropriate to trial the use of an adult-sized duodenoscope with the intention of maximizing function, but in whom patient/scope mismatch is most likely to occur. In addition, the prone position typically used during ERCP can compromise chest excursion, resulting in hypoventilation, and can make airway rescue technically challenging. Pulse oximetry and hemodynamic monitoring should be routinely used and individuals comfortable with pediatric monitoring and rescue maneuvers should be present throughout the procedure.

Pediatric-Specific Equipment

Pediatric-specific equipment is rarely needed, even in the busiest pediatric centers. Standard adult diagnostic or therapeutic duodenoscopes can be used in most children weighing more than 10 to 15 kg (22–33 lbs), and whatever devices fit through their accessory channels may be used as well.[36] However, although using standard duodenoscopes in children is feasible, endoscopists must take care when passing the upper esophageal sphincter and pylorus. In addition, tracheal compression manifested by hypoxia or inability to ventilate can occur when larger scopes are passed in smaller patients.

Appropriate duodenoscope selection is critical to allow for a safe and effective procedure, but unfortunately, there is little literature available to help guide the endoscopist. Descriptions of diagnostic ERCP in the setting of neonatal cholestasis exclusively use pediatric duodenoscopes with outer diameters ranging from 7.5 to 8.6 mm.[8,12,25–28] Outside of these settings, most case series cite utilization of a similarly sized duodenoscope for children less than 1 year of age.

Between October 2006 and July 2015, the authors' group performed 385 pediatric ERCPs at their pediatric referral center in Dallas, with immediate access to both pediatric and adult duodenoscopes. In 11 children less than 1 year of age (all also <10 kg) who underwent primarily therapeutic ERCP, a pediatric duodenoscope with an outer diameter of 7.5 mm (Olympus PJF 160; Olympus America, Center Valley, PA) was the scope of choice and successfully used in 9 patients. In 2 patients, a larger duodenoscope with an outer diameter of 10.6 mm was first attempted, but failed to allow for appropriate positioning within the duodenum, resulting in duodenal perforation in one patient. In 27 ERCPs performed in children between 10 and 15 kg, a duodenoscope with an outer diameter of 10.6 mm or larger was used as the scope of choice with success in 93% of cases. In all children greater than 15 kg, a duodenoscope with an outer diameter of at least 10.6 mm was used. Combining the available literature with the authors' experience, the authors think that pediatric duodenoscopes are the instrument of choice for patients less than 10 kg, whereas adult duodenoscopes should be considered for patients greater than 10 kg, because the larger working channel allows for a greater selection of accessories.

Pediatric duodenoscopes are available for loan on a case-by-case basis, or for purchase if warranted. These scopes currently measure approximately 7.5 mm outer diameter and use a 2.0-mm accessory channel. The smaller accessory channel makes pediatric duodenoscopes more challenging to use because triple lumen catheters are not accepted. Double-lumen sphincterotomes, extraction baskets, and retrieval balloons, which can be used with a 2.0-mm channel, are commercially available from many manufacturers of endoscopic devices, and small stents, up to 5-Fr diameter, are accepted.

ADVERSE EVENTS

Clarifying the incidence of risk factors for ERCP-associated AEs has been the subject of numerous prospective multicenter adult studies, and early pediatric-specific literature on this topic is now emerging. **Table 2** lists the most commonly reported AEs in pediatric ERCP,[5–22] which seem consistent with reports from the adult literature.[37]

The low volume of pediatric ERCP and the infrequent nature of ERCP-related AEs make it difficult for pediatric-specific studies to take place. Other than reports of incidences from small single-center retrospective experiences, which often use nonstandardized methods of reporting, no pediatric-specific work on identification of risk factors or strategies to mitigate risk have taken place. This finding forces endoscopists to use data generated from adult patients as best as they can, although this literature is also limited.

Recently, a standardized manner of reporting all endoscopic-associated AEs has been proposed[38] with the goal of facilitating a more accurate understanding of specific procedural risks. According to this lexicon, an AE is defined as any event that results in one or more of the following:

- An inability to complete the planned procedure
- Unplanned admission to the hospital
- Prolongation of an existing hospital stay
- Another unplanned procedure
- Subsequent medical consultation

To help gauge the impact of an AE, each should be further characterized in terms of the following:

- *Type*, using standardized definitions
- *Timing*, in relation to the procedure: preprocedure, intraprocedural, early postprocedural (<14 days), late postprocedural (>14 days)

Table 2
Adverse events associated with pediatric endoscopic retrograde cholangiopancreatography

Event	Definition[38]	Incidence (%)
Pancreatitis	Typical pain + Amylase and/or lipase >3× ULN	3–11
Pain	New or increased abdominal pain not related to PEP or other AE	1–2
Bleeding	Evidence of GI bleeding + hemoglobin drop >2 g	1–2
Perforation	Evidence of air or luminal contents outside GI tract	<1
Cholangitis	Fever >38°C + >24 h after procedure + worsening cholestasis	<1
Fever without a source	Fever >38°C + >24 h after procedure without obvious source	<1

Abbreviation: ULN, upper limit of normal.

- *Likelihood of attribution*: definite, probable, possible, unlikely
- *Severity*: mild, moderate, severe

At this time, it is recommended that all endoscopists performing ERCP in children monitor and report AEs associated with the procedure using this standardized approach.[38] In turn, it may be possible to gain a more accurate understanding of pediatric-specific ERCP-associated AEs.

Pancreatitis

Post-ERCP pancreatitis (PEP) is the most common AE following ERCP and can result in significant morbidity and health care costs.[37] As a result, it has been the subject of multiple large multicenter adult studies, which have also been well chronicled.[39] The relatively high incidence of PEP has also allowed for several smaller-scale pediatric studies.[9,20,21] **Box 2** shows risk factors that have been most commonly identified as associated with the development of PEP in both children and adults. Pediatric studies suggest that having a history of chronic pancreatitis at the time of the procedure may be protective and reduce the likelihood of developing PEP.[20,21]

There is evidence that adult patients at high risk for developing PEP warrant prophylaxis.[40–42] However, although a multitude of interventions have been studied, few interventions have been shown to be consistently effective. The interventions most often used to prevent PEP included utilization of prophylactic pancreatic duct stenting[40,41] and administration of rectal indomethacin suppository at the time of the procedure.[42] Recent meta-analyses have shown prophylactic pancreatic stenting to be highly effective at preventing PEP, particularly in high-risk patients wherein the

---

Box 2
Factors most commonly associated with development of post-endoscopic retrograde cholangiopancreatography pancreatitis

Patient factors

- Suspected Sphincter of Oddi Dysfunction
- Age less than 60 years
- Normal bilirubin
- Previous history of PEP

Procedural factors

- Pancreatic duct injection[a]
- Pancreatic sphincterotomy[a]
- Pancreatic guidewire placement
- Pancreatic tissue sampling
- Difficult or failed cannulation
- Precut sphincterotomy after difficult cannulation
- Balloon dilation of native papilla
- Dorsal duct cannulation in pancreatic divisum

[a] Pediatric-specific data available.
Adapted from Freeman ML. Complications of endoscopic retrograde cholangiopancreatography: avoidance and management. Gastrointest Endosc Clin N Am 2012;22(3):571; with permission.

number needed to treat may be lower than 8.[41] In addition, although appropriate patient selection remains somewhat controversial, placement of prophylactic stents in high-risk patients has been shown to be a cost-effective strategy.[43] Similarly, a recent large-scale multicenter randomized trial has shown that rectal indomethacin administered at the time of ERCP significantly decreased rates of PEP when compared with placebo (9.2 vs 16.9%), corresponding to a relative risk reduction of 56% and a number needed to treat to prevent one episode of pancreatitis, 13.[42] Given the costs and ease of administration of this safe and simple intervention, it has quickly gained popularity among endoscopists performing the procedure.

Despite the strong evidence supporting these preventative measures, questions remain as to whether the same protective effect will be seen in children. Indeed, a recent retrospective study has suggested prophylactic pancreatic duct stenting may not have the same protective effect in pediatric patients and in fact may be harmful.[21] Similar studies looking at pancreatic stenting in general (not necessary for prevention of pancreatitis) also support this claim.[9,20] Although this data are relatively weak compared with the abundance of literature demonstrating the efficacy of pancreatic stenting in adult patients, endoscopists who choose to continue using pancreatic stenting as a prophylactic technique in pediatric patients should do so with caution and careful monitoring.

Similarly, there are no studies evaluating the efficacy of rectal indomethacin in children. Although many endoscopists routinely administer rectal indomethacin to pediatric patients deemed to be at high risk given the strength of evidence in the adult literature, appropriate dosing for smaller children has not been determined and it is not clear that manipulating rectal indomethacin suppositories can result in reliable dosing. Despite these limitations, a reasonable indomethacin dosing strategy in pediatrics proposed by the authors is presented in **Box 3**, which would result in approximately 1 to 2 mg/kg dose. As with prophylactic stenting, those who use rectal indomethacin as a preventative strategy should do so with caution and careful monitoring given the lack of pediatric-specific data.

Bleeding, Perforation, and Infection

Significant gastrointestinal (GI) bleeding following ERCP is typically only encountered in patients who have undergone sphincterotomy and can occur up to 2 weeks following the procedure. Risk factors for post-ERCP-related bleeding as identified by large studies in adult populations are presented in **Box 4**.[44–46] Sphincterotomy is considered an endoscopic technique that places patients at higher risk for bleeding, thus anticoagulation therapy should be adjusted according to previously published guidelines.[47] As with other endoscopic procedures, use of aspirin or nonsteroidal anti-inflammatory drugs is not significantly associated with postprocedural bleeding. Appropriate patient selection and careful technique are currently considered the best ways to prevent significant bleeding associated with ERCP.

When significant bleeding does occur, standard endoscopic hemostatic techniques are usually effective in achieving hemostasis. Injection of 1:10,000 epinephrine is the

---

Box 3
Proposed rectal indomethacin dosing for post-endoscopic retrograde cholangiopancreatography pancreatitis prophylaxis in pediatric patients

>50 kg	100 mg (2 × 50 mg suppositories)
25–50 kg	50 mg (1 × 50 mg suppository)
<25 kg	25 mg (1/2 a 50 mg suppository)

> **Box 4**
> **Factors associated with post-endoscopic retrograde cholangiopancreatography bleeding**
>
> - Sphincterotomy, particularly precut sphincterotomy
> - Coagulopathy before the procedure
> - Anticoagulation within 3 days following the procedure
> - Cholangitis before the procedure
> - Bleeding during the procedure
> - Stenosis of the ampulla of Vater
> - Low case volume of endoscopist (<52 ERCPs annually)
> - Procedure performed at small center

most commonly described method of achieving hemostasis after sphincterotomy. Although not effective monotherapy in the setting of peptic ulcer bleeds, it appears to be effective monotherapy for sphincterotomy bleeds, achieving initial hemostasis in greater than 96% of patients with rebleeding rates less than 5% reported in 2 studies.[48,49] When dilute epinephrine is not effective, coaptive thermocoagulation, argon plasma coagulation, and application of hemostatic clips have all been described as being effective modalities of achieving hemostasis.[50–53] Angiography and surgery are rarely required for refractory bleeding but are also highly effective. When applying endoscopic hemostasis techniques near the papilla, one must take care to identify and avoid the pancreatic and biliary orifice so as not to inadvertently obstruct them with interventional maneuvers.

Perforation is considered an uncommon complication following ERCP and thus remains inadequately studied. Nevertheless, there is a risk of perforation of the GI lumen, penetration of the ductal systems, typically with a guidewire or catheter, as well as perforation after sphincterotomy with extension through the duodenal wall.[39] Sphincterotomy-related perforations are the most common perforation encountered.[54] Field experts have suggested that needle-knife sphincterotomy and management of sphincter of Oddi dysfunction may increase the risk of sphincterotomy-associated perforation because control and extent of sphincterotomy may be more difficult to manage in these settings.[39] It is likely that luminal perforations will be more commonly encountered in patients with surgically altered anatomy or smaller children, wherein scope/size mismatch is likely to occur, as discussed previously. Management of perforations will be dictated by their location and extent as well as local expertise. Although endoscopists are more frequently attempting to manage acute luminal perforations endoscopically, surgical intervention is still typically sought in the pediatric population. Penetrations of the ductal system can be managed endoscopically in a manner similar to that in which bile duct leaks are approached in which the pressure gradient generated by the sphincter is obliterated by stenting or sphincterotomy, encouraging appropriate ductal drainage. Endoscopic management is typically successful at managing sphincterotomy-related perforations, as is clipping of the site or placement of temporary drains or covered metal stents, which drain the bile duct and occlude the leak.[54]

Cholangitis may occur following ERCP, particularly if complete biliary drainage is not obtained after the procedure. Risk factors for ERCP-associated cholangitis as identified by large adult-based study include (1) combined percutaneous endoscopic procedure; (2) stenting of malignant strictures; and (3) failed biliary access or drainage.[44]

Although meta-analyses have failed to show any significant clinical benefit of routine prophylactic antibiotic use in ERCP,[55,56] the ASGE has recommended consideration of prophylaxis in cases in which ductal drainage (eg, primary sclerosing cholangitis, hilar strictures) is anticipated to be incomplete, or transpapillary drainage of pancreatic cysts or pseudocyst is to be attempted.[57] It remains common practice, although inadequately studied, to consider antibiotic prophylaxis in patients shown to be at higher risk for developing infectious complications after ERCP, including patients requiring biliary interventions after liver transplantation, stenting in the setting of biliary malignancy, and situations in which a combined percutaneous-endoscopic approach is undertaken.

Unintentional introduction and transmission of exogenous infectious agents during ERCP has captured significant recent attention.[58,59] The complex design of duodenoscopes renders them difficult to disinfect, thus predisposing them to bacterial colonization and subsequent biofilm formation. Duodenoscope-associated transmission of New Delhi metallo-β-lactamase *Escherichia coli* has been described in adult populations even in the setting of strict adherence to recommended high-level disinfection techniques.[58] In addition, the US Food Drug Administration has been receiving an increasing number of medical device reports associating the transmission of multi-drug-resistant bacterial infections with duodenoscope exposure, leading them to issue a recent safety alert.[59] Although the absolute risk remains extremely low, and no pediatric cases of multi-drug-resistant organism transmission have been published following duodenoscope exposure, these are concerning developments and will undoubtedly be an area of active future research.

The Future of Pediatric Endoscopic Retrograde Cholangiopancreatography

The utilization of pediatric ERCP will likely continue to increase as new indications are identified and access to the procedure is increased. In addition, its role will continue to evolve, particularly as additional experience is gained with alternative and often complementary diagnostic modalities such as *endoscopic ultrasound* and magnetic resonance cholangiopancreatography. Although previously published case series have provided a basic understanding of the feasibility and clinical utility of the procedure in the pediatric population, the pediatric literature does not enjoy the same rigor that has been available to advanced endoscopists caring for adult patients. To date, pediatric-specific investigations of ERCP have been traditionally hampered by the relatively small volume of cases performed at any single site coupled with a lack of organized forums to foster and support collaborative research in this arena. Fortunately, there is evidence that this environment seems to be changing.

Recently a formal pediatric ERCP special interest group was formed by the North America Society for Pediatric Gastroenterology, Hepatology, and Nutrition to provide a forum for endoscopists performing ERCP in children to share experiences and identify knowledge gaps.[60] In addition, several high-volume pediatric endoscopists performing ERCPs from around the world are now collaborating through a multicenter pediatric ERCP database, which seems well positioned to longitudinally evaluate technical and clinical outcomes as a result of pediatric ERCPs.[61] Supportive environments and collaborations such as these should be fostered with the goal of obtaining a more complete understanding of the unique role ERCP plays in the evaluation and treatment of pediatric pancreaticobiliary pathologic abnormality.

SUMMARY

ERCP continues to see increasing utilization within the pediatric population and its role continues to evolve. Although primarily used as a therapeutic modality as in adult patients, there are applications unique to the pediatric population that warrant further study. Technical and clinical outcomes are likely similar between pediatric and adult patients undergoing the procedure for particular indications, although potential significant size and physiologic differences between these 2 populations may warrant adjustments in patient preparation and equipment selection. To date, the published pediatric experience suggests that the data yielded by emerging multicenter pediatric-specific studies will be critical to improving patient selection and optimizing technical and clinical outcomes. Fortunately, there seems to be some recent momentum to help support and implement such projects.

REFERENCES

1. Early DS, Ben-Menachem T, Decker GA, et al. Appropriate use of GI endoscopy. Gastrointest Endosc 2012;75(6):1127–31.
2. Adler DG, Lieb JG, Cohen J, et al. Quality indicators for ERCP. Am J Gastroenterol 2015;81(1):54–66.
3. Fox VL, Werlin SL, Heyman MB. Endoscopic retrograde cholangiopancreatography in children. Subcommittee on Endoscopy and Procedures of the Patient Care Committee of the North American Society for Pediatric Gastroenterology and Nutrition. J Pediatr Gastroenterol Nutr 2000;30(3):335–42. Available at: http://www.ncbi.nlm.nih.gov/pubmed/10749424.
4. Liguory C, Mougenot J-F, Andrade de Paulo G. Endoscopic Retrograde Cholangiopancreatography. In: Kleinman R, Goulet O, Mieli-Vergani G, et al, editors. Walker's pediatric gastrointestinal disease. 5th edition. Shelton (CT): People's Medical Publishing House-USA; 2008. p. 1329–40.
5. Varadarajulu S, Wilcox CM, Hawes RH, et al. Technical outcomes and complications of ERCP in children. Gastrointest Endosc 2004;60(3):367–71. Available at: http://www.ncbi.nlm.nih.gov/pubmed/15332025.
6. Rocca R, Castellino F, Daperno M, et al. Therapeutic ERCP in paediatric patients. Dig Liver Dis 2005;37(5):357–62.
7. Cheng CL, Fogel EL, Sherman S, et al. Diagnostic and therapeutic endoscopic retrograde cholangiopancreatography in children: a large series report. J Pediatr Gastroenterol Nutr 2005;41(4):445–53. Available at: http://www.ncbi.nlm.nih.gov/pubmed/16205513.
8. Petersen C, Meier PN, Schneider A, et al. Endoscopic retrograde cholangiopancreaticography prior to explorative laparotomy avoids unnecessary surgery in patients suspected for biliary atresia. J Hepatol 2009;51(6):1055–60.
9. Iqbal CW, Baron TH, Moir CR, et al. Post-ERCP pancreatitis in pediatric patients. J Pediatr Gastroenterol Nutr 2009;49(4):430–4.
10. Vegting IL, Tabbers MM, Taminiau JA, et al. Is endoscopic retrograde cholangiopancreatography valuable and safe in children of all ages? J Pediatr Gastroenterol Nutr 2009;48(1):66–71.
11. Jang JY, Yoon CH, Kim KM. Endoscopic retrograde cholangiopancreatography in pancreatic and biliary tract disease in Korean children. World J Gastroenterol 2010;16(4):490–5.
12. Keil R, Snajdauf J, Rygl M, et al. Diagnostic efficacy of ERCP in cholestatic infants and neonates–a retrospective study on a large series. Endoscopy 2010;42(2):121–6.
13. Otto AK, Neal MD, Slivka AN, et al. An appraisal of endoscopic retrograde cholangiopancreatography (ERCP) for pancreaticobiliary disease in children: our institutional experience in 231 cases. Surg Endosc 2011;25(8):2536–40.

14. Shteyer E, Wengrower D, Benuri-Silbiger I, et al. Endoscopic retrograde cholangiopancreatography in neonatal cholestasis. J Pediatr Gastroenterol Nutr 2012; 55(2):142–5.
15. Troendle DM, Barth BA. ERCP can be safely and effectively performed by a pediatric gastroenterologist for choledocholithiasis in a pediatric facility. J Pediatr Gastroenterol Nutr 2013;57(5):655–8.
16. Halvorson L, Halsey K, Darwin P, et al. The safety and efficacy of therapeutic ERCP in the pediatric population performed by adult gastroenterologists. Dig Dis Sci 2013;58(12):3611–9.
17. Agarwal J, Nageshwar Reddy D, Talukdar R, et al. ERCP in the management of pancreatic diseases in children. Gastrointest Endosc 2014;79(2):271–8.
18. Enestvedt BK, Tofani C, Lee DY, et al. Endoscopic retrograde cholangiopancreatography in the pediatric population is safe and efficacious. J Pediatr Gastroenterol Nutr 2013;57(5):649–54.
19. Saito T, Terui K, Mitsunaga T, et al. Role of pediatric ERCP in an era stressing less-invasive imaging modalities. J Pediatr Gastroenterol Nutr 2014;59(2):204–9.
20. Giefer MJ, Kozarek RA. Technical outcomes and complications of pediatric ERCP. Surg Endosc 2015. [Epub ahead of print].
21. Troendle DM, Abraham O, Huang R, et al. Factors associated with post-ERCP pancreatitis and the effect of pancreatic duct stenting in a pediatric population. Gastrointest Endosc 2015;81(6):1408–16.
22. Hiramatsu T, Itoh A, Kawashima H, et al. Usefulness and safety of endoscopic retrograde cholangiopancreatography in children with pancreaticobiliary maljunction. J Pediatr Surg 2015;50(3):377–81.
23. Pant C, Sferra TJ, Barth BA, et al. Trends in endoscopic retrograde cholangiopancreatography in children within the United States, 2000-2009. J Pediatr Gastroenterol Nutr 2014;59(1):57–60.
24. Moyer V, Freese DK, Whitington PF, et al, North American Society for Pediatric Gastroenterology, Hepatology and Nutrition. Guideline for the evaluation of cholestatic jaundice in infants: recommendations of the North American Society for Pediatric Gastroenterology, Hepatology and Nutrition. J Pediatr Gastroenterol Nutr 2004;39(2):115–28.
25. Wilkinson ML, Mieli-Vergani G, Ball C, et al. Endoscopic retrograde cholangiopancreatography in infantile cholestasis. Arch Dis Child 1991;66(1):121–3.
26. Guelrud M, Jaen D, Mendoza S, et al. ERCP in the diagnosis of extrahepatic biliary atresia. Gastrointest Endosc 1991;37(5):522–6.
27. Ohnuma N, Takahashi T, Tanabe M, et al. The role of ERCP in biliary atresia. Gastrointest Endosc 1997;45(5):365–70.
28. Shanmugam NP, Harrison PM, Devlin J, et al. Selective use of endoscopic retrograde cholangiopancreatography in the diagnosis of biliary atresia in infants younger than 100 days. J Pediatr Gastroenterol Nutr 2009;49(4):435–41.
29. Lakhole A, Liu QY. Sa1659 ERCP can be performed effectively and safely by an independent pediatric gastroenterologist at a freestanding children's hospital. Gastrointest Endosc 2015;81(5):AB298.
30. Troendle D, Fishman DS, Fox VL, et al. Su1759 the management of patients requiring ERCP at pediatric centers: a US Survey. Gastrointest Endosc 2014; 79(5):AB287.
31. Chutkan RK, Ahmad AS, Cohen J, et al. ERCP core curriculum. Gastrointest Endosc 2006;63(3):361–76.
32. Shahidi N, Ou G, Telford J, et al. When trainees reach competency in performing ERCP: a systematic review. Gastrointest Endosc 2015;81(6):1337–42.

33. Kapral C, Duller C, Wewalka F, et al. Case volume and outcome of endoscopic retrograde cholangiopancreatography: results of a nationwide Austrian benchmarking project. Endoscopy 2008;40(8):625–30.

34. Testoni PA, Mariani A, Giussani A, et al. Risk factors for post-ERCP pancreatitis in high- and low-volume centers and among expert and non-expert operators: a prospective multicenter study. Am J Gastroenterol 2010;105(8):1753–61.

35. ASGE Standards of Practice Committee, Lightdale JR, Acosta R, et al. Modifications in endoscopic practice for pediatric patients. Gastrointest Endosc 2014; 79(5):699–710.

36. ASGE Technology Committee, Barth BA, Banerjee S, et al. Equipment for pediatric endoscopy. Gastrointest Endosc 2012;76(1):8–17.

37. ASGE Standards of Practice Committee, Anderson MA, Fisher L, et al. Complications of ERCP. Gastrointest Endosc 2012;75(3):467–73.

38. Cotton PB, Eisen GM, Aabakken L, et al. A lexicon for endoscopic adverse events: report of an ASGE workshop. Gastrointest Endosc 2010;71(3):446–54.

39. Freeman ML. Complications of endoscopic retrograde cholangiopancreatography: avoidance and management. Gastrointest Endosc Clin N Am 2012;22(3): 567–86.

40. Mazaki T, Masuda H, Takayama T. Prophylactic pancreatic stent placement and post-ERCP pancreatitis: a systematic review and meta-analysis. Endoscopy 2010;42(10):842–53.

41. Choudhary A, Bechtold ML, Arif M, et al. Pancreatic stents for prophylaxis against post-ERCP pancreatitis: a meta-analysis and systematic review. Gastrointest Endosc 2011;73(2):275–82.

42. Elmunzer BJ, Scheiman JM, Lehman GA, et al. A randomized trial of rectal indomethacin to prevent post-ERCP pancreatitis. N Engl J Med 2012;366(15): 1414–22.

43. Das A, Singh P, Sivak MV Jr, et al. Pancreatic-stent placement for prevention of post-ERCP pancreatitis: a cost-effectiveness analysis. Gastrointest Endosc 2007;65(7):960–8.

44. Freeman ML, Nelson DB, Sherman S, et al. Complications of endoscopic biliary sphincterotomy. N Engl J Med 1996;335(13):909–18.

45. Masci E, Toti G, Mariani A, et al. Complications of diagnostic and therapeutic ERCP: a prospective multicenter study. Am J Gastroenterol 2001;96(2):417–23.

46. Loperfido S, Angelini G, Benedetti G, et al. Major early complications from diagnostic and therapeutic ERCP: a prospective multicenter study. Gastrointest Endosc 1998;48(1):1–10.

47. ASGE Standards of Practice Committee, Anderson MA, Ben-Menachem T, et al. Management of antithrombotic agents for endoscopic procedures. Gastrointest Endosc 2009;70(6):1060–70.

48. Leung JW, Chan FK, Sung JJ, et al. Endoscopic sphincterotomy-induced hemorrhage: a study of risk factors and the role of epinephrine injection. Gastrointest Endosc 1995;42(6):550–4.

49. Wilcox CM, Canakis J, Monkemuller KE, et al. Patterns of bleeding after endoscopic sphincterotomy, the subsequent risk of bleeding, and the role of epinephrine injection. Am J Gastroenterol 2004;99(2):244–8.

50. Sherman S, Hawes RH, Nisi R, et al. Endoscopic sphincterotomy-induced hemorrhage: treatment with multipolar electrocoagulation. Gastrointest Endosc 1992;38(2):123–6.

51. Kuran S, Parlak E, Oguz D, et al. Endoscopic sphincterotomy-induced hemorrhage: treatment with heat probe. Gastrointest Endosc 2006;63(3):506–11.

52. Oviedo JA, Barrison A, Lichtenstein DR. Endoscopic argon plasma coagulation for refractory postsphincterotomy bleeding: report of two cases. Gastrointest Endosc 2003;58(1):148–51.

53. Baron TH, Norton ID, Herman L. Endoscopic hemoclip placement for post-sphincterotomy bleeding. Gastrointest Endosc 2000;52(5):662.

54. Paspatis GA, Dumonceau J-M, Barthet M, et al. Diagnosis and management of iatrogenic endoscopic perforations: European Society of Gastrointestinal Endoscopy (ESGE) Position Statement. Endoscopy 2014;46(8):693–711.

55. Harris A, Chan AC, Torres-Viera C, et al. Meta-analysis of antibiotic prophylaxis in endoscopic retrograde cholangiopancreatography (ERCP). Endoscopy 1999; 31(9):718–24.

56. Bai Y, Gao F, Gao J, et al. Prophylactic antibiotics cannot prevent endoscopic retrograde cholangiopancreatography-induced cholangitis: a meta-analysis. Pancreas 2009;38(2):126–30.

57. Banerjee S, Shen B, Baron TH, et al. Antibiotic prophylaxis for GI endoscopy. Gastrointest Endosc 2008;67(6):791–8.

58. Epstein L, Hunter JC, Arwady MA, et al. New Delhi metallo-β-lactamase-producing carbapenem-resistant escherichia coli associated with exposure to duodenoscopes. JAMA 2014;312(14):1447–55.

59. FDA. FDA Safety Communications. Available at: http://www.fda.gov/MedicalDevices/Safety/AlertsandNotices/ucm434871.htm. Accessed March 4, 2015.

60. NASPGHAN ERCP SIG. NASPGHAN Off Website. Available at: http://www.naspghan.org/content/121/en/. Accessed July 27, 2015.

61. Troendle DM, Liu QY, Kim KM, et al. 853 ERCP in younger vs older children: initial report from the multicenter pediatric ERCP database initiative. Gastrointest Endosc 2015;81(5):AB173.

Role of Endoscopic Ultrasound in Pediatric Disease

Arathi Lakhole, MD[a], Quin Y. Liu, MD[b],*

KEYWORDS

- Pediatric endoscopic ultrasound • Fine-needle aspiration • Pancreatitis
- Choledocholithiasis • Endoscopic cystgastrostomy • Autoimmune pancreatitis

KEY POINTS

- The application of endoscopic ultrasound (EUS) in children is growing, but remains limited because of lack of availability in pediatric centers and pediatric gastroenterologists trained in this advanced endoscopic procedure.
- Special technical considerations must be considered when performing EUS in very small children.
- Performing EUS before ERCP may represent a promising means of avoiding unnecessary ERCP in children with suspected choledocholithiasis.
- Further studies are required to evaluate the diagnostic and therapeutic potential of EUS in children.

INTRODUCTION

Endoscopic ultrasound (EUS) is a procedure that uses an ultrasound transducer built into the tip of a flexible endoscope to obtain high-resolution images of the gastrointestinal (GI) mucosal layer and adjacent organs, such as lymph nodes, pancreas, bile duct, liver, mediastinum, and kidneys. EUS is widely used in adults, especially in the diagnosis and treatment of pancreaticobiliary disease and in GI malignancy staging. Diagnosis with fine-needle aspiration (FNA) or core-needle biopsy (CNB) can be performed along with therapeutic procedures, such as injections, celiac plexuses neurolysis, and pancreatic or biliary fluid collection drainage.

Disclosure Statement: The authors have nothing to disclose.
[a] Division of Gastroenterology, Hepatology and Nutrition, Children's Hospital Los Angeles, 4650 Sunset Boulevard, Mailstop #78, Los Angeles, CA 90027, USA; [b] Division of Gastroenterology, Hepatology, and Nutrition, Children's Hospital Los Angeles, Keck School of Medicine of USC, 4650 Sunset Boulevard, Mailstop #78, Los Angeles, CA 90027, USA
* Corresponding author.
E-mail address: QLiu@chla.usc.edu

Gastrointest Endoscopy Clin N Am 26 (2016) 137–153
http://dx.doi.org/10.1016/j.giec.2015.08.001
1052-5157/16/$ – see front matter © 2016 Elsevier Inc. All rights reserved.

Although EUS is a well establish procedure in adult populations, experience in children is more limited (**Table 1**).[1-7] Nevertheless, the application of EUS in children has been growing, with most literature describing its use in pancreaticobiliary diseases. In addition, uses for EUS have expanded in other pediatric diseases, including congenital GI anatomic anomalies, pyloric stenosis, inflammatory bowel disease (IBD), vascular lesions, and liver disease.

There are two types of EUS imaging: radial and curvilinear (**Fig. 1**). The radial echoendoscope allows a 360° view, perpendicular to the transducer. This gives an image similar to that seen on axial images of a computed tomography (CT) scan. A curvilinear array (CLA) echoendoscope provides a 180° view, parallel to the transducer.

Although both EUS modalities are equally suitable for diagnostic imaging, most CLA echoendoscopes are designed with a working channel and elevator (similar to a duodenoscope) to allow for FNA, CNB, and other therapeutic instruments to be used under real-time sonographic visualization.

High-resolution EUS probes are also available to be used through the working channel of gastroscopes, colonoscopes, and duodenoscopes. These probes are available at frequencies ranging from 12 to 30 MHz and provide higher detailed imaging of individual GI layers compared with the radial or CLA echoendoscopes. Therefore EUS probes are frequently used to study mucosal and submucosal lesions. The trade-off of these high-frequency probes providing such high-resolution images is the reduced depth of penetration and visualization (**Fig. 2**).

All EUS transducers described previously also provide Doppler flow, which can be used to differentiate vessels from ducts, and vascular lesions from solid masses or cysts.

Special Technical Considerations

Standard EUS endoscopes are relatively large and at times challenging to intubate the esophagus, especially in smaller patients. Echoendoscope tip sizes vary depending on the manufacturer, with diameters range from 11.4 to 13.9 mm. Most echoendoscopes provide an oblique endoscopic view that requires a semiblind esophageal intubation, although newer forward-viewing EUS endoscopes are now available and have been described in the literature.[8-10] The length of the angled echoendoscope tips is also longer than those of standard gastroscopes.

It is important to recognize that esophageal intubation of a small child with a standard EUS scope carries an increased risk of cervical esophageal perforation. Nevertheless, there are studies reporting successful EUS with "standard" echoendoscopes in children 6 months to 3 years of age.[2,6] Radial echoendoscopes with smaller insertion diameters are more technically feasible in smaller children, but the inability to perform FNA or CNB under direct sonographic visualization limits the radial echoendoscopes to diagnostic procedures.

In addition to the technical limitations of performing EUS in the smallest of pediatric patients, EUS is also not widely available in pediatric centers because of lack of formal training programs for pediatric gastroenterologists. Even in adult gastroenterology, EUS is performed by a minority of gastroenterologists and only recently has EUS become available in community hospitals. The availability of EUS for children is limited by the small number of adult gastroenterologists who are able to perform the procedure in children, and the very few pediatric gastroenterologists who have been appropriately trained to perform it.

INDICATIONS

Many indications for EUS exist and more continue to be studied (**Table 2**). This section discusses various GI indications for EUS in children, and is organized anatomically.

Table 1
Comparison of pediatric EUS studies

Study	Sample Size	Indications (# of Procedures)	Technical Success Rate	Impact	Complications
Scheers et al[4]	52 EUS 48 children (2–17 y)	• Pancreatic (30) • Biliary (22) • Therapeutic (13) • EUS-FNA (12)	100%	98% (51) procedures established definitive diagnosis or altered management	2 children with hemorrhagic complications
Al-Rashdan et al[3]	58 EUS 56 children (4–18 y)	• Pancreatic (28) • Mucosal/submucosal lesions (8) • Biliary (5) • Anal/rectal (4) • Therapeutic (5) • EUS-FNA (15)	100%	86% (44) procedures established definitive diagnosis or altered management	None
Attila et al[2]	40 EUS 38 children (3–17 y)	• Pancreatic (22) • Biliary (3) • Stomach (6) • Mediastinal (5) • Esophageal (1) • Rectal (1) • EUS-FNA (12)	100%	75% (9) patients FNA established definitive diagnosis	None
Cohen et al[5]	32 children (1.5–18 y)	• Pancreatic (15) • Biliary (4) • Esophagus (8) • Stomach (2) • Rectum (2) • EUS-FNA (7)	100%	44% (14) procedures established definitive diagnosis or altered management	None
Bjerring et al[6]	18 EUS 18 children (0.5–15 y)	• Tumor (9) • Pancreatic (2) • Biliary (2)	100%	78% (14) procedures established definitive diagnosis or altered management	None
Varadarajulu et al[1]	15 EUS 14 children (5–17 y)	• Pancreatic (6) • Biliary (5) • Abdominal pain of biliary etiology (3) • EUS-FNA (3)	100%	93% (13) procedures established definitive diagnosis or altered management	None
Roseau et al[7]	23 EUS 18 children (4–16 y)	• Upper digestive tract (17) • Anorectal (6)	100%	—	None

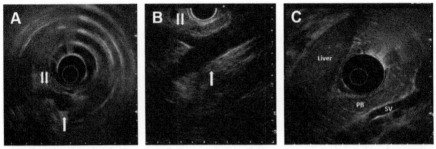

Fig. 1. (*A*) Radial EUS image, 360° view perpendicular to the transducer (*center of image*) of aorta (*single arrow*) and celiac artery (*double arrow*). (*B*) Curvilinear array EUS image at the same location, 180° view parallel to the transducer (*top-center of image*) of aorta (*single arrow*) and celiac artery (*double arrow*). (*C*) Radial EUS image with an axial view of the liver, body of pancreas (PB), and splenic vein (SV).

Esophagus

The most common indication for EUS of the esophagus is to evaluate the extent of esophageal tumors and periesophageal lymph nodes. Because of low incidence of esophageal tumors in children, EUS of the esophagus in children is generally used for other conditions beyond those associated with malignancy. In particular, there are some congenital anomalies for which EUS is helpful in establishing their definitive diagnosis. In addition, eosinophilic esophagitis (EoE), esophageal varices, and motility disorders may also represent conditions that may benefit from examination with EUS.

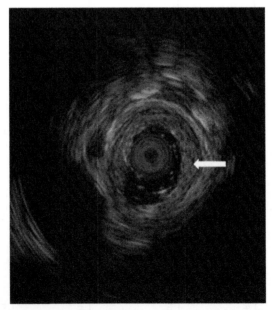

Fig. 2. EUS probe through a gastroscope working channel. A thickened esophageal mucosa layer is seen in greater detail (*arrow*).

Table 2	
Indications for EUS in pediatrics	
Diagnostic	**Therapeutic**
Pancreaticobiliary	• Endoscopic cystgastrostomy
• Recurrent/chronic pancreatitis	• Celiac plexus neurolysis
• Suspected biliary obstruction	• Direct biliary access
• Choledochal cyst	• Control of bleeding
• Autoimmune pancreatitis	
• Pancreas divisum	
• Malignant pancreatic/biliary lesions	
• Liver biopsy	
Esophageal	—
• Congenital esophageal stenosis	
• Eosinophilic esophagitis	
• Esophageal motility disorders	
• Esophageal varices	
Gastric/duodenal	—
• Duodenal duplication	
• Gastric varices	
• Submucosal lesions	
• Pyloric stenosis	
Intestinal	—
• Inflammatory bowel disease	
Anorectal	—
• Anorectal malformation	
• Fecal incontinence	
• Rectal varices	

Congenital esophageal stenosis

Congenital esophageal stenosis is an extremely rare congenital malformation. There are three subtypes: (1) fibromuscular, (2) tracheobronchial remnant (TBR), and (3) membranous web. Therapy typically includes dilation of the stenosis with surgery reserved for refractory dilations. In patients with the TBR subtype, dilation is usually ineffective despite repeated attempts, increasing a patient's risk for an esophageal perforation. Therefore surgical resection is traditionally preferred. Visualization of the TBR on CT or MRI is difficult, and hence EUS has been proposed to identify the TBR-type stenosis.

Bocus and colleagues[11] suggested using EUS and three-dimensional EUS in all patients with congenital esophageal stenosis to choose the correct therapeutic strategy. Additionally, EUS gives information about the nature and length of the stenosis and its relationship with surrounding structures to assist with surgical planning. A systematic literature review of 144 articles showed overall success rate of 90% when dilating with EUS guidance compared with 29% without EUS. Overall perforation rate with EUS was 7% compared with 24% without EUS.[12]

Eosinophilic esophagitis and gastroesophageal reflux

EoE is a relatively common allergic inflammatory process of the esophagus, with symptoms similar to gastroesophageal reflux disease (GERD). The diagnosis of EoE is based on endoscopic appearance and histopathology, but a clear diagnosis is challenging and difficult to distinguish from GERD if typical histologic characteristics are not present, especially in partially treated cases. Accurate diagnosis is important because the management for each differ.

EUS has been shown to help differentiate EoE from GERD. Dalby and colleagues[13] studied endoscopy with EUS, esophageal impedance, and pH measurements to characterize GERD and EoE. The authors showed increased thickness of the mucosal layers at the distal and proximal esophagus in patients with EoE compared with GERD and control subjects. Another study by Fox and colleagues[14] investigated anatomic alterations on EUS in children with EoE compared with healthy children and demonstrated that children with EoE had significantly increased thickness of the esophageal wall and its mucosa, submucosa, and muscularis propria layers compared with control subjects.

Gastroesophageal varices and portal hypertension

EUS can be used for early detection and diagnosis of esophageal varices and also to provide endoscopic therapy for EUS-guided sclerotherapy. McKiernan and coworker[15] performed esophagogastroduodenoscopy (EGD) and EUS in the evaluation 16 children undergoing small bowel intestinal transplantation to help determine if those children also required a combined liver transplant by evaluating for early gastroesophageal varices as a marker for moderate hepatic fibrosis. In seven patients, gastroesophageal varices not seen on EGD were noted on EUS. Based on those findings, the authors suggest that invasive liver biopsy can be avoided in those patients with EUS-proved varices (who otherwise would have undergone a liver biopsy based on EGD without varices) and that EUS is superior to EGD in detecting variceal lesions in children.

Motility disorders

Esophageal motility disorders typically present with symptoms of dysphagia, heartburn, chest pain, and vomiting. Primary esophageal dysmotility is rare in pediatrics. Diagnosis is made with manometry, which provides pressure recordings. Krishnan and colleagues[16] evaluated the use of EUS in patients with esophageal motility disorder and discovered that 15% of patients diagnosed with esophageal motility disorders actually had anatomic abnormalities (eg, external vascular compression, intramural mass, congenital muscular ring) contributing to their symptoms and leading to a change in management. This may be of particular relevance in pediatrics because underlying congenital anomalies should be considered in the differential diagnosis given the rare incidence of primary esophageal dysmotility in this population.

Stomach and Duodenum

Duodenal duplication

Duodenal duplication is a rare congenital anomaly located in close relation to the medial wall of the duodenum. Symptoms of duodenal duplication include duodenal obstruction, bleeding, and pancreatitis. Usually treatment is surgical resection, but endoscopic resection has been suggested. Romeo and colleagues[17] used an EUS probe to characterize the anatomy of duodenal duplication with the goal of optimizing surgical management. If the common wall separating the duodenum involved the biliary or pancreatic ductal system, then general surgical treatment was recommended. If the pancreatic or biliary ductal systems were not involved, endoscopic resection of the duodenal common wall was performed to treat the duplication cyst. In this way, EUS was used to guide treatment of duodenal duplication. The authors also showed that endoscopic resection was associated with shorter hospital stays.

Pyloric stenosis

Pyloric stenosis typically presents in the neonatal period with projectile vomiting and sometimes a firm hard pylorus palpable on physical examination. Abdominal ultrasound and upper GI barium studies are useful to establish this diagnosis, but it is not uncommon for the infant's clinical history, physical examination, laboratory, or radiographic studies to be equivocal. Khan[18] reported the use of a high-resolution EUS probe in an infant with an unusual clinical presentation for pyloric stenosis, but a transabdominal ultrasound suggestive of the diagnosis. Khan[18] was able to use the EUS probe to determine the pylorus to have a normal wall thickness, thereby helping the infant to avoid an unnecessary surgery. High-resolution EUS probes may allow for more precise wall thickness measurements compared with transabdominal ultrasound, as was described in this case report.

Submucosal and vascular lesions

GI submucosal lesions have been reported in children, although such lesions are much more common in adults.[19] Submucosal lesions are difficult to assess by standard endoscopy because there is generally a normal overlying mucosal surface and standard endoscopic biopsy forceps may not penetrate the mucosal layer to adequately obtain tissue samples. EUS can be used to assess a submucosal lesion to determine its size, origin, and extent of involvement to the intestinal layers and surrounding structures. It can also be of help in better characterizing the lesion (ie, cystic, solid, echogenicity). Furthermore, EUS Doppler can be used to determine if a lesion is vascular, because if it is not or if the risk of bleeding is minimal, FNA can be performed to diagnose the lesion. Despite the rarity of submucosal lesions in children, the use of EUS-FNA in children for submucosal lesions has been reported to be done successfully and safely.[2,3]

Inflammatory bowel disease

The diagnosis of IBD is based on clinical history, laboratory results, endoscopy, and histology. In certain patients, the diagnosis or the differentiation of ulcerative colitis (UC) or Crohn disease (CD) may be challenging. Ellrichmann and colleagues[10] used EUS to differentiate UC from CD and assess disease activity. In this cohort, the investigators associated increased total wall thickness with a high positive predictive value for active IBD. In this way, they reported that EUS could be used to differentiate active UC from CD, and to quantify the degree of colonic inflammation. Yoshizawa and colleagues[20] showed that EUS is useful to determine the depth of intestinal inflammation in UC, predict the response to medical treatment, and determine need for surgery.

EUS may also have use in the evaluation of perianal CD. In a study by Rosen and colleagues,[21] EUS was used to guide management of perianal CD in children. Setons were placed in those patients with complex fistulizing disease. Serial EUS examinations were performed in patients with setons to monitor fistula healing and inflammation, and also to help guide medical versus surgical intervention. In those patients with persistent inflammation seen on EUS, seton treatment was continued, whereas those without inflammation had setons removed. The authors showed that time for recurrence was longer for those who were followed with EUS examinations rather than physical examination only, and that an algorithm for rectal EUS was helpful for effectively guiding management in children and adult patients with perianal CD.[21,22]

Anorectal

Anorectal endoscopy is well established in adults for the evaluation of polyps, submucosal lesions, IBD, fecal incontinence, and rectal cancer staging. In pediatrics, there are several studies that have evaluated the use of anorectal EUS to assess the internal anal sphincter for constipation and anorectal malformations.[23,24] Jones and colleagues[24] evaluated anal sphincters in normal children versus those with surgery for congenital anorectal malformations and showed that EUS provided information of the postanorectoplasty sphincter anatomy that helped determine if surgical revision of the anorectoplasty was required before closure of a colostomy. Another single-center experience with pediatric rectal EUS for a range of indications (congenital malformation, perianal fistulizing disease, rectal prolapse) suggested that EUS was effective, safe (with no early or late complications), and provided information that altered clinical management in all patients who underwent testing.[25]

EUS has also been demonstrated to be superior to standard colonoscopy in identifying rectal varices in children. Yachha and colleagues,[26] in children with portal hypertension, found rectal varices by endoscopy in only 35% compared with 76% by rectal EUS showing the increased sensitivity of EUS in diagnosing rectal varices.

Pancreaticobiliary

Pancreas

As in adults, the largest indication for pediatric EUS is for the evaluation and management of pancreaticobiliary disease.[2–5] Similar to lesions of the esophagus and stomach, EUS can fully evaluate the size, location, and extent of the lesion in terms of its involvement with surrounding structures, and stage malignant tumors. EUS can characterize lesions and most importantly obtain tissue diagnosis with either FNA or CNB (**Fig. 3**).

Malignant pancreaticobiliary lesions in children are extremely rare, but have been reported.[27,28] Children can present with abdominal pain, pancreatitis, and jaundice if a pancreatic mass at the head of the pancreas leads to common bile duct obstruction. Although malignancy must be ruled out in any child with a pancreatic tumor, of greater suspicion in the pediatric population is autoimmune pancreatitis (AIP) presenting as a solid mass of the pancreas.[29] Such a lesion can also present as recurrent acute pancreatitis or chronic pancreatitis.

To best guide management in children with pancreatic tumors, either EUS-FNA or CNB should be first performed to obtain tissue for diagnostic purposes. Both have been shown to be technically feasible, and can allow adequate tissue for biopsy diagnosis of AIP.[30,31]

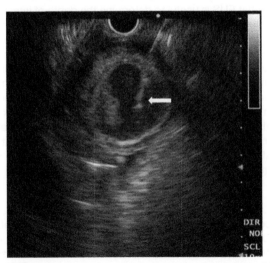

Fig. 3. FNA (*arrow*) of a peripancreatic cystic lesion in a 16-year-old girl presenting with pancreatitis.

In particular, EUS-FNA has been shown to be useful in the diagnosis and differentiation of the subtypes of AIP.[30] Nevertheless, biopsy specimens, as opposed to aspirate specimens for cytology, are preferred to obtain adequate tissue for diagnosis.

To this end, one small care series by Fujii and colleagues[32] demonstrated the use of EUS-CNB in nine children with suspicion of AIP. In this study, EUS had a diagnostic yield of 86% with one patient with AIP having nondiagnostic pathology. Mizuno and colleagues[33] demonstrated EUS-CNB to be superior to FNA for the diagnosis of AIP, whereas Jung and colleagues[31] also showed preferable utility of EUS-CNB compared with endoscopic retrograde cholangiopancreatography (ERCP) and ampullary biopsy. Neither study suggested an increased risk of adverse events. Using EUS-FNA or CNB to confirm a diagnosis of AIP in a child presenting with a pancreatic solid mass can help avoid more invasive surgical biopsies and unnecessary surgical resection in favor of effective medical treatment for AIP.

Biliary tree

The incidence of choledocholithiasis as an acquired biliary disease is rising in children. Determining if ERCP is indicated can be challenging when laboratory values are concerning for choledocholithiasis, but imaging studies are inconclusive. Even the American Society of Gastrointestinal Endoscopy guidelines to stratify the presence of choledocholithiasis in adult patients places the highest probability based on laboratory values and imaging studies at only greater than 50%.[34]

Biliary dilation on transabdominal ultrasound can be particularly difficult to interpret in young children, in large part because bile duct sizes for certain age groups are difficult to standardize and transabdominal ultrasound cannot always visualize the distal intrapancreatic portion of the common bile duct. Availability of CT and magnetic resonance cholangiopancreatography (MRCP) may be useful in determining the presence of choledocholithiasis, but CT exposes children to potentially harmful ionizing radiation and MRCP requires a cooperative child from movement or sedation to obtain clear images.

EUS under one anesthesia encounter can provide real-time evidence of biliary stone or sludge. EUS can visualize the entire extrahepatic bile duct and has been shown to be very accurate in detecting biliary stones with a sensitivity of 94% and a specificity of 95% (**Fig. 4**).[35] With the use of EUS in children with ambiguous laboratory studies and

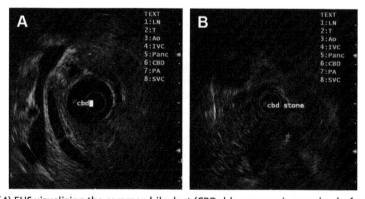

Fig. 4. (*A*) EUS visualizing the common bile duct (CBD; *blue measuring markers*) of a 12-year-old girl who presented with suspicion of choledocholithiasis. No stone was visualized on EUS and the patient proceeded to a cholecystectomy. (*B*) CBD stone (*blue measuring markers*) and sludge in an 11-year-old girl who then had an ERCP done under the same anesthesia.

imaging studies, it is possible to rule out choledocholithiasis, thereby avoiding unnecessary ERCP and its associated risks (**Fig. 5**).[4]

EUS can also be used to evaluate children with choledochal cysts. Although MRCP and ERCP are more often used for surgical planning of cyst resection and may be better suited to determine the subtype of choledochal cyst, EUS can be used to evaluate the extent of a choledochal cyst into the pancreas and liver parenchyma for surgical planning.[36]

Pancreatitis

The incidence of childhood pancreatitis has been rising,[37,38] with a significant proportion of patients suffering from recurrent pancreatitis without an identifiable cause. In this subset of children with "idiopathic" recurrent acute pancreatitis (IRAP), in which traditional imaging, laboratory, and genetic evaluations are unremarkable, EUS can be used. Ardengh and colleagues[39] incorporated EUS for evaluation of adults with IRAP and found 27 of 36 (75%) patients had microlithiasis on surgical histology, with EUS identifying 25 of the 27 cases with an overall EUS accuracy of 83.2%. Although not at the same prevalence, previous studies have also shown that EUS can be used to identify a biliary cause (along with other causes, such as tumors and pancreatic divisum) in patients with IRAP.[40–44] EUS may have higher yield identifying biliary cause for IRAP and should be considered in those patients, especially with gallbladder in situ (**Fig. 6**).[45]

EUS has also been compared with MRCP for the evaluation of patients with IRAP.[46–48] Although both modalities seem comparable in their ability to identify etiologies of pancreatitis and may complement each other in establishing diagnoses, evidence suggests that EUS is better for identifying biliary etiologies, whereas MRCP is better for identifying pancreatic anomalies (eg, tumors, cyst, divisum).

The normal variant of pancreatic divisum is a controversial cause of pancreatitis. Regardless of its role in pancreatitis, EUS can identify or confirm the presence of divisum accurately with sensitivities, specificities, positive predictive values, and negative predictive values of 100%, 97%, 86%, and 100%, respectively, with an overall accuracy of 97%.[49,50] Greater accuracy is achieved with the CLA echoendoscope, which normally can visualize the pancreatic duct from the head to the body in continuity. In those patients with pancreas divisum, either the pancreatic duct at the head is not visualized or the duct cannot be traced from the head to the body.

Criteria for the diagnosis of chronic pancreatitis with EUS findings have also been proposed,[51] but have not been validated in pediatrics.

Liver

Liver biopsy of the left lobe of the liver is possible during EUS examination. This can be done with the CLA echoendoscope in the stomach or duodenum. Johal and colleagues[52] demonstrated the feasibility and safety of EUS liver biopsy in children in a small case series with a 19-gauge FNA needle. Although more invasive than a percutaneous liver biopsy, EUS-guided liver biopsy can be considered in children who require endoscopy and liver biopsy, thereby enabling performance of both procedures during the same anesthetic. EUS liver biopsy may also be considered in patients with chronic liver disease requiring endoscopy for evaluation of esophageal varices. Another group who may benefit are post–liver transplant patients who require ERCP for evaluation of bile duct-to-duct surgical anastomosis for liver enzyme abnormalities. In those patients where ERCP determines that a biliary stricture is not present, one could consider obtaining an EUS-guided liver biopsy under the same anesthetic for evaluation of liver graft rejection.

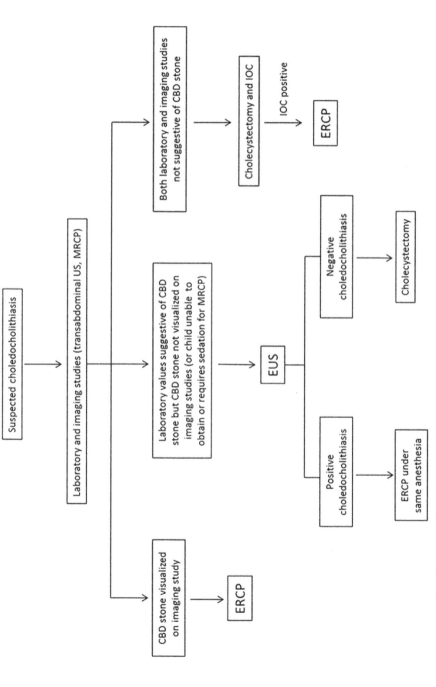

Fig. 5. Proposed algorithm for using EUS in the management of suspected choledocholithiasis in children. IOC, intraoperative cholangiogram.

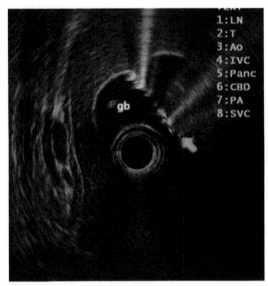

Fig. 6. EUS image of a gallbladder (gb) with shadowing microlithiasis (*green arrow*) in a 12-year-old girl with history of recurrent acute pancreatitis. Previous transabdominal ultrasound and CT scans failed to visualized the microlithiasis seen on EUS.

THERAPEUTIC ENDOSCOPIC ULTRASOUND
Endoscopic Cystgastrostomy

Drainage of fluid collections and pancreatic pseudocysts with the creation of a cystgastrostomy is now predominantly done endoscopically. Varadarajulu and colleagues[53] showed endoscopic cystgastrostomy as effective and safe as surgical cystgastrotomy and also associated with shorter hospital stays. With EUS, the cyst can be fully evaluated and then accessed with an FNA needle to collect fluid and sonographically visualize guidewire placement and even stent deployment.

Endoscopic cystgastrostomy is well established in adults. Although its use in pediatrics is not extensively described, in our experience and in reports from other centers, endoscopic cystgastrostomy is technically feasible and safe in appropriately selected patients. In a retrospective pediatric study from Belgium, 12 children had successful EUS cystgastrostomy with one complication of cystgastrostomy site bleeding that was endoscopically treated. Another study from Dallas, Texas was successful in the drainage of 10 children with pancreatic pseudocyst without complications.[4,54]

Celiac Plexus Neurolysis

Pain management for patients with chronic pancreatitis can be challenging. An increasingly used option is EUS-guided celiac plexus neurolysis (CPN). With this technique, the celiac plexus is easily visualized with EUS to be accessible at the celiac artery take-off from the aorta (see **Fig. 1B**), usually when the echoendoscope is just distal to the gastroesophageal junction, along the lesser curvature. Specialized fenestrated EUS needles are available for the injection of the desired regimen (bupivacaine or alcohol).

Nevertheless, it is important to recognize that although EUS-CPN has been described in children,[2,3] its effectiveness for treating chronic idiopathic pancreatitis is suboptimal (51%–59%) compared with its effectiveness with reducing pain associated with pancreatic cancer (72%–80%).[55,56] In addition, pain relief with CPN for chronic pancreatitis has not been found to be sustainable and requires repeated treatments.

Endoscopic Ultrasound–Guided Biliary Access

Therapeutic EUS is used to establish biliary access if access from the major papilla is not possible. This advanced technique is used when the duodenoscope cannot be advanced to the major papilla secondary to duodenal anatomic abnormalities (eg, duodenal stricture or obstructing tumor) or a high-grade biliary stricture preventing retrograde access from the major papilla. In this scenario, the CLA echoendoscope can identify the biliary tree and the FNA needle can puncture into the bile duct usually through the first portion of the duodenum. Once guidewire access is established, a covered metal stent can be placed across the duodenum and into the bile duct to create a duodenocholedochostomy for biliary drainage. Use of this antegrade approach has been described in a pediatric patient, but from a transgastric approach creating a gastrocholedochostomy.[4] Complications related to this technique include bile leaks and bile peritonitis.[57,58]

Other Therapeutic Indications

The role of therapeutic EUS continues to evolve. Similar to establishing biliary access, EUS pancreatic duct access from the gastric wall is achievable. Other applications include its use to deliver brachytherapy, radiofrequency, and injection ablation for tumors.[59] For patients with portal hypertension, treatment of gastric varices with EUS-guided cyanoacrylate injection or coil placement is of potential.[60]

COMPLICATIONS

As in all endoscopic procedures, complications related to EUS include bleeding, infection, and perforation (**Table 3**). Perforation rates with EUS have been found to be similar to rates of standard endoscopy.[61] Cervical esophageal perforation is of particular concern when performing EUS in children because of the large EUS endoscope size, semioblique view, longer flexible tip, and the smaller size of children.

Risk of infection and bacteremia associated with EUS-FNA is also low and comparable with diagnostic endoscopy.[62] Prophylactic antibiotics are not recommended with routine EUS-FNA or CNB of solid lesion or organs. Although the overall risk of infection to cystic lesions with FNA is low with or without antibiotics,[63,64] expert recommendations are to provide prophylactic antibiotics when aspirating a cystic lesion.

EUS also has the known risk of pancreatitis. This risk is present when patients undergo FNA of pancreatic lesions with rates ranging from 0.44% to 2%.[65,66] Bile peritonitis is also a small risk not related to standard endoscopy but unique to EUS.

Table 3 Adverse events	
Event	**Reported Incidence (American Society of Gastrointestinal Endoscopy)[61]**
Infection/bacteremia	0.4%–1%
Hemorrhage	0.1%–4%
Cervical esophageal perforation	0.02%–0.07%
Pancreatitis	0%–2%
Bile peritonitis	—

Although discussed as a risk with EUS for biliary access, bile peritonitis has also been reported after EUS with FNA of a pancreatic head mass.[67]

SUMMARY

EUS has been shown to be safe, effective, and integral in the management of children with pancreaticobiliary or luminal diseases. Although the standard radial array or CLA echoendoscopes can be used in most children for diagnostic and therapeutic EUS, the smaller size of pediatric oropharynx coupled with the large size of these EUS endoscopes limits its availability from the smallest of children. Nevertheless, EUS can be technically performed in pediatric patients of all sizes, and in turn can be used to guide the management of a spectrum of pediatric diseases from EoE, IBD, and pancreaticobiliary disorders. Although most studies to date have shown the utility of EUS for diagnostic purposes, it is expected that more extensive studies over time will help to better characterize the role, effectiveness, and safety of therapeutic EUS in children.

REFERENCES

1. Varadarajulu S, Wilcox CM, Eloubeidi MA. Impact of EUS in the evaluation of pancreaticobiliary disorders in children. Gastrointest Endosc 2005;62(2):239–44.
2. Attila T, Adler DG, Hilden K, et al. EUS in pediatric patients. Gastrointest Endosc 2009;70(5):892–8.
3. Al-Rashdan A, LeBlanc J, Sherman S, et al. Role of endoscopic ultrasound for evaluating gastrointestinal tract disorders in pediatrics: a tertiary care center experience. J Pediatr Gastroenterol Nutr 2010;51(6):718–22.
4. Scheers I, Ergun M, Aouattah T, et al. The diagnostic and therapeutic role of endoscopic ultrasound in pediatric pancreaticobiliary disorders. J Pediatr Gastroenterol Nutr 2015;61(2):238–47.
5. Cohen S, Kalinin M, Yaron A, et al. Endoscopic ultrasonography in pediatric patients with gastrointestinal disorders. J Pediatr Gastroenterol Nutr 2008;46(5):551–4.
6. Bjerring OS, Durup J, Qvist N, et al. Impact of upper gastrointestinal endoscopic ultrasound in children. J Pediatr Gastroenterol Nutr 2008;47(1):110–3.
7. Roseau G, Palazzo L, Dumontier I, et al. Endoscopic ultrasonography in the evaluation of pediatric digestive diseases: preliminary results. Endoscopy 1998;30(5):477–81.
8. Iwashita T, Nakai Y, Lee JG, et al. A newly developed forward viewing echoendoscope - a comparative study to standard echoendoscope in imaging of abdominal organs and a feasibility of EUS-guided interventions. J Gastroenterol Hepatol 2011;27:362–7.
9. Voermans RP, Ponchon T, Schumacher B, et al. Forward-viewing versus oblique-viewing echoendoscopes in transluminal drainage of pancreatic fluid collections: a multicenter, randomized, controlled trial. Gastrointest Endosc 2011;74(6):1285–93.
10. Ellrichmann M, Wietzke-Braun P, Dhar S, et al. Endoscopic ultrasound of the colon for the differentiation of Crohn's disease and ulcerative colitis in comparison with healthy controls. Aliment Pharmacol Ther 2014;39(8):823–33.
11. Bocus P, Realdon S, Eloubeidi MA, et al. High-frequency miniprobes and 3-dimensional EUS for preoperative evaluation of the etiology of congenital esophageal stenosis in children (with video). Gastrointest Endosc 2011;74(1):204–7.
12. Terui K. Endoscopic management for congenital esophageal stenosis: a systematic review. World J Gastrointest Endosc 2015;7(3):183.

13. Dalby K, Nielsen RG, Kruse-Andersen S, et al. Gastroesophageal reflux disease and eosinophilic esophagitis in infants and children. A study of esophageal pH, multiple intraluminal impedance and endoscopic ultrasound. Scand J Gastroenterol 2010;45(9):1029–35.

14. Fox VL, Nurko S, Teitelbaum JE, et al. High-resolution EUS in children with eosinophilic "allergic" esophagitis. Gastrointest Endosc 2003;57(1):30–6.

15. McKiernan PJ, Sharif K, Gupte GL. The role of endoscopic ultrasound for evaluating portal hypertension in children being assessed for intestinal transplantation. Transplantation 2008;86(10):1470–3.

16. Krishnan K, Lin C-Y, Keswani R, et al. Endoscopic ultrasound as an adjunctive evaluation in patients with esophageal motor disorders subtyped by high-resolution manometry. Neurogastroenterol Motil 2014;26(8):1172–8.

17. Romeo E, Torroni F, Foschia F, et al. Surgery or endoscopy to treat duodenal duplications in children. J Pediatr Surg 2011;46(5):874–8.

18. Khan K. High-resolution EUS to differentiate hypertrophic pyloric stenosis. Gastrointest Endosc 2008;67(2):375–6.

19. Muniyappa P, Kay M, Feinberg L, et al. The endoscopic appearance of a gastrointestinal stromal tumor in a pediatric patient. J Pediatr Surg 2007;42(7):1302–5.

20. Yoshizawa S, Kobayashi K, Katsumata T, et al. Clinical usefulness of EUS for active ulcerative colitis. Gastrointest Endosc 2007;65(2):253–60.

21. Rosen MJ, Moulton DE, Koyama T, et al. Endoscopic ultrasound to guide the combined medical and surgical management of pediatric perianal Crohn's disease. Inflamm Bowel Dis 2010;16(3):461–8.

22. Rosen MJ, Schwartz DA. A 31-year-old patient with colitis and perianal disease. Clin Gastroenterol Hepatol 2010;8(1):10–4.

23. Keshtgar AS, Ward HC, Clayden GS, et al. Thickening of the internal anal sphincter in idiopathic constipation in children. Pediatr Surg Int 2004; 20(11–12):817–23.

24. Jones NM, Smilgin-Humphreys M, Sullivan PB, et al. Paediatric anal endosonography. Pediatr Surg Int 2003;19(11):703–6.

25. Morinville VD, Paquin SC, Sahai AV. Safety, feasibility, and usefulness of rectal endoscopic ultrasonography for pediatric anal and perianal complaints. J Pediatr Gastroenterol Nutr 2010;51(1):93–5.

26. Yachha SK, Dhiman RK, Gupta R, et al. Endosonographic evaluation of the rectum in children with extrahepatic portal venous obstruction. J Pediatr Gastroenterol Nutr 1996;23(4):438–41.

27. Park M, Koh KN, Kim BE, et al. Pancreatic neoplasms in childhood and adolescence. J Pediatr Hematol Oncol 2011;33(4):295–300.

28. Shorter NA, Glick RD, Klimstra DS, et al. Malignant pancreatic tumors in childhood and adolescence: the Memorial Sloan-Kettering experience, 1967 to present. J Pediatr Surg 2002;37(6):887–92.

29. Friedlander J, Quiros JA, Morgan T, et al. Diagnosis of autoimmune pancreatitis vs neoplasms in children with pancreatic mass and biliary obstruction. Clin Gastroenterol Hepatol 2012;10(9):1051–5.e1.

30. Ishikawa T, Itoh A, Kawashima H, et al. Endoscopic ultrasound-guided fine needle aspiration in the differentiation of type 1 and type 2 autoimmune pancreatitis. World J Gastroenterol 2012;18(29):3883–8.

31. Jung JG, Lee JK, Lee KH, et al. Comparison of endoscopic retrograde cholangiopancreatography with papillary biopsy and endoscopic ultrasound-guided pancreatic biopsy in the diagnosis of autoimmune pancreatitis. Pancreatology 2015;15(3):259–64.

32. Fujii LL, Chari ST, El-Youssef M, et al. Pediatric pancreatic EUS-guided Trucut biopsy for evaluation of autoimmune pancreatitis. Gastrointest Endosc 2013;77(5): 824–8.

33. Mizuno N, Bhatia V, Hosoda W, et al. Histological diagnosis of autoimmune pancreatitis using EUS-guided Trucut biopsy: a comparison study with EUS-FNA. J Gastroenterol 2009;44(7):742–50.

34. Maple JT, Ben-Menachem T, Anderson MA, et al. The role of endoscopy in the evaluation of suspected choledocholithiasis. Gastrointest Endosc 2010;71(1): 1–9.

35. Tse F, Liu L, Barkun AN, et al. EUS: a meta-analysis of test performance in suspected choledocholithiasis. Gastrointest Endosc 2008;67(2):235–44.

36. Liu QY, Nguyen V. Endoscopic approach to the patient with congenital anomalies of the biliary tract. Gastrointest Endosc Clin N Am 2013;23(2):505–18.

37. Nydegger A, Heine RG, Ranuh R, et al. Changing incidence of acute pancreatitis: 10-year experience at the Royal Children's Hospital, Melbourne. J Gastroenterol Hepatol 2007;22(8):1313–6.

38. Morinville VD, Barmada MM, Lowe ME. Increasing incidence of acute pancreatitis at an American pediatric tertiary care center: is greater awareness among physicians responsible? Pancreas 2010;39(1):5–8.

39. Ardengh JC, Malheiros CA, Rahal F, et al. Microlithiasis of the gallbladder: role of endoscopic ultrasonography in patients with idiopathic acute pancreatitis. Rev Assoc Med Bras 2010;56(1):27–31.

40. Tandon M, Topazian M. Endoscopic ultrasound in idiopathic acute pancreatitis. Am J Gastroenterol 2001;96(3):705–9.

41. Yusoff IF, Raymond G, Sahai AV. A prospective comparison of the yield of EUS in primary vs. recurrent idiopathic acute pancreatitis. Gastrointest Endosc 2004; 60(5):673–8.

42. Norton SA, Alderson D. Endoscopic ultrasonography in the evaluation of idiopathic acute pancreatitis. Br J Surg 2000;87(12):1650–5.

43. Liu CL, Lo CM, Chan JK, et al. EUS for detection of occult cholelithiasis in patients with idiopathic pancreatitis. Gastrointest Endosc 2000;51(1):28–32.

44. Frossard JL, Sosa-Valencia L, Amouyal G, et al. Usefulness of endoscopic ultrasonography in patients with "idiopathic" acute pancreatitis. Am J Med 2000; 109(3):196–200.

45. Wilcox CM, Varadarajulu S, Eloubeidi M. Role of endoscopic evaluation in idiopathic pancreatitis: a systematic review [A figure is presented]. Gastrointest Endosc 2006;63(7):1037–45.

46. Thevenot A, Bournet B, Otal P, et al. Endoscopic ultrasound and magnetic resonance cholangiopancreatography in patients with idiopathic acute pancreatitis. Dig Dis Sci 2013;58(8):2361–8.

47. Ortega AR, Gómez-Rodríguez R, Romero M, et al. Prospective comparison of endoscopic ultrasonography and magnetic resonance cholangiopancreatography in the etiological diagnosis of "idiopathic" acute pancreatitis. Pancreas 2011;40(2):289–94.

48. Mariani A, Arcidiacono PG, Curioni S, et al. Diagnostic yield of ERCP and secretin-enhanced MRCP and EUS in patients with acute recurrent pancreatitis of unknown aetiology. Dig Liver Dis 2009;41(10):753–8.

49. Lai R, Freeman ML, Cass OW, et al. Accurate diagnosis of pancreas divisum by linear-array endoscopic ultrasonography. Endoscopy 2004;36(8):705–9.

50. Rana SS, Bhasin DK, Sharma V, et al. Role of endoscopic ultrasound in the diagnosis of pancreas divisum. Endosc Ultrasound 2013;2(1):7–10.

51. Catalano MF, Sahai A, Levy M, et al. EUS-based criteria for the diagnosis of chronic pancreatitis: the Rosemont classification. Gastrointest Endosc 2009; 69(7):1251–61.
52. Johal AS, Khara HS, Maksimak MG, et al. Endoscopic ultrasound-guided liver biopsy in pediatric patients. Endosc Ultrasound 2014;3(3):191–4.
53. Varadarajulu S, Bang JY, Sutton BS, et al. Equal efficacy of endoscopic and surgical cystogastrostomy for pancreatic pseudocyst drainage in a randomized trial. Gastroenterology 2013;145(3):583–90.e1.
54. Jazrawi SF, Barth BA, Sreenarasimhaiah J. Efficacy of endoscopic ultrasound-guided drainage of pancreatic pseudocysts in a pediatric population. Dig Dis Sci 2011;56(3):902–8.
55. Puli SR, Reddy JBK, Bechtold ML, et al. EUS-guided celiac plexus neurolysis for pain due to chronic pancreatitis or pancreatic cancer pain: a meta-analysis and systematic review. Dig Dis Sci 2009;54(11):2330–7.
56. Kaufman M, Singh G, Das S, et al. Efficacy of endoscopic ultrasound-guided celiac plexus block and celiac plexus neurolysis for managing abdominal pain associated with chronic pancreatitis and pancreatic cancer. J Clin Gastroenterol 2010;44(2):127–34.
57. Itoi T, Itokawa F, Sofuni A, et al. Endoscopic ultrasound-guided choledochoduodenostomy in patients with failed endoscopic retrograde cholangiopancreatography. World J Gastroenterol 2008;14(39):6078–82.
58. Park DH, Jang JW, Lee SS, et al. EUS-guided biliary drainage with transluminal stenting after failed ERCP: predictors of adverse events and long-term results. Gastrointest Endosc 2011;74(6):1276–84.
59. Abu Dayyeh BK, Levy MJ. Therapeutic endoscopic ultrasound. Gastroenterol Hepatol (N Y) 2012;8(7):450–6.
60. Romero-Castro R, Ellrichmann M, Ortiz-Moyano C, et al. EUS-guided coil versus cyanoacrylate therapy for the treatment of gastric varices: a multicenter study (with videos). Gastrointest Endosc 2013;78(5):711–21.
61. Early DS, Acosta RD, Chandrasekhara V, et al. Adverse events associated with EUS and EUS with FNA. Gastrointest Endosc 2013;77(6):839–43.
62. Hirota WK, Petersen K, Baron TH, et al. Guidelines for antibiotic prophylaxis for GI endoscopy. Gastrointest Endosc 2003;58(4):475–82.
63. Guarner-Argente C, Shah P, Buchner A, et al. Use of antimicrobials for EUS-guided FNA of pancreatic cysts: a retrospective, comparative analysis. Gastrointest Endosc 2011;74(1):81–6.
64. Lee LS, Saltzman JR, Bounds BC, et al. EUS-guided fine needle aspiration of pancreatic cysts: a retrospective analysis of complications and their predictors. Clin Gastroenterol Hepatol 2005;3(3):231–6.
65. Gress F, Michael H, Gelrud D, et al. EUS-guided fine-needle aspiration of the pancreas: evaluation of pancreatitis as a complication. Gastrointest Endosc 2002;56(6):864–7.
66. Wang KX, Ben QW, Jin ZD, et al. Assessment of morbidity and mortality associated with EUS-guided FNA: a systematic review. Gastrointest Endosc 2011;73(2):283–90.
67. Chen HY, Lee CH, Hsieh CH. Bile peritonitis after EUS-guided fine-needle aspiration. Gastrointest Endosc 2002;56(4):594–6.

Advances in Pediatric Small Bowel Imaging

Tom K. Lin, MD

KEYWORDS

- Enteroscopy • Balloon-assisted • Double-balloon • Single-balloon • Children
- Pediatric • Small bowel

KEY POINTS

- Deep small bowel enteroscopy using balloon-assisted techniques provides an innovative, minimally invasive modality for diagnosing and treating small bowel diseases in children.
- Balloon-assisted enteroscopy in children has been proved to be safe and effective.
- Specific pediatric indications for balloon-assisted enteroscopy include the diagnosis and management of obscure GI bleeding, evaluation of suspected Crohn disease or established inflammatory bowel disease, and the management of polyposis syndromes.

INTRODUCTION

In the twenty-first century, it is currently possible to image, diagnose, and therapeutically treat diseases of the small bowel in children in a safe and minimally invasive manner. Although the various technologies that can accomplish small bowel imaging and allow therapeutic treatment have only been recently available to pediatrics, to some extent there has been a steady march toward these approaches over the past century. Radiologic imaging of the small bowel has been available dating back to the discovery of X-rays in 1895 by Wilhelm Roentgen. This advancement was a tremendous step forward to improving the evaluation of internal organs, including the gut. However, traditional radiologic studies have been grossly limited by their inability to tissue sample or to allow treatment when an abnormality is identified. Early on, the assessment required to confirm a diagnosis was left to invasive surgical resection and tissue sampling. Percutaneous sampling of intra-abdominal abnormalities was developed as an improvement on open surgical procedures for diagnostic purposes, whereas therapeutic capability continued to rely on surgical methods. In the 1990s, the advent of wireless capsule endoscopy (WCE) introduced another tool that could be used to noninvasively visualize the full length of the small bowel.

Disclosure Statement: The author has nothing to disclose.
Cincinnati Children's Hospital Medical Center, 3333 Burnet Avenue, MLC 2010, Cincinnati, OH 45229, USA
E-mail address: tom.lin@cchmc.org

Gastrointest Endoscopy Clin N Am 26 (2016) 155–168
http://dx.doi.org/10.1016/j.giec.2015.09.004   **giendo.theclinics.com**
1052-5157/16/$ – see front matter © 2016 Elsevier Inc. All rights reserved.

Although a remarkable innovation, WCE has also had its own set of limitations, including perhaps most importantly, a lack of therapeutic capability.

In 2001, Yamamoto and colleagues[1] described the first balloon-assisted enteroscopy (BAE) device, double-balloon enteroscopy (DBE; FUJIFILM Medical Systems, Wayne, NJ), named for its unique system using two attached inflatable balloons and an overtube over an endoscope. Additional devices have since been developed and are commercially available, including single-balloon enteroscopy (SBE; Olympus, Tokyo, Japan) (**Figs. 1** and **2**) and spiral enteroscopy (SE; Endo-Ease Discovery SB, Spirus Medical, Stoughton, MA) (**Fig. 3**). The BAE systems (DBE and SBE) have proven diagnostic and therapeutic benefits in the adult population, with similar identified advantages in children.[2–8] The earliest published experience on the use of BAE in children was in 2006 and 2007.[9,10] To date, SE has not been described in pediatrics, and indeed may have limited usage in children because of the relative larger size of the overtube thus restricting its application in smaller patients.

This comprehensive overview looks at pediatric enteroscopy and its defined diagnostic and therapeutic applications to date. We compare and contrast how enteroscopy in children differs from its use in adults, in terms of its indications and its therapeutic potential.

OVERVIEW OF ENTEROSCOPY

The development of balloon-assisted enteroscopes has revolutionized the minimally invasive approach to treating small bowel disorders in children and adult patients. To date, three technologies exist (DBE, SBE, and SE). Yamamoto and colleagues[1] first described the double-balloon technique in 2001 that was followed by the introduction of the single balloon[11] and spiral[12] technologies.

Irrespective of the technology used, the process of enteroscopy is the same: progressive pleating of the small bowel over the enteroscope with gradual greater depths of advancement of the scope tip deep into the small bowel. Full small bowel visualization has been described as technically feasible in adult and pediatric series.[2,6,13,14] This has been accomplished unidirectionally (antegrade alone) and also in the combined approach of antegrade and retrograde examinations.

It is important to recognize that complete small bowel visualization in many cases is not required, and should not necessarily be the objective of all enteroscopy

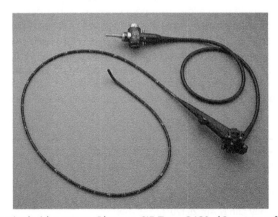

Fig. 1. Small intestinal videoscope: Olympus SIF Type Q180. (*Courtesy of* Olympus, Tokyo, Japan; with permission.)

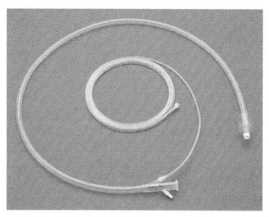

Fig. 2. Single-use splinting tube: ST-SB1. (*Courtesy of* Olympus, Tokyo, Japan; with permission.)

procedures. Of greater importance is whether the primary indication for the procedure has been met by the length of visualized small bowel. Has the abnormality viewed by WCE been identified? Is an encountered hemorrhagic lesion the solitary source of the patient's gastrointestinal (GI) bleeding or are there additional lesions downstream? How numerous is the small bowel polyp burden in a child with Peutz-Jeghers syndrome (PJS)? Such questions may not be easily answered, and the decision as to when to stop the procedure is often left to the degree of clinical suspicion.

To date, DBE has been more described as useful in pediatrics, which is likely less because of a greater advantage of DBE over the alternate technologies, but more because of the longer duration DBE has been commercially available in comparison with SBE (2001 for DBE vs 2007 for SBE). There has been limited literature on the application of SBE in children,[8,15–18] and no published pediatric literature on use of SE. Current consensus holds that although SE has been shown to have comparable safety and efficacy with BAE methods,[19] it is likely to be restricted in use to older adolescents, who are generally large enough to safely tolerate the SE overtube outer diameter of 16 mm.

ENTEROSCOPY TECHNIQUE

The DBE system is available in variable sized models (**Table 1**) and incorporates two separate latex balloons located at the distal ends of the enteroscope and overtube.

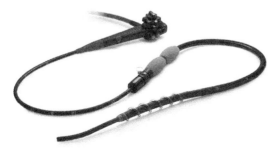

Fig. 3. Discovery sb. (*Courtesy of* Spirus Medical, Stoughton, MA; with permission.)

Table 1
Enteroscope and overtube specifications

	OD (mm)	Working Length (cm)	Total Length (cm)	Accessory Channel (mm)	Overtube Material
DBE					
EN-450P5	8.5	200	230	2.2	—
TS-12140 overtube	12.2	135	145	—	Latex
EN-450T5	9.4	200	230	2.8	—
TS-13140 overtube	13.2	135	145	—	Latex
EC-450BI5	9.4	152	182	2.8	—
TS-13101 overtube	13.2	95	105	—	Latex
SBE					
SIF-Q180	9.2	200	234.5	2.8	—
ST-SB1 overtube	13.2	132	140	—	Silicone
Spiral enteroscopy (Discovery sb)	16	—	118	N/A	PVC

Abbreviations: N/A, not applicable; OD, outer diameter; PVC, polyvinyl chloride.

The balloons are inflatable to a maximum pressure of 45 mm Hg. As described by Yamamoto and colleagues[1] and others,[20] the balloons are inflated and deflated in alternate fashion resulting in deep insertion of the enteroscope.

The SBE system uses a single silicone inflatable balloon fitted at the tip of the overtube only (see **Fig. 2**). A similar push-pull technique is used along with previously described tip deflection or hooking technique of the enteroscope to anchor the instrument in place, as the overtube is advanced followed by a subsequent reduction and pleating of the bowel over the shaft of the scope (**Fig. 4**).[20]

For both techniques, balloon inflation should be performed at a distance safely beyond the ampulla to minimize a patient's risk of developing pancreatitis (author's opinion). Although direct trauma to the ampulla has been theorized to be just one of the mechanisms for the complication of pancreatitis,[4,21,22] the definitive process remains unclear and careful attention by the endoscopist may not completely eliminate the risk.

All endoscopic therapeutic modalities can be applied during BAE, including hemostasis (electrocautery, argon plasma coagulation, endoclip, injection), polypectomy, stricture dilation, and stenting.[13] Therapeutic interventions during enteroscopy should generally be performed when a lesion is first encountered. This avoids the potential misidentification of iatrogenic mucosal trauma as a pre-existing lesion when in fact it resulted from the procedure itself. This includes treatment of arteriovenous malformations and polypectomies, although concern for disrupting a newly treated lesion with the continuation of the enteroscopy exists.

Specific clinical scenarios may represent indications for attempts at complete enteroscopic small bowel examination. This may entail performance of an antegrade and retrograde enteroscopy during two separate anesthesia sessions to optimize the total length of small bowel visualized.[23] This approach may also be beneficial by alleviating operator fatigue and limiting bowel distention from prolonged insufflation.

In the author's opinion, performing a standard colonoscopy before passage of a retrograde enteroscope has the benefit of providing the endoscopist a "roadmap" of the colon. A redundant sigmoid colon may be encountered allowing the provider the anticipation that enteroscope passage may be a greater challenge. The initial

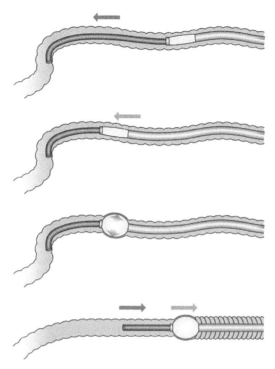

Fig. 4. Operational method of the single-balloon enteroscopy system. (*Courtesy of* Olympus, Tokyo, Japan; with permission.)

passage of a colonoscope also allows a preassessment of the mucosa should the patient not have had a prior colonoscopy, or should new lesions have developed since the last endoscopic evaluation. Initial passage of the colonoscope may also assist in straightening out portions of the colon that would otherwise be difficult to negotiate with the more flexible enteroscope.

During BAE, standard endoscopic maneuvers, including torque, may be significantly restricted with the overtube in place. In addition, insufflation may be partly hindered because of escape of air through a gap that exists between the enteroscope and the overtube.

In patients with a history of abdominal surgery and possible intestinal adhesion formation, there may be appropriate concern for increased risk for perforation or other complication from BAE. Because of the characteristic "push-pull" technique of BAE, care must be undertaken to the smooth advancement and reduction of the enteroscope and overtube, with attention to any significant resistance that may be encountered. This emphasizes the important roles of all participants in the successful performance of BAE, including the coproceduralist handling the overtube, and the need for all members of the team to be vested in the care and safety of the patient.

PATIENT PREPARATION AND PROCEDURAL SEDATION

Fasting is most often all that is required before an antegrade BAE approach. A retrograde approach necessitates a standard pediatric colonoscopy preparation to optimize visualization and procedural success. A recent report outlines various options for bowel preparation for pediatric colonoscopy and may be useful in preparing patients for retrograde BAE.[24]

Although many BAE adult series report the safe and effective use of endoscopist-administered intravenous anesthesia, the choice of sedation for enteroscopy in children is often more variable.[6,8,14,25,26] For standard endoscopy and colonoscopy, a 2005 survey of pediatric gastroenterologists found a roughly equivalent distribution of sedation methods used among endoscopist-administered intravenous sedation, general anesthesia, and anesthesiologist-administered propofol.[27] A more recent report on the sedation methods for pediatric endoscopy suggests several patient-specific factors that should be assessed when considering the choice of sedation including patient age, developmental stage, and the overall health status of the child as defined by the American Society of Anesthesiologists.[28]

For pediatric enteroscopy, use of general anesthesia seems to be more common,[8,14] and may be better suited for the inherent prolonged duration of these procedures. A pediatric Japanese study advocated general anesthesia usage in children undergoing BAE who are younger than 14 years of age, but with the authors indicating that DBE can successfully and safely be performed with endoscopist-administered moderate intravenous sedation in the older adolescent.[6] Regardless of the method of sedation, the endoscopist should choose the available option that is most suitable to their practice, while taking into consideration patient comorbid conditions and the main goal of maximizing patient safety.

INDICATIONS

There are several accepted indications for the performance of BAE in children, including diagnosis and management of obscure GI bleeding (OGIB), inflammatory bowel disease, and polyposis syndromes (**Box 1**).

Obscure Gastrointestinal Bleeding

The role of deep enteroscopy, including BAE, in diagnosing and managing OGIB has been well substantiated and has recently been recognized by endoscopic societies.[29] In adult patients, more than half of all enteroscopies are performed for OGIB.[30] The

---

Box 1
Primary indications for enteroscopy in children

Obscure GI bleeding

Polyposis syndromes

Biliary stricture (eg, Roux-en-Y hepaticojejunostomy post liver transplantation)

Diarrhea

Inflammatory bowel disease/Crohn disease

Foreign body retrieval

Celiac disease (refractory)

Abdominal pain (unexplained)

Protein-losing enteropathy

Vascular malformations (eg, BRBNS)

Abbreviation: BRBNS, blue rubber bleb nevus syndrome.

two largest pediatric series to date of DBE procedures identified OGIB to be the second most common procedure indication.[6,14] When exclusive to this specific indication, the reported adult diagnostic yield has been up to 81%.[31] In pediatrics, the diagnostic yield for OGIB has been found to be 70%.[6] Identified sources of bleeding in children include polyps, ulcers, varices, strictures, and arteriovenous malformations (**Fig. 5**). Additional reports have described identification of Meckel diverticulum (**Fig. 6**) as a source for GI bleeding in children.[32,33]

Inflammatory Bowel Disease/Crohn Disease

There is a growing body of literature reporting the benefits of small bowel enteroscopy in patients with known or suspected diagnosis of Crohn disease (CD).[15,18,34–37] In the adult and pediatric studies, use of BAE in patients with suspected CD has been shown to be of use in confirming the diagnosis; in other cases the enteroscopic findings have effectively ruled it out. When used in children with established CD, findings of significant small bowel inflammation during BAE have been shown to prompt an escalation of medical therapy favorably impacting the course of their disease.[18,37] Successful therapeutic applications have also been described, specifically balloon dilation of small bowel CD strictures.[18,35]

CD may still be suspected when other conventional diagnostic testing has been inconclusive. In a small pediatric series by Di Nardo and colleagues,[18] 12 of 16 pediatric-aged patients with suspected small bowel CD were confirmed to have CD after undergoing SBE. Of these patients with SBE-confirmed CD, WCE was diagnostic in only 30%. Although a small patient cohort, this study demonstrates the potential diagnostic limitations for CD with WCE.

A similar scenario exists for patients with indeterminate colitis being considered for total proctocolectomy. Such patients may benefit from BAE before considering surgery, especially if there are negative findings from other studies, and CD continues to be considered as a possible diagnosis. Indeed, magnetic resonance enterography (MRE) may also have a lower sensitivity for detecting small bowel activity CD compared with BAE, as shown by de Ridder and colleagues.[15] In this pediatric cohort of 20 patients (ages 8–18 years old) with known or suspected CD, the investigators

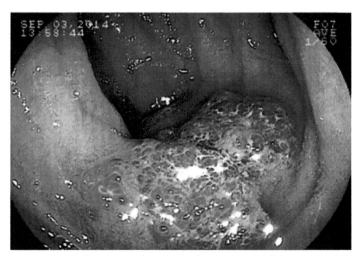

Fig. 5. Jejunal venous malformation. (*Courtesy of* Quin Liu, Children's Hospital Los Angeles, Los Angeles, USA.)

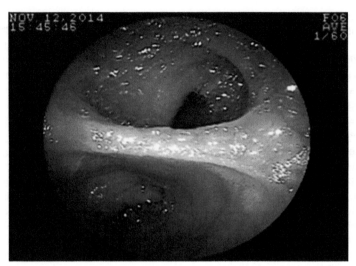

Fig. 6. Meckel diverticulum. (*Courtesy of* Quin Liu, Children's Hospital Los Angeles, Los Angeles, USA.)

identified three patients with isolated jejunal lesions missed by MRE. Moreover, in a recent predominantly adult study that compared MRE findings directly with those on BAE, MRE was found to have a high sensitivity for detecting active small bowel lesions but a low sensitivity for stenoses.[38]

Polyposis Syndromes

Therapeutic enteroscopy has been shown to play an invaluable role in the treatment of children with hereditary polyposis syndromes. Among the polyposis syndromes, PJS patients have been the most described population to benefit the most from BAE, although other populations of children with polyposis syndromes including familial adenomatous polyposis and Cowden disease have also been reported to have had successful intervention with enteroscopy.[6,7,14,16]

Significant morbidity in children with PJS can come from small bowel intussusception necessitating emergent laparotomy that may require a partial bowel resection. Incorporating BAE in the surveillance algorithm for these patients seems to ameliorate such complications.[16] In a report of their institutional experience with SBE management in children with PJS, Bizzarri and colleagues[16] describe successfully removing a combination of 53 pedunculated and sessile polyps from 10 children over 24 months. The one significant complication encountered during this series was a postpolypectomy perforation after resection of a large 6-cm jejunal polyp.

In a similarly sized cohort of 14 patients, Urs and colleagues[14] reported their institutional experience performing 28 DBE procedures in children with PJS undergoing a total of 52 polypectomies, and described some polyps to be as large as 5 cm. In this study, there were no reported complications and the authors' recommended biannual endoscopic surveillance with removal of polyps when found to be greater than 1.5 cm diameter. Additional small case series of children with PJS undergoing BAE also document successful small bowel polyp removal and substantiate the ability of BAE to enable the safe removal of large polyps that would otherwise have a high probability for intussusception.[6,7,26] At this time it seems clear that BAE has had a positive impact on this unique patient population; nevertheless, the optimal timing and size-threshold for removing such polyps has yet to be determined.

Roux-en-Y Altered Anatomy

In recent years, the numbers of patients with Roux-en-Y altered anatomy has greatly increased in line with the greater numbers of gastric bypass and complex liver surgeries (eg, liver transplantation) that are being performed by surgical colleagues. This altered GI anatomy can present a unique set of challenges to the endoscopist, specifically when access to the afferent limb is needed for pancreaticobiliary disease. Bilioenteric anastomotic strictures, recurrent cholangitis, and choledocholithiasis seem to be the more common therapeutic indications for BAE encountered in patients with Roux-en-Y anatomy.[39] Although the successful percutaneous access and treatment of biliary diseases in children with Roux-en-Y anatomy has been described,[40] patients and families often find this to be an undesirable option. Accessibility for endoscopic retrograde cholangiopancreatography (ERCP) has previously been found to be demanding and less technically feasible.[41,42] However, with evolving experience using BAE, significant success in performing ERCP has been achieved in adult and pediatric patients with Roux-en-Y anatomy.[6,43-45]

Nishimura and colleagues[6] reported on their performance of 43 DBE-assisted ERCP procedures on 23 children (age range, 4–17 years) requiring treatment of biliary anastomotic strictures post liver transplantation with Roux-en-Y hepaticojejunostomy. In this study, the hepaticojejunostomy could not be reached in eight of the children, who were then described to undergo percutaneous transhepatic dilatation or other intervention. Thirteen (57%) children were reported to have successful endoscopic therapy, with the remaining two children needing percutaneous transhepatic dilatation because of failed biliary cannulation. Technical success has been equal to that seen in adult patients, with a diagnostic success rate ranging from 60% to 100% and a similar therapeutic success rate.[39] Likely, with greater experience in performing enteroscopy in children with altered GI anatomy, therapeutic endoscopists will attain higher technical success rates.

Supplemental endoscopic techniques for increasing BAE-assisted ERCP success have previously been described.[46,47] These tips focus on the use of DBE, and include use of a transparent cap or hood on the end of the enteroscope allowing for favorable spacing between the hepaticojejunostomy or papilla of Vater, injection of olive oil through the working channel to allow for smoother passage of devices with less drag, and the use of a shorter enteroscope (eg, DBE EC-450BI5) that can facilitate use of conventional ERCP devices.

Effective intubation of the afferent limb of the Roux-en-Y anastomosis also can pose a challenge for an endoscopist. Techniques to ensure technical success have been described to mark the limb that has already been accessed, by application of an endoclip or a mucosal tattoo.[46] A novel method using carbon dioxide enterography was recently described in an adult patient that allowed the investigators the early identification of the afferent loop of a Roux-en-Y anastomosis for biliary investigation, thereby improving procedural efficiency.[48] For those post-Roux-en-Y gastric bypass patients who fail BAE, a laparoscopy-assisted ERCP may be an alternative approach.[49]

COMPLICATIONS

Reported complication rates in adults are 0.8% to 4.8%, with the higher rate resulting from therapeutic interventions.[50,51] Current evidence suggests that BAE in children is similarly safe, because there have been limited reports of major complications. The few significant adverse events reported in children undergoing BAE have included abscess development, postpolypectomy bleeding, and intestinal perforation.[6,26,52] The two largest available pediatric series found a complication rate of 2.7% (3 of 113 procedures) and 1.1% (1 of 92 procedures).[6,14] Comparative complications associated with the performance of BAE in adult and pediatric patients are listed in **Table 2**.

Early experience with BAE in children identified postprocedural abdominal pain and discomfort to be common occurrences that typically were self-limiting and mild.[6,7] This complication of BAE seems to be less common in more recent publications, which may be because of the growing number of institutions incorporating carbon dioxide (CO_2) insufflation in their endoscopy units. Carbon dioxide is more readily absorbed from the bowel, and has been shown to cause less postprocedural pain and bowel distention during colonoscopy. To date, there has been inconsistent benefits reported when CO_2 is used for ERCP and BAE,[53] and this should be a focus for future studies. Nonetheless, the use of CO_2 insufflation has been advocated for patients with altered GI anatomy based on the rare occurrence of a fatal air embolism.[54]

TRAINING AND COMPETENCE

No formal, accredited training program for learning to perform BAE in either adults and/or children currently exists. Several courses and conferences are held periodically, which may provide an opportunity for attendees to gain hands-on introduction to the technique, but such limited exposure is insufficient to provide the necessary training in a technique that entails a steep learning curve. In the absence of specific training curriculum, the achievement of procedural competence is often gained from hands-on exposure under the tutelage of an already accomplished therapeutic endoscopist skilled in BAE. Based on available adult literature, the learning curve for antegrade DBE procedures has been estimated to be approximately 10 cases[55] with a similar procedure volume for all enteroscopy techniques (including SBE and SE) suggested in a more recent publication.[56] Because the retrograde approach is believed to be more technically challenging due to the need for ileocecal valve intubation, a greater number of cases (estimated at 20–30) is often needed to gain the appropriate skill to independently perform these procedures safely and successfully.[20,57] The use of fluoroscopy for the first several cases of antegrade and retrograde intubation is helpful to the endoscopist to improve their conceptualization of the push-pull technique and to assist in the recognition of looping that may impede scope advancement.

It has been expressed that performing BAE in children is technically more difficult than in adults.[6] Whether an endoscopist should achieve a level of proficiency on adult patients before performing such procedures in children has yet to be determined.

Table 2	
Enteroscopy complications	
Adult Complications	**Pediatric Complications**
Acute pancreatitis	Perforation
Perforation	GI bleeding
GI bleeding	Hypotension
Mallory-Weiss syndrome	Intra-abdominal abscess (unclear relation)
Sedation related (eg, aspiration pneumonia)	
Intussusception	
Air embolism (rare)	

SPECIAL CONSIDERATIONS

The old adage that "children are just small adults" has long been shown to be inaccurate. Unfortunately, endoscopic technology for use in pediatric patients often lags behind that of adult patients, and adult endoscopic equipment may often be too large for the smallest of children. Thankfully, the inflatable balloons available on the DBE and SBE systems are air pressure monitored and can safely accommodate the smaller luminal size of the small bowel in children as young as 3 (retrograde) and 4 years of age.[6,10,37] In fact, in one series, BAE was described to be safely performed in a 12-month-old, 7.92-kg child without complication.[14] In contrast, Uchida and colleagues[37] has suggested that use of the smaller DBE enteroscope (DBE enteroscope EN-450P5, see **Table 1**) by the antegrade approach may be too large for children 3 years of age. Nonetheless, until smaller instruments are developed, special considerations need to be made when younger children undergo BAE.

Furthermore, because of the technical demands of BAE, such procedures should be performed during fully staffed hospital shifts, and ideally avoided after standard hours or on the weekends, when adequate staff and assistance may be limited.

SUMMARY

Small bowel enteroscopy, specifically BAE, has established itself as a valuable, minimally invasive modality in the treatment of small bowel disorders in adults and children. The diagnostic and therapeutic success rate in children is comparable with those found in adult studies. As the knowledge of the use and indications of BAE grows, the use of BAE in children will continue to advance. In the future, central obstacles to overcome include gaining an improved understanding of the safety of performing BAE in children, a broader availability to expert facilities skilled in the performance of this procedure, and well-defined training guidelines to ensure future competent providers. Development of smaller instruments capable of being used in smaller children will further expand the application of BAE to the pediatric age group.

REFERENCES

1. Yamamoto H, Sekine Y, Sato Y, et al. Total enteroscopy with a nonsurgical steerable double-balloon method. Gastrointest Endosc 2001;53(2):216–20.
2. Gross SA, Stark ME. Initial experience with double-balloon enteroscopy at a U.S. center. Gastrointest Endosc 2008;67(6):890–7.
3. Tsujikawa T, Saitoh Y, Andoh A, et al. Novel single-balloon enteroscopy for diagnosis and treatment of the small intestine: preliminary experiences. Endoscopy 2008;40(1):11–5.
4. Heine GD, Hadithi M, Groenen MJ, et al. Double-balloon enteroscopy: indications, diagnostic yield, and complications in a series of 275 patients with suspected small-bowel disease. Endoscopy 2006;38(1):42–8.
5. Domagk D, Mensink P, Aktas H, et al. Single- vs. double-balloon enteroscopy in small-bowel diagnostics: a randomized multicenter trial. Endoscopy 2011;43(6): 472–6.
6. Nishimura N, Yamamoto H, Yano T, et al. Safety and efficacy of double-balloon enteroscopy in pediatric patients. Gastrointest Endosc 2010;71(2):287–94.
7. Lin TK, Erdman SH. Double-balloon enteroscopy: pediatric experience. J Pediatr Gastroenterol Nutr 2010;51(4):429–32.
8. Barth BA, Channabasappa N. Single-balloon enteroscopy in children: initial experience at a pediatric center. J Pediatr Gastroenterol Nutr 2010;51(5):680–4.

9. Xu CD, Deng CH, Zhong J, et al. Application of double-balloon push enteroscopy in diagnosis of small bowel disease in children. Zhonghua Er Ke Za Zhi 2006; 44(2):90–2 [In Chinese].

10. Leung YK. Double balloon endoscopy in pediatric patients. Gastrointest Endosc 2007;66(Suppl 3):S54–6.

11. Hartmann D, Eickhoff A, Tamm R, et al. Balloon-assisted enteroscopy using a single-balloon technique. Endoscopy 2007;39(Suppl 1):E276.

12. Akerman PA, Agrawal D, Cantero D, et al. Spiral enteroscopy with the new DSB overtube: a novel technique for deep peroral small-bowel intubation. Endoscopy 2008;40(12):974–8.

13. Yamamoto H, Kita H, Sunada K, et al. Clinical outcomes of double-balloon endoscopy for the diagnosis and treatment of small-intestinal diseases. Clin Gastroenterol Hepatol 2004;2(11):1010–6.

14. Urs AN, Martinelli M, Rao P, et al. Diagnostic and therapeutic utility of double-balloon enteroscopy in children. J Pediatr Gastroenterol Nutr 2014;58(2): 204–12.

15. de Ridder L, Mensink PB, Lequin MH, et al. Single-balloon enteroscopy, magnetic resonance enterography, and abdominal US useful for evaluation of small-bowel disease in children with (suspected) Crohn's disease. Gastrointest Endosc 2012; 75(1):87–94.

16. Bizzarri B, Borrelli O, de'Angelis N, et al. Management of duodenal-jejunal polyps in children with Peutz-Jeghers syndrome with single-balloon enteroscopy. J Pediatr Gastroenterol Nutr 2014;59(1):49–53.

17. Oliva S, Pennazio M, Cohen SA, et al. Capsule endoscopy followed by single balloon enteroscopy in children with obscure gastrointestinal bleeding: a combined approach. Dig Liver Dis 2015;47(2):125–30.

18. Di Nardo G, Oliva S, Aloi M, et al. Usefulness of single-balloon enteroscopy in pediatric Crohn's disease. Gastrointest Endosc 2012;75(1):80–6.

19. Morgan D, Upchurch B, Draganov P, et al. Spiral enteroscopy: prospective U.S. multicenter study in patients with small-bowel disorders. Gastrointest Endosc 2010;72(5):992–8.

20. Gerson LB, Flodin JT, Miyabayashi K. Balloon-assisted enteroscopy: technology and troubleshooting. Gastrointest Endosc 2008;68(6):1158–67.

21. Groenen MJ, Moreels TG, Orlent H, et al. Acute pancreatitis after double-balloon enteroscopy: an old pathogenetic theory revisited as a result of using a new endoscopic tool. Endoscopy 2006;38(1):82–5.

22. Honda K, Mizutani T, Nakamura K, et al. Acute pancreatitis associated with peroral double-balloon enteroscopy: a case report. World J Gastroenterol 2006;12(11):1802–4.

23. Teshima CW, Aktas H, van Buuren HR, et al. Retrograde double balloon enteroscopy: comparing performance of solely retrograde versus combined same-day anterograde and retrograde procedure. Scand J Gastroenterol 2011;46(2): 220–6.

24. Pall H, Zacur GM, Kramer RE, et al. Bowel preparation for pediatric colonoscopy: report of the NASPGHAN endoscopy and procedures committee. J Pediatr Gastroenterol Nutr 2014;59(3):409–16.

25. Liu W, Xu C, Zhong J. The diagnostic value of double-balloon enteroscopy in children with small bowel disease: report of 31 cases. Can J Gastroenterol 2009; 23(9):635–8.

26. Thomson M, Venkatesh K, Elmalik K, et al. Double balloon enteroscopy in children: diagnosis, treatment, and safety. World J Gastroenterol 2010;16(1):56–62.

27. Lightdale JR, Mahoney LB, Schwarz SM, et al. Methods of sedation in pediatric endoscopy: a survey of NASPGHAN members. J Pediatr Gastroenterol Nutr 2007;45(4):500–2.

28. Fredette ME, Lightdale JR. Endoscopic sedation in pediatric practice. Gastrointest Endosc Clin N Am 2008;18(4):739–51.

29. Fisher L, Lee Krinsky M, Anderson MA, et al. The role of endoscopy in the management of obscure GI bleeding. Gastrointest Endosc 2010;72(3):471–9.

30. Xin L, Liao Z, Jiang YP, et al. Indications, detectability, positive findings, total enteroscopy, and complications of diagnostic double-balloon endoscopy: a systematic review of data over the first decade of use. Gastrointest Endosc 2011;74(3):563–70.

31. Zhong J, Ma T, Zhang C, et al. A retrospective study of the application on double-balloon enteroscopy in 378 patients with suspected small-bowel diseases. Endoscopy 2007;39(3):208–15.

32. Chen SM, Sheu JN, Wu TT, et al. Double-balloon enteroscopy for bleeding Meckel's diverticulum in a child younger than 4 years of age. Gastrointest Endosc 2009;70(2):398–400.

33. Zheng CF, Huang Y, Tang ZF, et al. Double-balloon enteroscopy for the diagnosis of Meckel's diverticulum in pediatric patients with obscure GI bleeding. Gastrointest Endosc 2014;79(2):354–8.

34. Rahman A, Ross A, Leighton JA, et al. Double-balloon enteroscopy in Crohn's disease: findings and impact on management in a multicenter retrospective study. Gastrointest Endosc 2015;82(1):102–7.

35. Despott EJ, Gupta A, Burling D, et al. Effective dilation of small-bowel strictures by double-balloon enteroscopy in patients with symptomatic Crohn's disease (with video). Gastrointest Endosc 2009;70(5):1030–6.

36. Di Nardo G, Aloi M, Oliva S, et al. Investigation of small bowel in pediatric Crohn's disease. Inflamm Bowel Dis 2012;18(9):1760–76.

37. Uchida K, Yoshiyama S, Inoue M, et al. Double balloon enteroscopy for pediatric inflammatory bowel disease. Pediatr Int 2012;54(6):806–9.

38. Takenaka K, Ohtsuka K, Kitazume Y, et al. Comparison of magnetic resonance and balloon enteroscopic examination of the small intestine in patients with Crohn's disease. Gastroenterology 2014;147(2):334–42.e3.

39. Moreels TG. Altered anatomy: enteroscopy and ERCP procedure. Best Pract Res Clin Gastroenterol 2012;26(3):347–57.

40. Racadio JM, Kukreja K. Pediatric biliary interventions. Tech Vasc Interv Radiol 2010;13(4):244–9.

41. Elton E, Hanson BL, Qaseem T, et al. Diagnostic and therapeutic ERCP using an enteroscope and a pediatric colonoscope in long-limb surgical bypass patients. Gastrointest Endosc 1998;47(1):62–7.

42. Gostout CJ, Bender CE. Cholangiopancreatography, sphincterotomy, and common duct stone removal via Roux-en-Y limb enteroscopy. Gastroenterology 1988;95(1):156–63.

43. Shimatani M, Matsushita M, Takaoka M, et al. Effective "short" double-balloon enteroscope for diagnostic and therapeutic ERCP in patients with altered gastrointestinal anatomy: a large case series. Endoscopy 2009;41(10):849–54.

44. Shah RJ, Smolkin M, Yen R, et al. A multicenter, U.S. experience of single-balloon, double-balloon, and rotational overtube-assisted enteroscopy ERCP in patients with surgically altered pancreaticobiliary anatomy (with video). Gastrointest Endosc 2013;77(4):593–600.

45. Itokawa F, Itoi T, Ishii K, et al. Single- and double-balloon enteroscopy-assisted endoscopic retrograde cholangiopancreatography in patients with Roux-en-Y

plus hepaticojejunostomy anastomosis and Whipple resection. Dig Endosc 2014; 26(Suppl 2):136–43.

46. Hatanaka H, Yano T, Tamada K. Tips and tricks of double-balloon endoscopic retrograde cholangiopancreatography (with video). J Hepatobiliary Pancreat Sci 2015;22(6):E28–34.

47. Shimatani M, Takaoka M, Okazaki K. Tips for double balloon enteroscopy in patients with Roux-en-Y reconstruction and modified child surgery. J Hepatobiliary Pancreat Sci 2014;21(4):E22–8.

48. Fukuba N, Moriyama I, Ishihara S, et al. Carbon dioxide enterography: a useful method for double-balloon enteroscopy-assisted ERCP. Endoscopy 2014; 46(Suppl 1 UCTN):E587–8.

49. Schreiner MA, Chang L, Gluck M, et al. Laparoscopy-assisted versus balloon enteroscopy-assisted ERCP in bariatric post-Roux-en-Y gastric bypass patients. Gastrointest Endosc 2012;75(4):748–56.

50. Mensink PB, Haringsma J, Kucharzik T, et al. Complications of double balloon enteroscopy: a multicenter survey. Endoscopy 2007;39(7):613–5.

51. Aktas H, de Ridder L, Haringsma J, et al. Complications of single-balloon enteroscopy: a prospective evaluation of 166 procedures. Endoscopy 2010;42(5): 365–8.

52. Spahn TW, Kampmann W, Eilers M, et al. Small-bowel perforation after endoscopic resection of a Peutz-Jeghers polyp in an infant using double-balloon enteroscopy. Endoscopy 2007;39(Suppl 1):E217.

53. Wang WL, Wu ZH, Sun Q, et al. Meta-analysis: the use of carbon dioxide insufflation vs. room air insufflation for gastrointestinal endoscopy. Aliment Pharmacol Ther 2012;35(10):1145–54.

54. Yamamoto H. Be aware of the fatal risk of air embolism. Dig Endosc 2014; 26(1):23.

55. Mehdizadeh S, Ross A, Gerson L, et al. What is the learning curve associated with double-balloon enteroscopy? Technical details and early experience in 6 U.S. tertiary care centers. Gastrointest Endosc 2006;64(5):740–50.

56. Schafer ME, Lo SK. Navigating beyond the ligament of Treitz: an introduction to learning enteroscopy. Gastrointest Endosc 2010;71(6):1029–32.

57. Mehdizadeh S, Han NJ, Cheng DW, et al. Success rate of retrograde double-balloon enteroscopy. Gastrointest Endosc 2007;65(4):633–9.

Advances in Pediatric Gastrostomy Placement

Maireade E. McSweeney, MD, MPH[a],*, C. Jason Smithers, MD[b]

KEYWORDS

- Gastrostomy • Percutaneous endoscopic gastrostomy • Gastrojejunostomy
- Enteral feeding • Laparoscopic gastrostomy • Complications • Children

KEY POINTS

- Percutaneous endoscopic gastrostomy (PEG) is a common method of establishing an indwelling gastrostomy tube that can support infants and children with a host of complex medical issues.
- PEG placement is generally safe, but can be associated with a range of intraprocedural and postprocedural complications, with most occurring within the first year of placement.
- Laparoscopic gastrostomy is a burgeoning, minimally invasive method for gastrostomy tube placement that may avoid the routine need for exchange to a balloon-based device.
- Regardless of method of placement, a focus on long-term pediatric enteral tube care represents a critical component of improving outcomes of gastrostomy tubes in children.

BACKGROUND

Placement of gastrostomy tubes were first developed as a method for enteral feeding in children and adults in the late nineteenth and early twentieth century.[1] Initial gastrostomies were established via open surgical approaches, such as the Stamm gastrostomy procedure, which still remains a commonly used method for primary gastrostomy tube placement in the United States and internationally.[1]

With ongoing advances in surgical techniques and the increasing demand for less invasive methods of enteral access, newer gastrostomy techniques have emerged as feasible and safe in children. In 1980, percutaneous endoscopic gastrostomy

Disclosure Statement: All authors have no conflicts of interest and no funding resources to disclose.
[a] Division of Gastroenterology and Nutrition, Department of Medicine, Boston Children's Hospital, Harvard Medical School, 300 Longwood Avenue, Boston, MA 02115, USA; [b] Department of General Surgery, Boston Children's Hospital, Harvard Medical School, 300 Longwood Avenue, Boston, MA 02115, USA
* Corresponding author. Division of Pediatric Gastroenterology and Nutrition, Boston Children's Hospital, 300 Longwood Avenue, Boston, MA 02115.
E-mail address: maireade.mcsweeney@childrens.harvard.edu

Gastrointest Endoscopy Clin N Am 26 (2016) 169–185
http://dx.doi.org/10.1016/j.giec.2015.09.001
1052-5157/16/$ – see front matter © 2016 Elsevier Inc. All rights reserved.

(also known as the PEG procedure) was codeveloped by a pediatric surgeon, M.W.L. Gauderer, and a gastroenterologist, J.L. Ponsky, as a novel, minimally invasive endoscopic-based technique for primary gastrostomy tube placement.[2] Since its development, the PEG procedure has been adopted by both adult and pediatric surgeons, gastroenterologists, and radiologists, as a method of gastrostomy tube placement that can be performed in a variety of settings. It also has quickly become one of the most common approaches to primary gastrostomy tube placement in infants and children.[3–7]

Within pediatrics, the PEG procedure has proved effective in a variety of patient populations with complex medical needs. In particular, it has been shown to be safe to perform in small infants, even those weighing less than 6 kg, and in patients with complex neurologic disability, congenital heart disease, cancer, or other complex medical comorbidities.[2,3,8–11] The PEG procedure has also proved beneficial in that helps to minimize exposure to anesthesia, requires a less invasive surgical approach, may occur outside of operating room settings, and is associated with both rapid postoperative recovery times and initiation of enteral feedings. In addition, PEG stomas are considered likely to spontaneously close, when and if a patient elects to remove the gastrostomy tube.[12–14]

PERCUTANEOUS ENDOSCOPIC GASTROSTOMY PROCEDURE

The classic PEG procedure uses a pull technique.[2] At the start of the procedure, after a standardized antiseptic skin preparation is applied to the abdomen and antibiotics are provided to the patient, a gastroscope is inserted through the patient's mouth and into the stomach. Gastric distension is then performed by air insufflation, which in turn inflates the anterior gastric wall up against the abdominal wall. Transillumination of the abdominal wall by the lighted gastroscope is then visualized externally in the mid-epigastrium to guide placement, and a small stab abdominal incision is performed through which a needle, followed by a guide wire, are passed. This wire is then snared by the gastroscope, pulled out in a retrograde fashion from the stomach, through the esophagus, into the mouth, and released. A PEG tube is then tied to this wire, lubricated, and pulled back down through the mouth, esophagus, and stomach, affixing the gastric and abdominal walls together. The gastroscope is then reintroduced to confirm intragastric position of the PEG tube, and an external bumper is applied to secure the tube against the skin.[5,15,16]

As a primary tube, a PEG will typically be left in place for a minimum of 6 weeks to 6 months, after which time it may be permanently removed, or exchanged for a skin-level or other balloon-based gastrostomy if the patient continues to require an indwelling tube. A PEG exchange can be accomplished by 1 of 2 basic methods: (1) performing a percutaneous pull, or (2) performing an endoscopic exchange of the PEG tube via endoscopic snaring and retrograde removal of the PEG inner bolster.[17] The latter generally involves general anesthesia and allows for easy visual confirmation of the new intragastric position of the gastrostomy tube using the endoscope; whereas a percutaneous pull may require minimal or even no sedation, and is most safely immediately followed by fluoroscopy to confirm the intragastric position of the new tube.[17]

Complications of Percutaneous Endoscopic Gastrostomy

Since its original description, the PEG procedure has been widely adopted. In turn, multiple PEG-related complications have been documented (**Box 1**).[3,15,18,19] Published retrospective rates of complications associated with the PEG procedure have

---

Box 1
List of reported complications associated with PEG procedure

- Intraprocedural
  - Esophageal injury or perforation
  - Other abdominal visceral injury
  - Pneumoperitoneum
  - Hemoperitoneum
  - Gastrocolocutaneous fistula
  - Peritonitis

- Postprocedural
  - Bowel or gastric volvulus
  - Abdominal wall bleeding
  - Gastric bleeding or ulceration
  - Buried bumper syndrome
  - Gastric outlet obstruction
  - PEG tract disruption with tube exchange
  - PEG tube dislodgement
  - PEG tube malfunction (tube clogging, breakage, and so forth)

- Stoma-related
  - Abscess
  - Cellulitis
  - Peristomal leakage
  - Peristomal pain
  - Granulation tissue
  - Stomal gastric herniation

- Patient feeding intolerance
  - Ileus
  - Gastroparesis
  - Exacerbation of gastroesophageal reflux disease
  - Aspiration
  - Post-PEG placement diarrhea

---

varied, ranging from 4% to almost 50%, and likely reflect varied definitions of PEG-related complications (**Table 1**).[3,4,6,7,12,18,20–26] One recent prospective study of 103 patients undergoing PEG placement by surgeons at a single institution reported a total major complication rate of 14%.[27]

Various reports of complications have categorized and defined complications according to whether the complication occurs perioperatively or postoperatively. There have also been widely different definitions of early versus late postoperative complications. **Table 1** lists reported complication rates according to individual study definitions.[3,4,7,18,25,26] Other investigators have categorized complications based on whether the complication was related to the procedure versus the tube, whether it involved a stoma-related issue, or was related to patient feeding intolerance or change in clinical status (eg, worsening gastroesophageal reflux disease, aspiration pneumonia).[4,7,8,12,18–20,25,26]

PEG complications have also been defined as minor or major (**Table 2**).[6,21–24,28] Major complications, or those that are severe in nature, are often defined as adverse patient events requiring urgent evaluation, hospitalization, or repeat surgical or other interventional procedures.[18,21,28] The authors' group performed a long-term outcome study of a cohort of patients who received PEGs at Boston Children's Hospital from April 1999 through December 2000 (n = 138) and followed them up to 10 years. In this retrospective survival analysis, which focused on time from placement to a first

Table 1
Pediatric literature examining early versus late complication rates after PEG placement

Authors,[Ref.] Year	No. of PEGs	Complication Rate	Early Complications	Late Complications
Lalanne et al,[25] 2014 France	368	Early (≤7 d after PEG placement): 43% Late (>7 d after PEG placement): 56%	Sepsis, aspiration pneumonia, failure of PEG placement, gastric bleeding, cellulitis, local erythema, wound infection, transient ileus, pain, leakage, pneumoperitoneum	Surgical closure of stoma, gastric ulcer, cutaneous necrosis, intragastric buried or extruded tube, catheter migration, gastrocolic fistula, cellulitis, granulation tissue, erythema, leakage, wound infection, other
Park et al,[7] 2011 Korea	32	Overall complication rate: 47% Early (<48 h): 25% Late (>48 h): 22%	Pneumoperitoneum, pneumomediastinum, paralytic ileus, atelectasis	Wound infection, worsening gastroesophageal reflux disease, gastrocolic fistula
Fortunato et al,[3] 2010 Baltimore, MD	747	Overall complication rate: 12% Early (during hospitalization for PEG): 3.7% Late (after hospital discharge): 20%	Gastric separation, wound infection, pneumoperitoneum, cutaneous necrosis, failure of PEG placement	Gastrocolic fistula, wound infection, granulation tissue, pressure necrosis, wound infection
Sathesh-Kumar et al,[12] 2009 England	172	Overall complication rate: 28%	PEG infection, leakage, bowel obstruction due to tube migration, fever of unknown origin, chest infection	PEG infection, buried bumper, worsening gastroesophageal reflux disease, tube migration, gastrocutaneous fistula, gastrocolic fistula, overgrowth of gastric mucosa

Study	N	Complication rate	Major complications	Minor complications
Avitsland et al,[4] 2006 Norway	121	Early (<30 d postop.): 12% Late (>30 d postop.): not reported	Stoma-related infection, pneumonia, tube dislodgment	Stoma infection, tube dislodgment, skin problems, pain, leakage, granulation tissue, gastrocolonic fistula, internal bumper in esophagus (with a tracheoesophageal fistula)
Segal et al,[26] 2001 France	110	Late complication rate (>6 d after placement): 44% (26% patients had at least one complication)	Not reported	Intragastric buried/extruded button, granulation tissue, pseudotumoral proliferative gastric mucosa, mucosal ulceration, cutaneous necrosis, gastrocolic fistula, delay of stoma closure postremoval, subcostal neuralgia, peritonitis
Fox et al,[18] 1997 Boston, MA	137	Overall complication rate: 12.4% Early (<2 wk after placement): 7.3% Late (>2 wk after placement): 5.1%	Cellulitis, gastrocolic fistula, duodenal hematoma, pneumoperitoneum	Cellulitis, fasciitis, gastrocolic fistula, gastric perforation, catheter migration

Abbreviation: PEG, percutaneous endoscopic gastrostomy.

Table 2
Pediatric retrospective reviews examining major versus minor complication rates after PEG placement

Authors,[Ref.] Year	No. of PEGs	Complication Rate	Major Complications	Minor Complications
McSweeney et al,[21] 2015 Boston, MA	591	Major: 10.5% Minor: 16.5%	Cellulitis requiring hospitalization, tract disruption with PEG exchange, surgical resection of granulation tissue, perforation of colon/viscera, pneumoperitoneum, other	Infection treated with oral antibiotics, PEG dislodgment, other minor complications
McSweeney et al,[28] 2013 Boston, MA	138	Overall major complication rate: 11%	Cellulitis requiring hospitalization, surgical resection of granulation tissue, tube dislodgment, intraoperative PEG complication	Not reported
Vervloessem et al,[22] 2009 Belgium	448 PEGs and 19 lap-PEGs	Overall major complication rate: 12.6%	Any complication requiring repeat surgery/endoscopy, treatment antibiotics, blood transfusion, leading to death	Not reported
Zamakhshary et al,[23] 2005 Canada	93 PEGs and 26 lap-PEGs	Overall complication rate: 14% (7.7% lap-PEGs)	Transcolonic tube placement, failed PEG tube placement, peritonitis, tract disruption with PEG exchange	Nonspecific complications noted (including aspiration pneumonia, persistent fistula on tube removal, excessive granulation tissue requiring surgical debridement)
van der Merwe et al,[24] 2003 South Africa	70	Overall complication rate: 6%	Esophageal perforation, significant stomal complication, submucosal bumper migration (buried bumper syndrome), sepsis	Not reported
Khattak et al,[6] 1998 England	130	Major: 17.5% Minor: 22.5%	Development or exacerbation of gastroesophageal reflux, severe stoma complications, peritonitis (early or later with PEG exchange), failed PEG tube placement, gastrocolocutaneous fistula, intestinal obstruction, major hemorrhage, external migration of inner bolster, sepsis, death	Peristomal leakage, infection, granulation tissue, recurrent chest infections, pain, PEG tube related problems, feeding intolerance, difficulty in teaching parent to use gastrostomy, single-episode hematemesis, retained inner bolster

Abbreviation: lap-PEG, laparoscopically assisted PEG.

major complication; most major PEG-related complications were postprocedural, and tended to occur within the first 6 months to 1 year of placement (**Fig. 1**).[28] The cumulative incidence rate of patients having a major complication was 9.4% at 6 months (95% confidence interval [CI] 5.3%–16.4%), 10.4% (95% CI 6%–17.6%) at 1 year, and 15% (95% CI 8.9%–24.5%) by 65 months (5.4 years; see **Fig. 1**).

In addition, despite several initiatives focused on standardizing PEG tube placement at the author's institution, including use of a consistent 2-person placement technique, regular administration of intraoperative antibiotics, and exchange after 6 months, the group has repeatedly and reported a steady 11% to 12% major complication rate and 16% minor complication rate over the last 20 years.[18,21,28] Most recently the authors have implemented a standardized postoperative PEG-monitoring protocol for patients being discharged home, based on hopes that a focus on postplacement care will decrease complications; however, the outcomes of such protocols remain to be seen.

Risk Factors for Complications of Percutaneous Endoscopic Gastrostomy in Children

Several studies have explored risk factors for developing PEG complications in children, including age, comorbidities, and methods of placement.[3,21,22] In addition, Vervloessem and colleagues[21,22] have suggested that the presence of a preoperative ventriculoperitoneal shunt may be a risk factor for PEG tube complications. The authors' group recently reviewed a total of 591 PEG placements at Boston Children's

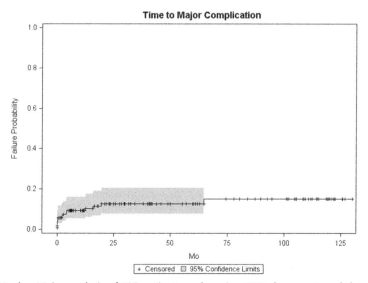

Fig. 1. Kaplan-Meier analysis of 138 patients undergoing PEG placement, and the proportion going on to experience a major complication over a 10-year follow-up period. The shaded area represents the 95% confidence interval (CI). The cumulative incidence rate of patients having a major complication was 15% (95% CI 8.9%–24.5%) by 65 months (5.4 years), with most complications taking place within the first 6 to 12 months of PEG placement. (*Adapted from* McSweeney ME, Jiang H, Deutsch AJ, et al. Long-term outcomes of infants and children undergoing percutaneous endoscopy gastrostomy tube placement. J Pediatr Gastroenterol Nutr 2013;57(5):666; with permission.)

Hospital over 5 years and assessed for risk factors for development of major complications within 6 months of PEG placement.[21] In this study younger age, American Society of Anesthesiologists (ASA) grade III, and presence of a neurologic disorder were found to be protective against developing a major PEG procedural complication, perhaps because of higher intensity of postprocedural and long-term monitoring (**Fig. 2**).[21] Nevertheless, the presence of a ventriculoperitoneal shunt was found in this cohort, as had been described previously, to be a risk factor for PEG-associated major complications (see **Fig. 2**).[21,22] Therefore, the authors agree that the presence of a ventriculoperitoneal shunt in a child should warrant consideration for exploration of alternative methods to PEG for gastrostomy tube placement.

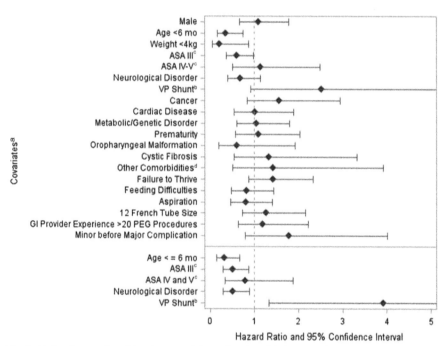

Fig. 2. Univariate and multivariate models evaluating risk factors of major complications after PEG placement. [a] Covariates listed above the horizontal line are risk factors studied in univariate Cox proportional hazards regression models. Covariates listed below the horizontal line are risk factors achieving significance at $P \leq .05$ level in multivariate Cox proportional hazards regression model. All horizontal lines represent the hazard ratio with associated 95% CI. Covariates are defined as having (versus not having) the above listed characteristics (the only exception is ASA variables whereby patients with ASA I–II were used as the reference group). Diamonds represent point estimates of the hazard ratio. [b] 95% CI for the hazard ratio in univariate and multivariate models were too wide because of the small sample size of patients with ventriculoperitoneal (VP) shunt, hence the upper limit was truncated in the plot. The upper limit for 95% CI was 6.96 in the univariate Cox model and 11.66 in the multivariate Cox model ($P<.05$). [c] ASA = reference group ASA grades I and II. [d] Other comorbidities included renal, immunodeficiency, and gastrointestinal disorders. (*Adapted from* McSweeney ME, Kerr J, Jiang H, et al. Risk factors for complications in infants and children with percutaneous endoscopic gastrostomy tubes. J Pediatr 2015;166(6):1517.e1; with permission.)

Exchange and Removal of Percutaneous Endoscopic Gastrostomy

The process of exchanging a PEG for a balloon-based gastrostomy tube, although simple in theory, has also been well described to be fraught with complications.[4,17,21,23,28] One major complication directly associated with using a percutaneous pull method is tract disruption at the time of exchange.[4,17,21,23,28] In the authors' study, the rate of tract disruption during percutaneous pull of the PEG was found to be approximately 2% across all 5 years of patient follow-up.[21] Owing to the potential for this complication, and the well-described "silent nature" of the disruption, it has been strongly recommended that fluoroscopic confirmation be performed to confirm intragastric position of the new gastrostomy tube whenever a percutaneous PEG pull is performed.[4,17,21,23,28]

As an alternative approach, the endoscopic PEG-exchange method is often thought to be more beneficial in that it has a decreased risk of tract disruption or trauma, and allows for visual confirmation of the new position of the gastrostomy tube after the exchange has taken place. It should also be noted that many parents describe increased stoma-related issues of pain and worsened granulation tissue following a traumatic PEG exchange, and the endoscopic approach theoretically helps avoid this. Of course, the major downside of the endoscopic method is its need for a second general anesthetic. In children who often have complex medical issues and who are at high risk for complications of general anesthesia, this may not be a small concern.

In adults, the "cut-and-push" method, which allows for spontaneous passage of the PEG internal bolster, has been used.[29] This method is not typically recommended in pediatric patients because of the potentially higher risk of esophageal perforation or retained PEG pieces, which has been reported to lead to nonhealing gastrocutaneous fistulas or symptoms of gastric outlet obstruction from PEG components.[17,30] Complications of the cut-and-push method have been reported to take place in children almost immediately after the exchange, or even months after initial PEG exchange or removal. In turn, either percutaneous PEG pull or endoscopic removal remains the preferred method for PEG exchange in children.[30]

PEG removal with no tube replacement (also known as permanent PEG removal) via either method is generally associated with spontaneous stoma healing. A 2004 report by El-Rifai and colleagues[14] of 296 PEG tubes and 16 surgically placed gastrostomies found that only 8 of 28 permanently removed PEGs resulted in a nonhealing stoma site 1 month after removal and required surgical closure. In this study, there were no differences in patients' underlying disease status, age, and weight at gastrostomy insertion or removal; moreover, patients' gastrostomy size, length, and presence of stomal infection or granulation tissue were found not to affect the healing of the gastrocutaneous fistula.[14] The only major predictor of a persistent gastrocutaneous fistula after tube removal was the length of time the gastrostomy or PEG tube had been in place (with patients with nonhealing stoma sites having a gastrostomy in place for 39 ± 19 months, versus closed stoma sites having been in place for 22 ± 23 months; $P<.03$).[14]

Alternative Percutaneous Endoscopic Gastrostomy Techniques

With ongoing reported complication rates associated with PEG placement, and its common need in children for exchange to a skin-level or balloon-based gastrostomy device, alternatives to the classic PEG pull placement technique have been developed.[23,31,32] One of the first advances in the mid-1990s was the "one-step PEG."[33,34] The one-step PEG procedure uses a push method of button placement over a guide wire through an abdominal incision.[33] Using the one-step technique, a gastrostomy button is deployed in the stomach, and its intragastric position is confirmed by endoscopy.[33] This method offers the benefit of endoscopically placing a low-profile, skin-level device during the first gastrostomy procedure; thereby avoiding the need for future endoscopic or percutaneous exchange.[31] There may also be decreased health care costs using this procedure.[32–34]

However, complications after one-step PEGs have been reported to occur at rates similar to those of traditional PEG procedures.[35,36] Reported complications after one-step PEGs have included cellulitis, formation of granulation tissue, skin breakdown, stoma leakage, tract dilation, and gastrostomy migration.[32–37] Tract migration is one of the major complications reported with one-step PEGs, as it can be associated with cellulitis, peritonitis, and eventual gastrostomy removal and replacement.[32–34] With any one-step PEG, careful measurements of stoma length must be obtained at the time of placement to decrease the risk of tract disruptions during short-term and long-term postoperative periods. The development of technical expertise in placing one-step PEGs has been found to reduce the associated complication rate.[32]

Depending on available resources and staffing at various institutions, other methods for percutaneous gastrostomy tube placement have been implemented. In particular, image-guided placement of percutaneous gastrostomy and gastrojejunostomy tubes by interventional radiologists using fluoroscopy has been described, along with complication rates in pediatric patients comparable with those of traditional PEGs.[38,39] In one series of 253 image-guided gastrostomy or gastrojejunostomy tube placements at the Hospital for Sick Children in Toronto, a 5% major complication rate and 73% minor complication rate were found.[38] A 2007 review of 378 PEGs placed in adults using endoscopic versus fluoroscopic methods reported a higher rate of complications with fluoroscopic-assisted PEGs compared with endoscopy-assisted PEGs.[40]

In certain clinical situations patients may demonstrate gastric feeding intolerance, and require postpyloric feeding after PEG placement. Recent investigations have reported using a percutaneous endoscopic gastrojejunostomy tube placement technique after primary PEG placement.[41,42] One recent case series also discussed use of a primary one-step percutaneous gastrojejunostomy in 3 infants with gastric feeding intolerance.[43]

LAPAROSCOPIC GASTROSTOMY TUBE PLACEMENT

Over the last 10 years, there has been renewed interest among general surgeons in exploring refinements in laparoscopically assisted gastrostomy tube insertion techniques.[8,22,44,45] The main overall advantages of a laparoscopic technique is that it allows direct visualization of the stomach, eliminating the potential risk of accidental colon interposition and perforation during placement, and removes the need for secondary exchange to a skin-level or balloon-based device 3 to 6 months later.[23,36] Generally speaking, the laparoscopic approach to gastrostomy tube insertion is considered to be associated with fewer intraoperative major complications, including less risk of tract disruption and perforation of other abdominal viscera.[8,22,44,45]

In turn, some investigators have noted that if there is concern for upper gastrointestinal tract obstruction or other complicated anatomic conditions (ie, hepatomegaly), non-PEG techniques, such as laparoscopy, should be considered as a preferred method of gastrostomy placement.[8] On the other hand, nonlaparoscopic methods of gastrostomy placement, such as the PEG procedure, may still need to considered in certain patient populations, including: (1) severely obese patients, because of increased abdominal girth and tissue placing excessive traction on laparoscopically placed tubes; (2) patients with an immobile stomach; or (3) patients who may not tolerate prolonged anesthesia times or have significant underlying respiratory conditions.[8,23,45]

Different techniques for laparoscopically placed gastrostomy tubes have been reported.[22,23,46] Of note, some investigators have also reported performance of a traditional PEG procedure along with each, to ensure appropriate introduction of the PEG tube and to aid in the approximation of the stomach with the abdominal wall.[22]

Laparoscopic Techniques

There are 3 commonly used methods of laparoscopic gastrostomy tube placement, the first of which can be described as a laparoscopically assisted mini-open technique. In the mini-open technique, an umbilical trocar is placed for camera insertion and allows for inspection of the abdominal cavity, and for choosing the most appropriate gastrostomy location in relation to the abdominal wall and stomach. A small incision is then made and sutures are secured to the posterior rectus sheath by a careful open exposure. The chosen site of the stomach is delivered through this small incision, and fascial sutures are then secured to the stomach in a Stamm-like fashion. A purse string can also be placed at an individual surgeon's discretion. The gastrostomy tube is then directly placed, with most patients and surgeons opting for placement of a skin-level, balloon-based gastrostomy tube.

The mini-open technique provides a secure gastrostomy tube site and tract, with an extremely low rate of traction disruption, and removes the need for any future gastrostomy exchanges under anesthesia. A downside of this method is that it involves the creation of a slightly larger skin opening at the gastrostomy stoma, which may inadvertently lead to increased leakage and granulation tissue. It also requires a relatively longer total operative time, especially for larger patients with a thicker abdominal wall.[47]

The second popular method of laparoscopic gastrostomy placement is based on a Seldinger technique. Using the Seldinger technique an umbilical trocar for camera inspection is also used, and the most optimal sites of the abdominal wall and stomach are chosen similarly to the mini-open method. However, in this approach only a very small abdominal stab incision is used, and gastric suspending sutures are placed on either side that traverse the abdominal wall and remain external to the patient. The stomach is then accessed by an introducer needle followed by a guide wire. The stoma tract is serially dilated, and a gastrostomy tube is then placed over the guide wire. The external suspending sutures are then tied over the sides of the gastrostomy tube to secure the tube in place. These external sutures are later removed in 3 to 10 days following the procedure after the stoma tract has had time to mature.

The Seldinger technique for gastrostomy tube placement is faster than the mini-open technique, and may be less prone to initial site leakage and granulation tissue. However, the stomach fixation is less secure, especially after external suture removal. In addition, the external sutures can create skin pressure necrosis sores within a very short time. Finally, it should be recognized that placement of dressings under the gastrostomy tube is not straightforward when the sutures are in place.[48]

A third option that has become increasingly widespread over the past several years is similar to the Seldinger technique just described, except that smaller suspending sutures are used. In addition, the smaller suspending sutures are placed through tiny skin incisions that allow them to be tied in the subcutaneous space, and therefore to remain permanently in the patient, without need for removal. This modified approach to the Seldinger procedure combines the benefits of using the smallest possible incision for the gastrostomy tube itself, which minimizes postoperative leakage and granulation tissue formation, and provides permanent suture stomach fixation to the abdominal wall without incurring the risk of pressure sores created by external suspension sutures. In turn, the modified approach allows for performance of laparoscopic gastrostomy tube placement in as little as 15 to 20 minutes, and with surgical experience can begin to approach the short operative times achievable by the PEG technique.[49]

All of the laparoscopically based methods offer similar benefits in that they allow for direct visualization of the stomach and other abdominal organs. Issues such as hepatomegaly, ventriculoperitoneal shunts, pacemakers, and other obstacles can be easily accommodated. Laparoscopy also offers diagnostic benefits beyond those necessary for the gastrostomy tube procedure itself, and surgical teams may sometimes encounter additional congenital gastrointestinal abnormalities during a gastrostomy tube placement which in turn can be simultaneously repaired. For example, surgeons may diagnose and repair umbilical and inguinal hernias, intestinal malrotation, pyloric stenosis, and omphalomesenteric remnants, in addition to potentially providing further clarification of malrotation and malfixation in the setting of heterotaxy syndromes.

One final benefit of laparoscopically assisted gastrostomy tube methods may be in their potential to facilitate the placement of postpyloric feeding tubes should intragastric feedings fail. To this end, any of the aforementioned methods of laparoscopic placement that use internal stomach fixation sutures can be used to permit early safe wire exchange of the gastrostomy tube for a gastrojejunostomy tube (ie, within a few days or weeks of the initial gastrostomy tube placement) without concern for tract disruption. In addition, the performance of primary laparoscopic gastrojejunostomy tube placement has been reported, and is a straightforward modification of the laparoscopically assisted gastrostomy placement with the addition of fluoroscopy.[50]

Percutaneous Endoscopic Gastrostomy Versus Laparoscopic Technique

To date, most studies have suggested that major complication rates with laparoscopically assisted techniques, including laparoscopically assisted gastrostomy or PEG placement, may be lower than those of the traditional PEG pull procedure, whereas minor postoperative complication rates may be similar.[23,27,44,45] For example, Liu and colleagues[45] retrospectively compared open gastrostomy tube techniques with PEG procedures and with laparoscopically placed gastrostomies, and found that PEGs had a higher risk of developing early complications when compared with laparoscopically placed tubes. Unfortunately, the risk of late complications, which often represent most of the complications in a cohort, was comparable between patients who had undergone PEG versus laparoscopic placement.[45] As laparoscopic techniques continue to be developed and refined, further studies are needed to compare both short-term and long-term outcomes, including postoperative minor complications, among the various methods.

FUTURE OF GASTROSTOMY PLACEMENT

Regardless of the method used, placement of gastrostomy tubes continues to remain a common procedure in infants and children, as health care options for children with complex medical conditions continues to advance and children with significant health care needs are surviving longer. In 2014, Fox and colleagues[51] looked at the Kids' Inpatient Database and found that the rates of gastrostomy placement in the United States increased dramatically over a decade, from 16.6 procedures per 100,000 hospitalized children in 1997 to 18.5 per 100,000 hospitalized children in 2009. The rate of increase in performance of the procedure was especially notable in infants younger than 1 year **(Fig. 3)**. Of interest, the investigators also found significant regional

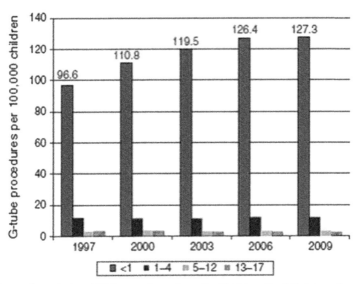

Fig. 3. Rates of surgical and PEG procedures from the Kids' Inpatient Database by age category (1–17 years old) in study years. (*From* Fox D, Campagna EJ, Friedlander J, et al. National trends and outcomes of pediatric gastrostomy tube placement. J Pediatr Gastroenterol Nutr 2014;59(5):585; with permission.)

variations across the United States in both the frequency and preferred method of gastrostomy tube placement.[51] Moreover, longer postoperative lengths of stay and higher costs were associated with gastrostomies performed by surgeons in comparison with PEGs, although they were unable to associate the exact surgical method used (open versus laparoscopically assisted gastrostomies) at the patient level. In their analysis, Fox and colleagues[51] again found an overall similarity in immediate postprocedural complication rates regardless of the method of placement (surgical versus endoscopic) used.

The long-term data from the authors' institution that focused on the cohort of 138 consecutive patients undergoing PEG placement from April 1999 to December 2000 showed that approximately half were still likely to have an indwelling enteral tube in place 10 years later (**Fig. 4**).[28] This finding substantiated anecdotal reports of the lengthy time that many pediatric patients may remain enterally dependent, requiring ongoing, long-term gastrostomy tube care. Health services research into children with complex medical issues has suggested that patients with indwelling feeding devices are at risk of having more hospital readmissions.[52] Such children may also be at high risk for requiring additional medical resources and services in pediatric emergency departments.[52,53]

Therefore, in addition to continually improving methods of gastrostomy tube placement, pediatric gastroenterologists and surgeons must also focus on identifying opportunities to mitigate the risk of long-term gastrostomy-related complications. For example, future studies may identify the best means of aiding parents of infants and children with complex medical issues to maintain the gastrostomy tube without experiencing troublesome complications. At their institution, the authors have focused on implementing new educational initiatives and programs targeted to improve the long-term quality of care and coordination for infants and children who are gastrostomy tube dependent, by developing specific outpatient clinics and inpatient consultation

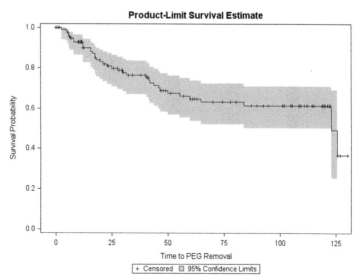

Fig. 4. Kaplan-Meier curve (in months) estimating the probability of 138 patients requiring ongoing enteral tube use after PEG placement during a 10-year follow-up period. The shaded area represents the 95% CI; median time to elective/permanent tube removal was 122.9 months or 10.2 years. (*Adapted from* McSweeney ME, Jiang H, Deutsch AJ, et al. Long-term outcomes of infants and children undergoing percutaneous endoscopy gastrostomy tube placement. J Pediatr Gastroenterol Nutr 2013;57(5):665; with permission.)

tube services.[54] The authors have also focused on developing a multidisciplinary staff with expertise, to help standardize and streamline the follow-up care for patients dependent on gastrostomy or gastrojejunostomy tubes.

In brief, although PEG and laparoscopic gastrostomy tube placement should overall be considered a safe and important procedure for children with complex medical needs, future research and quality improvement initiatives are still needed to improve and advance the care of gastrostomy-dependent pediatric patients.

REFERENCES

1. Minard G. The history of surgically placed feeding tubes. Nutr Clin Pract 2006; 21(6):626–33.
2. Gauderer MW, Ponsky JL, Izant RJ Jr. Gastrostomy without laparotomy: a percutaneous endoscopic technique. J Pediatr Surg 1980;15(6):872–5.
3. Fortunato JE, Troy AL, Cuffari C, et al. Outcome after percutaneous endoscopic gastrostomy in children and young adults. J Pediatr Gastroenterol Nutr 2010; 50(4):390–3.
4. Avitsland TL, Kristensen C, Emblem R, et al. Percutaneous endoscopic gastrostomy in children: a safe technique with major symptom relief and high parental satisfaction. J Pediatr Gastroenterol Nutr 2006;43(5):624–8.
5. Gauderer MW. Percutaneous endoscopic gastrostomy-20 years later: a historical perspective. J Pediatr Surg 2001;36(1):217–9.
6. Khattak IU, Kimber C, Kiely EM, et al. Percutaneous endoscopic gastrostomy in paediatric practice: complications and outcome. J Pediatr Surg 1998;33(1): 67–72.

7. Park JH, Rhie S, Jeong SJ. Percutaneous endoscopic gastrostomy in children. Korean J Pediatr 2011;54(1):17–21.
8. Fortunato JE, Cuffari C. Outcomes of percutaneous endoscopic gastrostomy in children. Curr Gastroenterol Rep 2011;13(3):293–9.
9. Green A, Shepherd EG, Erdman SH. Sedated percutaneous endoscopic gastrostomy (PEG) placement in the neonate. Gastroenterology 2011;140(5 (Supplement of 2011 DDW Abstracts)):S-687.
10. Corkins MR, Fitzgerald JF, Gupta SK. Feeding after percutaneous endoscopic gastrostomy in children: early feeding trial. J Pediatr Gastroenterol Nutr 2010; 50(6):625–7.
11. Szary NM, Arif M, Matteson ML, et al. Enteral feeding within three hours after percutaneous endoscopic gastrostomy placement: a meta-analysis. J Clin Gastroenterol 2011;45(4):e34–8.
12. Sathesh-Kumar T, Rollins H, Cheslyn-Curtis S. General paediatric surgical provision of percutaneous endoscopic gastrostomy in a district general hospital—a 12-year experience. Ann R Coll Surg Engl 2009;91(5):404–9.
13. Kobak GE, McClenathan DT, Schurman SJ. Complications of removing percutaneous endoscopic gastrostomy tubes in children. J Pediatr Gastroenterol Nutr 2000;30(4):404–7.
14. El-Rifai N, Michaud L, Mention K, et al. Persistence of gastrocutaneous fistula after removal of gastrostomy tubes in children: prevalence and associated factors. Endoscopy 2004;36(8):700–4.
15. Schrag SP, Sharma R, Jaik NP, et al. Complications related to percutaneous endoscopic gastrostomy (PEG) tubes. A comprehensive clinical review. J Gastrointestin Liver Dis 2007;16(4):407–18.
16. Loser C, Aschl G, Hebuterne X, et al. ESPEN guidelines on artificial enteral nutrition—percutaneous endoscopic gastrostomy (PEG). Clin Nutr 2005;24(5): 848–61.
17. Palmer GM, Frawley GP, Heine RG, et al. Complications associated with endoscopic removal of percutaneous endoscopic gastrostomy (PEG) tubes in children. J Pediatr Gastroenterol Nutr 2006;42(4):443–5.
18. Fox VL, Abel SD, Malas S, et al. Complications following percutaneous endoscopic gastrostomy and subsequent catheter replacement in children and young adults. Gastrointest Endosc 1997;45(1):64–71.
19. Gauderer MW. Percutaneous endoscopic gastrostomy: a 10-year experience with 220 children. J Pediatr Surg 1991;26(3):288–92 [discussion: 292–4].
20. Chang PF, Ni YH, Chang MH. Percutaneous endoscopic gastrostomy to set up a long-term enteral feeding route in children: an encouraging result. Pediatr Surg Int 2003;19(4):283–5.
21. McSweeney ME, Kerr J, Jiang H, et al. Risk factors for complications in infants and children with percutaneous endoscopic gastrostomy tubes. J Pediatr 2015; 166(6):1514–9.e1.
22. Vervloessem D, van Leersum F, Boer D, et al. Percutaneous endoscopic gastrostomy (PEG) in children is not a minor procedure: risk factors for major complications. Semin Pediatr Surg 2009;18(2):93–7.
23. Zamakhshary M, Jamal M, Blair GK, et al. Laparoscopic vs percutaneous endoscopic gastrostomy tube insertion: a new pediatric gold standard? J Pediatr Surg 2005;40(5):859–62.
24. van der Merwe WG, Brown RA, Ireland JD, et al. Percutaneous endoscopic gastrostomy in children—a 5-year experience. S Afr Med J 2003;93(10): 781–5.

25. Lalanne A, Gottrand F, Salleron J, et al. Long-term outcome of children receiving percutaneous endoscopic gastrostomy feeding. J Pediatr Gastroenterol Nutr 2014;59(2):172–6.

26. Segal D, Michaud L, Guimber D, et al. Late-onset complications of percutaneous endoscopic gastrostomy in children. J Pediatr Gastroenterol Nutr 2001;33(4): 495–500.

27. Brewster BD, Weil BR, Ladd AP. Prospective determination of percutaneous endoscopic gastrostomy complication rates in children: still a safe procedure. Surgery 2012;152(4):714–9 [discussion: 719–1].

28. McSweeney ME, Jiang H, Deutsch AJ, et al. Long-term outcomes of infants and children undergoing percutaneous endoscopy gastrostomy tube placement. J Pediatr Gastroenterol Nutr 2013;57(5):663–7.

29. Pearce CB, Goggin PM, Collett J, et al. The 'cut and push' method of percutaneous endoscopic gastrostomy tube removal. Clin Nutr 2000;19(2):133–5.

30. Yaseen M, Steele MI, Grunow JE. Nonendoscopic removal of percutaneous endoscopic gastrostomy tubes: morbidity and mortality in children. Gastrointest Endosc 1996;44(3):235–8.

31. Novotny NM, Vegeler RC, Breckler FD, et al. Percutaneous endoscopic gastrostomy buttons in children: superior to tubes. J Pediatr Surg 2009;44(6): 1193–6.

32. Jacob A, Delesalle D, Coopman S, et al. Safety of the one-step percutaneous endoscopic gastrostomy button in children. J Pediatr 2015;166(6):1526–8.

33. Treem WR, Etienne NL, Hyams JS. Percutaneous endoscopic placement of the "button" gastrostomy tube as the initial procedure in infants and children. J Pediatr Gastroenterol Nutr 1993;17(4):382–6.

34. Kozarek RA, Payne M, Barkin J, et al. Prospective multicenter evaluation of an initially placed button gastrostomy. Gastrointest Endosc 1995;41(2):105–8.

35. Evans JS, Thorne M, Taufiq S, et al. Should single-stage PEG buttons become the procedure of choice for PEG placement in children? Gastrointest Endosc 2006; 64(3):320–4 [quiz: 389–92].

36. Pattamanuch N, Novak I, Loizides A, et al. Single-center experience with 1-step low-profile percutaneous endoscopic gastrostomy in children. J Pediatr Gastroenterol Nutr 2014;58(5):616–20.

37. Gothberg G, Bjornsson S. One-step insertion of low-profile gastrostomy in pediatric patients vs pull percutaneous endoscopic gastrostomy: retrospective analysis of outcomes. JPEN J Parenter Enteral Nutr 2015. [Epub ahead of print].

38. Friedman JN, Ahmed S, Connolly B, et al. Complications associated with image-guided gastrostomy and gastrojejunostomy tubes in children. Pediatrics 2004; 114(2):458–61.

39. Nah SA, Narayanaswamy B, Eaton S, et al. Gastrostomy insertion in children: percutaneous endoscopic or percutaneous image-guided? J Pediatr Surg 2010;45(6):1153–8.

40. MacLean AA, Alvarez NR, Davies JD, et al. Complications of percutaneous endoscopic and fluoroscopic gastrostomy tube insertion procedures in 378 patients. Gastroenterol Nurs 2007;30(5):337–41.

41. El-Matary W. Percutaneous endoscopic gastrojejunostomy tube feeding in children. Nutr Clin Pract 2011;26(1):78–83.

42. Michaud L, Coopman S, Guimber D, et al. Percutaneous gastrojejunostomy in children: efficacy and safety. Arch Dis Child 2012;97(8):733–4.

43. Michaud L, Robert-Dehault A, Coopman S, et al. One-step percutaneous gastrojejunostomy in early infancy. J Pediatr Gastroenterol Nutr 2012;54(6):820–1.

44. Akay B, Capizzani TR, Lee AM, et al. Gastrostomy tube placement in infants and children: is there a preferred technique? J Pediatr Surg 2010;45(6):1147–52.
45. Liu R, Jiwane A, Varjavandi A, et al. Comparison of percutaneous endoscopic, laparoscopic and open gastrostomy insertion in children. Pediatr Surg Int 2013;29(6):613–21.
46. Naiditch JA, Lautz T, Barsness KA. Postoperative complications in children undergoing gastrostomy tube placement. J Laparoendosc Adv Surg Tech A 2010;20(9):781–5.
47. Rothenberg SS, Bealer JF, Chang JH. Primary laparoscopic placement of gastrostomy buttons for feeding tubes. A safer and simpler technique. Surg Endosc 1999;13(10):995–7.
48. Aprahamian CJ, Morgan TL, Harmon CM, et al. U-stitch laparoscopic gastrostomy technique has a low rate of complications and allows primary button placement: experience with 461 pediatric procedures. J Laparoendosc Adv Surg Tech A 2006;16(6):643–9.
49. Petrosyan M, Hunter C, Estrada J, et al. Subcutaneous fixation of gastrostomy tube is superior to temporary fixation. J Laparoendosc Adv Surg Tech A 2010; 20(2):207–9.
50. Onwubiko C, Bairdain S, Murphy AJ, et al. Laparoscopic gastrojejunostomy tube placement in infants with congenital cardiac disease. J Laparoendosc Adv Surg Tech A 2015. [Epub ahead of print].
51. Fox D, Campagna EJ, Friedlander J, et al. National trends and outcomes of pediatric gastrostomy tube placement. J Pediatr Gastroenterol Nutr 2014;59(5): 582–8.
52. Berry JG, Hall DE, Kuo DZ, et al. Hospital utilization and characteristics of patients experiencing recurrent readmissions within children's hospitals. JAMA 2011;305(7):682–90.
53. Saavedra H, Losek JD, Shanley L, et al. Gastrostomy tube-related complaints in the pediatric emergency department: identifying opportunities for improvement. Pediatr Emerg Care 2009;25(11):728–32.
54. Correa JA, Fallon SC, Murphy KM, et al. Resource utilization after gastrostomy tube placement: defining areas of improvement for future quality improvement projects. J Pediatr Surg 2014;49(11):1598–601.

Role of Endoscopy in Diagnosis and Management of Pediatric Eosinophilic Esophagitis

Amanda B. Muir, MD[a,b,1], Jamie Merves, MD[a,b,1], Chris A. Liacouras, MD[a,b,*]

KEYWORDS

- Eosinophilic esophagitis • Dilation • Food impaction • Food allergy • Dysphagia

KEY POINTS

- Endoscopy is currently the only way to diagnose eosinophilic esophagitis (EoE) and monitor disease activity.
- Food impaction occurs frequently in undiagnosed or chronic EoE, especially in the adult population, and may result in emergent endoscopic disimpaction.
- Stricture dilation in EoE may relieve symptoms of dysphagia but does not attenuate underlying inflammation.
- Endoscopic tools are being studied to find additional invasive biomarkers of disease activity.
- Less invasive techniques to diagnose and evaluate disease activity are currently being investigated.

INTRODUCTION

Eosinophilic esophagitis (EoE) is a chronic immune-mediated and antigen-mediated disorder characterized by an isolated eosinophilic infiltration of the esophagus resulting in esophageal dysfunction.[1] Although there are many causes of esophageal eosinophilia, EoE must be primarily distinguished from gastroesophageal reflux disease (GERD) and proton-pump inhibitor (PPI)–responsive esophageal eosinophilia

[a] Division of Gastroenterology, Hepatology, and Nutrition, The Children's Hospital of Philadelphia, 34th and Civic Center Boulevard, Philadelphia, PA 19104, USA; [b] Department of Pediatrics, Perelman School of Medicine, University of Pennsylvania, Philadelphia, PA 19104, USA
[1] Equal contributions.
* Corresponding author. The Children's Hospital of Philadelphia, 34th and Civic Center Boulevard, Philadelphia, PA 19104.
E-mail address: Liacouras@email.chop.edu

Gastrointest Endoscopy Clin N Am 26 (2016) 187–200
http://dx.doi.org/10.1016/j.giec.2015.08.006
1052-5157/16/$ – see front matter © 2016 Elsevier Inc. All rights reserved.

(PPI-REE). EoE is an emerging disorder associated with other allergic conditions[2] and currently affects approximately 56.7 per 100,000 people in the United States.[3] EoE pathophysiology is complex, involving a variety inflammatory cells and cytokines in a non–immunoglobulin E (IgE)-dependent allergic model.[4–6] EoE is primarily caused by the ingestion of one or more food antigens,[7,8] but may also be triggered by inhaled aeroantigens.[9] EoE and associated complications have a significant impact on patient quality of life[10] and patients with EoE in the United States have an annual health care cost of up to $1.4 billon.[11] EoE therapy is limited to dietary modification, steroids, and endoscopic dilatation.[1] At present, esophagogastroduodenoscopy (EGD) is the gold standard for diagnosis and disease monitoring.

EOSINOPHILIC ESOPHAGITIS DIAGNOSIS AND SURVEILLANCE

EoE requires a clinicopathologic diagnosis. EGD is often performed in children for a variety of reasons, including chronic reflux symptoms with or without a poor response to acid suppression therapy, feeding problems, poor growth, intermittent or persistent vomiting and regurgitation, chest or epigastric abdominal pain, gastric or duodenal ulcers, dysphagia, a history of food impaction, or any other chronic indication of esophageal or gastric dysfunction. Because the current gold standard for the diagnosis of EoE is histologic evidence of esophageal eosinophilia, when performing an EGD it is paramount to perform biopsies, even in the presence of normal-looking mucosa.[1]

Endoscopic Findings

Although there are no pathognomonic findings for EoE, esophageal edema, longitudinal furrows, mucosal fragility, whitish exudates, transient esophageal rings (feline folds), fixed esophageal rings (trachealization), diffuse esophageal narrowing, and small-caliber esophagus are its typical macroscopic findings (**Fig. 1**).[1] Up to one-third of children with EoE may have visually normal esophageal mucosa.[12]

A novel endoscopic classification and grading system called the EoE Endoscopic Reference Score (EREFS) was recently developed and validated in adults to define common nomenclature, severity description, and disease assessment among providers.[13] The EREFS score is generated based on the presence and/or severity of transient or fixed esophageal rings, exudates, furrowing, mucosal fragility (so-called crepe-paper esophagus), edema (and the associated vascular pattern), as well as stricture.[13] Although this system has good interobserver agreement between practitioners, a validated scoring system in children has yet to be established.

There are many past and present differences in EoE diagnostic practices between pediatric and adult gastroenterologists. For example, adult gastroenterologists have traditionally based the diagnosis of esophageal disorders primarily on symptoms and endoscopic findings, rather than histolopathology.[14] Alternatively, pediatric gastroenterologists have been trained to obtain mucosal biopsies in all diagnostic procedures, even if the mucosa is visually normal. The pediatric approach to diagnosis may be extremely important to identifying the presence of EoE, because it is common for patients of all ages to have a normal-appearing esophagus.[12]

Radiology

Although not recommended routinely for EoE diagnosis, imaging with upper gastrointestinal intestinal series (UGI) or esophagram should be recognized to be a useful test in patients with feeding problems, dysphagia, or food impaction to evaluate for anatomic and mucosal abnormalities such as narrowing, stricture, or formation of rings (**Fig. 2**).[1,15,16] In a cohort of 22 pediatric patients with EoE with strictures who

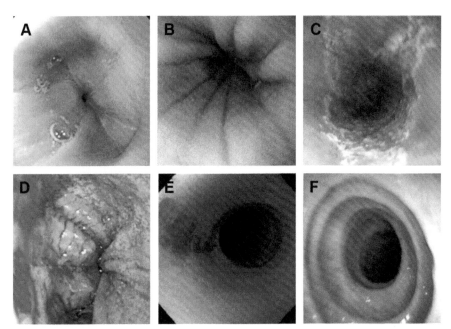

Fig. 1. Endoscopic findings of EoE. (*A*) Normal esophageal mucosa. (*B*) Esophageal furrowing. (*C*) Esophageal white mucosal plaques. (*D*) Esophageal mucosal fragility in a patient with EoE after biopsy. (*E*) Esophageal mucosal fragility with so-called crepe paper esophagus. (*F*) Esophageal trachealization. (*Courtesy of* [*C, E, F*] The International Gastrointestinal Eosinophilic Researchers (TIGERS) and Children's Digestive Health and Nutrition Foundation (CDHNF) slide set; and [*E*] Chris A. Liacouras, MD, Philadelphia, PA.)

underwent esophagram and endoscopy within 3 months of each other, 12 had esophageal strictures identified by esophagram alone and only 1 had a stricture identified by endoscopy but not esophagram.[16] Furthermore, 3 of 4 patients who received a barium pill had evidence of impaction or delayed pill transit.[16] Although not specific to EoE, these findings may provide valuable adjunctive monitoring and diagnostic information before performing an upper endoscopy. Characterizing a patients' anatomy may also be useful in preventing unwanted complications, including esophageal perforation. Patients with EoE may be at risk for perforation with instrumentation, and have been described as having crepe-paper esophagus.

Histology

EoE is a diagnosis that requires both clinical symptoms (isolated esophageal dysfunction) and abnormal histology, with greater than or equal to 15 esophageal eosinophils per high-power field in the most densely involved esophageal mucosal specimens. Eosinophils are not increased in any other part of the gastrointestinal tract. EoE often presents as a patchy disease, thus multiple biopsies are required. According to several recent guidelines, multiple biopsies should be obtained from both the mid/proximal and distal esophagus of patients who are being concomitantly treated with high-dose PPI therapy for 8 to 12 weeks before endoscopy.[1,15]

Common microscopic findings of EoE are shown in **Fig. 3**. Although the eosinophil is the predominant cell type seen on hematoxylin-eosin staining, additional microscopic findings, such as basal cell hyperplasia with resulting acanthosis, eosinophilic microabscess formation and layering, eosinophilic granules, dilated intercellular spaces, as

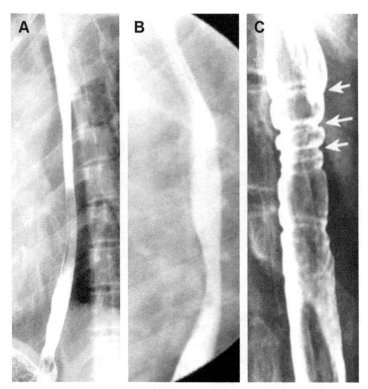

Fig. 2. Esophagram findings of EoE. (*A*) Diffuse esophageal narrowing. (*B*) Esophageal stricture with 2 pronounced areas of narrowing. (*C*) Esophageal rings indicated by white arrows. (*Courtesy of* [*A, C*] TIGERS and CDHNF slide set.)

well as thickened and dense lamina propria fibers, have also been reported.[1,17,18] In addition to eosinophils, the feature and predominant inflammatory cells of EoE, many other cell types, including mast cells, basophils, and both B and T lymphocytes, have been discovered in the inflammatory milieu.[1,17,19] A unique inflammatory cytokine and genetic profile has also been identified in human esophageal mucosal biopsies from patients with EoE.[20–22]

Recent guidelines have stressed the importance of making the distinction between esophageal eosinophilia and EoE. Esophageal eosinophilia is a descriptive term, whereas EoE is a disease and diagnosis. There are many causes of esophageal eosinophilia, including GERD; PPI-REE; bacterial, fungal, or parasitic infections; Crohn disease; primary immune deficiencies; other hypereosinophilic disorders; connective tissue disorders; and side effects of various medications.[23] There may be a some patients with EoE who do not meet the threshold of eosinophils for EoE diagnosis either because of inadequate biopsies and sampling error or partial treatment response, although these patients may have other characteristic histologic features.[1]

Eosinophilic Esophagitis Treatment

After establishing a diagnosis of EoE and initiating therapy, surveillance endoscopy is performed to evaluate for esophageal mucosal healing. At present, there are no other methods that can be used to evaluate the severity of esophageal inflammation. The frequency of endoscopic monitoring varies based on selected therapy. In general, it

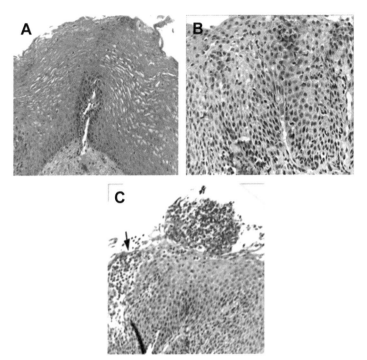

Fig. 3. Histology of the esophagus. (*A*) Normal esophagus (*B*) EoE esophagus with basal cell hyperplasia and eosinophilic infiltrate. (*C*) EoE esophagus with superficial layering of eosinophils (*black arrow*) and an eosinophilic abscess. Histologic evaluation of the esophagus by hematoxylin and eosin stain. (*Courtesy of* [*C*] TIGERS and CDHNF slide set.)

is recommended that repeat EGD with biopsy be performed to evaluate for response any time a therapy is initiated or altered, because clinical symptoms and histologic inflammation do not correlate.[24]

Dietary therapy

Dietary elimination of causative foods is an effective treatment strategy to address the inflammation associated with EoE and may reverse esophageal fibrosis.[25] Dietary elimination should be considered in all children diagnosed with EoE.[1] Dietary management strategies range from empiric elimination of 1 or more antigenic proteins (typically milk, wheat, soy, egg) to a targeted dietary elimination based on an allergy evaluation or the strict use of an elemental diet.[8,26,27] The use of an amino acid–based formula, thought to be the most efficacious of all EoE therapies, needs to be carefully considered secondary to the significant lifestyle changes and costs related to this therapy. The option chosen should be based on the likelihood of compliance and the patient's lifestyle and resources.[1] When any type of dietary therapy is chosen, consultation with a dietician should be considered to ensure appropriate nutrition in children on elimination diets.[1]

Endoscopy plays a major role in evaluating the effectiveness of dietary therapy. In many centers, follow-up endoscopy is typically performed 8 to 12 weeks after a change in dietary therapy to evaluate for histologic changes. Dietary therapy has been shown to significantly reverse endoscopic and histologic esophageal abnormalities.[8,25] Once remission is achieved, no further EGD with biopsies is required, unless and until symptoms recur and/or foods are reintroduced.

Corticosteroid therapy

Both systemic and topical corticosteroid therapies have been shown to be effective strategies for EoE management, and both may reverse fibrosis, although disease typically recurs upon discontinuation of either.[28] Although systemic corticosteroids can be considered in severe presentations,[1,29] swallowed topical corticosteroids are most commonly used as therapy for EoE[30–32] based on their lower bioavailability and risk of systemic side effects, although local fungal infection remains a concern.[33] Fluticasone is sprayed via a metered-dose inhaler directly into the mouth without a spacer and swallowed twice per day.[29,34] Budesonide can be administered as an oral viscous slurry.[33,35] Recommended dosing for these medications is outlined in recent guidelines.[1]

Similar to dietary therapy, EGD with biopsy is required not only after starting swallowed topical steroid therapy but also after changes in dosing. Although there are no established guidelines, most practitioners perform endoscopy no sooner than 8 to 12 weeks after steroid initiation to ensure response.

Eosinophilic Esophagitis Surveillance

How to decide when and how often to perform EGD with biopsy for surveillance of patients with a known diagnosis of EoE is currently not well understood. Because of the invasive nature of endoscopy, patient concerns, possible anesthesia side effects, and increased medical costs, some investigators argue to limit the number of endoscopies. In contrast, limiting these procedures can often delay therapeutic changes such as expanding a patient's diet or decreasing medication doses.

Moreover, although some physicians use patient symptoms to guide clinical management, the general lack of correlation between clinical symptoms and tissue inflammation in EoE has been well shown,[24] and this approach can often misguide therapeutic decision making. Although in a few cases clinical symptoms and histologic changes have been shown to coincide, this is not typical of most patients. Until less invasive diagnostic tools are available, physicians should recognize the limitations of clinical symptoms for guiding management, and make appropriate decisions regarding the timing of EGD with biopsy.

THERAPEUTIC ROLE OF ENDOSCOPY IN EOSINOPHILIC ESOPHAGITIS
Emergent Procedures in Eosinophilic Esophagitis

Food impaction accounts for up to 10% of pediatric esophageal foreign bodies[36] and is considered one of the classic disease presentations of EoE in adults.[37,38] Retrospective pediatric and adult studies suggest that approximately half of all food impactions requiring endoscopy are likely secondary to EoE.[38,39]

Patients with food impaction typically present with nausea, odynophagia, substernal chest pain, and salivation. Almost all food impactions are secondary to meat.[36,40] Nevertheless, all patients with suspected food impaction should undergo chest radiograph to rule out other radio-opaque foreign bodies and other complications of ingestion, such as pneumomediastinum and pneumothorax,[40] specifically in the pediatric population, in which patient history may be unreliable. In addition, surgical or otolaryngologic consultation should be considered for patients with proximal foreign bodies, which may be removed more successfully with a rigid endoscope rather than with a flexible instrument.

There has been recent controversy among gastroenterologists regarding whether or not to biopsy at the time of endoscopic food removal. Many patients who present with a food impaction may also have esophageal trachealization, furrows, or white plaques on the esophageal mucosa. In many of these cases, patients who present with impactions are not on a PPI, and physicians may erroneously presume that the endoscopic findings are pathognomonic for EoE. However, this is now appreciated to not be the case. A significant number of these patients respond effectively to treatment with PPI, and in turn have a diagnosis of PPI-REE. Thus, making a formal diagnosis of EoE during the initial EGD for a foreign body impaction in the absence of acid suppression can be challenging unless the EGD is repeated after the patient has been treated with high-dose PPI on a regular basis for 6 to 12 weeks. Regardless, biopsies should be obtained, if possible, during food disimpaction, because important information can be obtained and a biopsy that does not reveal features of EoE in PPI-naive patients may be helpful by suggesting a decreased likelihood of EoE.

Stricture Management and Dilations

Esophageal stricture is the most severe complication of EoE. Symptoms of stricture include dysphagia, delayed transit of food, and recurrent impaction. Recent evidence suggests that long-standing, untreated EoE leads to fibrostenosis.[41] Note that not all patients with severe, prolonged esophageal eosinophilia develop strictures. Alternatively, many patients with EoE who have esophageal strictures have developed coping mechanisms to deal with their symptoms, which can mask or further delay diagnosis. For example, patients may chew their food for a prolonged period of time or cut their food into very small pieces. They may also drink large quantities of water during meals in order to ease the passage of food, or they may take longer than an hour to eat a meal. Hence, diagnosis of stricture in EoE may require obtaining a specialized patient history that targets the identification of such behaviors.

EGD is not considered an adequate means of identifying esophageal strictures in EoE. Not only can an esophageal stricture or luminal narrowing be difficult to appreciate by EGD, but esophageal laceration can occur with passage of the scope, because of a small-caliber and/or crepe-paper appearance of the mucosa. An esophagram is helpful in patients with EoE who present with dysphagia or feeding difficulty and may diagnose strictures or narrowing more reliably.[16,42]

Esophageal stricture formation is rare in pediatric EoE compared with adults with the diagnosis, with the exact rate of this complication in children unknown.[12] Because esophageal narrowing and tissue inflammation have been shown to be reversible in children undergoing treatment of EoE,[43] dilation is most commonly recommended for symptomatic relief in patients who do not respond to medical therapy or who have irreversible stenotic lesions. In contrast, in adults with EoE, some physicians use dilation as a primary monotherapy.[44] Although this method of therapy may provide symptomatic relief, it is important to recognize that dilation does not treat the underlying esophageal inflammation in EoE and almost always needs to be repeated.

Before 2008, the rate of complications from esophageal dilation in patients with EoE was thought to be higher than in other benign esophageal conditions. For example, perforation rates were reported as high as 5%. However, in recent years larger-scale studies, some of which have included pediatric patients, have shown that the rate of perforation is considerably less than had been previously reported.[45] The most recent EoE consensus guidelines report only 3 perforations out of 839 performed dilations.[1] However, the guideline investigators also speculate that this decrease in perforations may reflect growing gastroenterologist experience with dilation in EoE.

To date, there are no standard dilation techniques for children and many of the practices are extrapolated from the adult literature. Bougie dilation and balloon pull-through techniques have both been successful in providing symptomatic relief in adults with esophageal stricture.[46] Although both dilation approaches are reported to be safe in adults,[47,48] their safety and efficacy have not been formally studied in the pediatric population.

Challenges with Eosinophilic Esophagitis Management

Although established consensus guidelines for EoE diagnosis and management are available,[1,15] there may be variation in interpretation of clinical history and histologic findings because the disease is patchy and many pathologists do not specify the size of a high-power field.[17] There is also significant variability in the practice among pediatric and adult providers.[49–52] For example, some providers do not recommend a PPI trial before endoscopy,[49] complicating the diagnostic distinction between GERD and PPI-REE, which may drastically change the management approach.

Another consideration in clinical management is the timing and interpretation of endoscopic evaluation in the context of a patient's treatment regimen for allergies, asthma, and other disorders. EoE is often comorbid with other allergic disorders, and reports of anecdotal experience have suggested that patients with allergic rhinitis may have a proximal esophageal eosinophilia that resolves with nasal corticosteroids. Nevertheless, at this time, there is no evidence to suggest any endoscopic or histologic benefit in EoE from nasal or inhaled steroids or antihistamines.

In addition, physicians must also always be aware of concomitant medication use. For example, systemic steroid therapy can induce clinical and pathologic remission of EoE.[53] Therefore, unless a patient is being treated primarily for EoE, patients taking systemic corticosteroids should undergo endoscopy at least 4 to 6 weeks after systemic steroid therapy to appropriately assess EoE disease status.

EMERGING METHODS OF DIAGNOSIS AND TREATMENT

Although established guidelines exist for EoE histologic diagnosis, there are current limitations of diagnosis and monitoring because EoE is a patchy disease and esophageal eosinophilia can result from other causes.[54,55] In addition, there has been some controversy over the variability in a diagnostic eosinophil count among investigators and pathologists both in eosinophil counts and high-power fields.[17] Histologic evaluation may diagnose EoE with 99% specificity, but only 80% sensitivity.[17,56] Additional review of biopsies, particularly those with borderline eosinophil counts, may result in increased sensitivity and more accurate EoE diagnosis.[56] Furthermore, unless deep esophageal mucosal biopsies are obtained with jumbo forceps, esophageal fibrosis and remodeling are difficult to detect in early stages before stricture formation. Emerging technologies in EoE include tissue biomarkers and methods, which may help to measure and monitor fibrosis, as well as further optimize disease diagnosis, monitoring, and management. These technological advances use both invasive and noninvasive approaches, and include new endoscopic instruments, such as Endo-FLIP, and use of less invasive tests, such as the cytosponge.

Molecular Analysis of Eosinophilic Esophagitis Tissue Samples

Gene expression profiling[57] using esophageal biopsies has led to development of a 96-gene panel, which may be available for future use to distinguish patients with active EoE from those in remission as well as from those with GERD, PPI-REE, and healthy controls.[58] RNA sequencing has identified transcriptional regulators involved in EoE and associated with the inflammatory milieu.[20] These methods have not yet been integrated into current standard of care for EoE, although molecular diagnostic techniques will likely enhance interpretation of esophageal biopsies, as well as EoE disease management in the future.

Endoscopic Ultrasonography

Although EoE is characterized by esophageal epithelial findings, evidence of dysmotility[59] and stricture formation in EoE suggest that the disorder extends to deeper layers than are evaluated by endoscopic biopsy, thus warranting further diagnostic methods. Endoscopic ultrasonography (EUS) evaluation of children and adults with EoE has provided further insight into the associated esophageal dysfunction and dysphagia. Expansion of the esophageal wall and individual tissue layers has been shown in children with EoE compared with healthy controls.[60] Functional studies performed in coordination with EUS have revealed esophageal longitudinal muscle dysfunction, as opposed to circular muscle function, which is typically detected with esophageal manometry.[61] Furthermore, the associated functional impairment improved with treatment.[61] Although EUS is not currently part of the EoE guidelines in children or adults, this diagnostic tool may provide further insight into future EoE management regarding fibrosis and esophageal motility.

EndoFLIP

EndoFLIP (endoluminal functional lumen imaging probe) uses high-resolution impedance palimetry to determine the pressure-geometry relationship or distensibility of hollow gastrointestinal organs, including the esophagus. The EndoFLIP catheter has an inflatable bag with pressure sensors (**Fig. 4**). The balloon is inserted into the esophagus while the patient is anesthetized and inflated with saline under endoscopic guidance. The catheter pressure sensors detect esophageal diameter and distensibility. A recent study using the EndoFLIP has shown decreased distensibility of the esophagus in adult patients with EoE compared with non-EoE controls. The impaired distensibility correlated with increased risk of food impaction and disease severity in the EoE population.[62]

Manometry

High-resolution manometry in adults with EoE has shown an increase in panesophageal pressurization and peristaltic dysfunction.[63] This increase may result because eosinophilic infiltration occurs not only in the epithelium of the EoE esophagus but also throughout the lamina propria and muscularis.[64] Feline esophageal smooth muscle strips displayed abrogated muscle contraction in the presence of eosinophil sonicates as well as EoE-associated cytokines, suggesting that inflammation hinders proper muscle function.[64] Further studies have correlated duration of disease with abnormal manometry studies[65] as well as the presence of fibrostenosis.[66] Although manometric evaluation may be useful to help explain dysphagia in this population, there are limited data to suggest manometry as a marker of disease activity. There is no current literature evaluating the motility of pediatric patients with EoE.

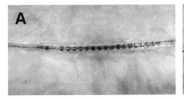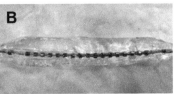

Fig. 4. EndoFLIP catheter. (*A*) EndoFLIP catheter deflated, and (*B*) inflated.

String Test and Cytosponge

The newest methods to evaluate EoE disease activity without endoscopy involve sampling of the esophageal milieu with a string[67] or tissue with a sponge.[68] The esophageal string test is an adaptation of the Enterotest, formerly used to diagnose gastrointestinal infection. A capsule with an internally coiled string is swallowed while the proximal end of the string is taped to the cheek and left in place for hours, sometimes overnight. The secretions obtained on the string from patients with active EoE have enhanced concentrations of eosinophil-derived proteins compared with inactive and control patients.[67]

Similarly, the cytosponge is a sponge within a capsule attached to a string. It is swallowed and after 5 minutes the capsule dissolves and the sponge is removed. The sponge is able to sample the epithelium and the tissue collected can be evaluated histologically for eosinophilia.[68]

Serum Testing

Although there are many serologic findings in the EoE population, none currently distinguish EoE from other atopic conditions. Serum peripheral eosinophilia, immuno-CAP testing, and IgE level do not correlate with active EoE. Larger-scale investigations of individual serum cytokines found no difference between patients with EoE and controls.[69,70] Levels of eosinophil-derived neurotoxin have been shown to be significantly increased in the serum of patients with active EoE but not in stool samples.[70] A specific serum micro-RNA (miRNA) signature pattern including induction of miR-21 and miR-223, and repression of miR-375 has been associated with EoE and is distinct from healthy control patients and those with noneosinophilic forms of esophagitis.[71,72] Furthermore, this signature nearly completely reverts to normal on disease remission.[71,72] Despite these findings, serum miRNA levels do not always reflect changes in esophageal biopsies[73] and further investigation is warranted to determine the clinical and diagnostic significance of miRNA dysregulation in EoE.

SUMMARY

Upper endoscopy with biopsies remains the cornerstone of diagnosis and surveillance in pediatric EoE. In making the diagnosis, it is critical to evaluate for other causes of esophageal eosinophilia, including PPI-REE. Children with known EoE should be considered to be on adequate therapy when there is remission of clinical symptoms and pathologic findings. Although there are many promising less invasive modalities emerging, histopatholgic examination of tissue is currently the only method of monitoring disease activity and fibrosis in pediatric and adult EoE.

REFERENCES

1. Liacouras CA, Furuta GT, Hirano I, et al. Eosinophilic esophagitis: updated consensus recommendations for children and adults. J Allergy Clin Immunol 2011;128(1):3–20.e26 [quiz: 21–2].
2. Jyonouchi S, Brown-Whitehorn TA, Spergel JM. Association of eosinophilic gastrointestinal disorders with other atopic disorders. Immunol Allergy Clin North Am 2009;29(1):85–97, x.
3. Dellon ES, Jensen ET, Martin CF, et al. Prevalence of eosinophilic esophagitis in the United States. Clin Gastroenterol Hepatol 2014;12(4):589–96.e1.
4. Merves J, Muir A, Modayur Chandramouleeswaran P, et al. Eosinophilic esophagitis. Ann Allergy Asthma Immunol 2014;112(5):397–403.

5. Mishra A. Mechanism of eosinophilic esophagitis. Immunol Allergy Clin North Am 2009;29(1):29–40, viii.
6. Clayton F, Fang JC, Gleich GJ, et al. Eosinophilic esophagitis in adults is associated with IgG4 and not mediated by IgE. Gastroenterology 2014;147(3):602–9.
7. Spergel JM, Brown-Whitehorn TF, Cianferoni A, et al. Identification of causative foods in children with eosinophilic esophagitis treated with an elimination diet. J Allergy Clin Immunol 2012;130(2):461–7.e5.
8. Markowitz JE, Spergel JM, Ruchelli E, et al. Elemental diet is an effective treatment for eosinophilic esophagitis in children and adolescents. Am J Gastroenterol 2003;98(4):777–82.
9. Sugnanam KK, Collins JT, Smith PK, et al. Dichotomy of food and inhalant allergen sensitization in eosinophilic esophagitis. Allergy 2007;62(11):1257–60.
10. Klinnert MD, Silveira L, Harris R, et al. Health-related quality of life over time in children with eosinophilic esophagitis and their families. J Pediatr Gastroenterol Nutr 2014;59(3):308–16.
11. Jensen ET, Kappelman MD, Martin CF, et al. Health-care utilization, costs, and the burden of disease related to eosinophilic esophagitis in the United States. Am J Gastroenterol 2015;110(5):626–32.
12. Liacouras CA, Spergel JM, Ruchelli E, et al. Eosinophilic esophagitis: a 10-year experience in 381 children. Clin Gastroenterol Hepatol 2005;3(12):1198–206.
13. Hirano I, Moy N, Heckman MG, et al. Endoscopic assessment of the oesophageal features of eosinophilic oesophagitis: validation of a novel classification and grading system. Gut 2013;62(4):489–95.
14. Schoepfer AM, Panczak R, Zwahlen M, et al. How do gastroenterologists assess overall activity of eosinophilic esophagitis in adult patients? Am J Gastroenterol 2015;110(3):402–14.
15. Dellon ES, Gonsalves N, Hirano I, et al. ACG clinical guideline: evidenced based approach to the diagnosis and management of esophageal eosinophilia and eosinophilic esophagitis (EoE). Am J Gastroenterol 2013;108(5):679–92 [quiz: 693].
16. Menard-Katcher C, Swerdlow MP, Mehta P, et al. Contribution of esophagram to the evaluation of complicated pediatric eosinophilic esophagitis. J Pediatr Gastroenterol Nutr 2015. [Epub ahead of print].
17. Collins MH. Histopathologic features of eosinophilic esophagitis and eosinophilic gastrointestinal diseases. Gastroenterol Clin North Am 2014;43(2):257–68.
18. Shah A, Kagalwalla AF, Gonsalves N, et al. Histopathologic variability in children with eosinophilic esophagitis. Am J Gastroenterol 2009;104(3):716–21.
19. Noti M, Kim BS, Siracusa MC, et al. Exposure to food allergens through inflamed skin promotes intestinal food allergy through the thymic stromal lymphopoietin-basophil axis. J Allergy Clin Immunol 2014;133(5):1390–9, 1399.e1–6.
20. Sherrill JD, Kiran KC, Blanchard C, et al. Analysis and expansion of the eosinophilic esophagitis transcriptome by RNA sequencing. Genes Immun 2014; 15(6):361–9.
21. Blanchard C, Mingler MK, Vicario M, et al. IL-13 involvement in eosinophilic esophagitis: transcriptome analysis and reversibility with glucocorticoids. J Allergy Clin Immunol 2007;120(6):1292–300.
22. Blanchard C, Stucke EM, Rodriguez-Jimenez B, et al. A striking local esophageal cytokine expression profile in eosinophilic esophagitis. J Allergy Clin Immunol 2011;127(1):208–17, 217.e1–7.
23. Mueller S. Classification of eosinophilic gastrointestinal diseases. Best Pract Res Clin Gastroenterol 2008;22(3):425–40.

24. Pentiuk S, Putnam PE, Collins MH, et al. Dissociation between symptoms and histological severity in pediatric eosinophilic esophagitis. J Pediatr Gastroenterol Nutr 2009;48(2):152–60.

25. Abu-Sultaneh SM, Durst P, Maynard V, et al. Fluticasone and food allergen elimination reverse sub-epithelial fibrosis in children with eosinophilic esophagitis. Dig Dis Sci 2011;56(1):97–102.

26. Kagalwalla AF. Dietary treatment of eosinophilic esophagitis in children. Dig Dis 2014;32(1–2):114–9.

27. Kagalwalla AF, Sentongo TA, Ritz S, et al. Effect of six-food elimination diet on clinical and histologic outcomes in eosinophilic esophagitis. Clin Gastroenterol Hepatol 2006;4(9):1097–102.

28. Helou EF, Simonson J, Arora AS. 3-yr-follow-up of topical corticosteroid treatment for eosinophilic esophagitis in adults. Am J Gastroenterol 2008;103(9):2194–9.

29. Schaefer ET, Fitzgerald JF, Molleston JP, et al. Comparison of oral prednisone and topical fluticasone in the treatment of eosinophilic esophagitis: a randomized trial in children. Clin Gastroenterol Hepatol 2008;6(2):165–73.

30. Teitelbaum JE, Fox VL, Twarog FJ, et al. Eosinophilic esophagitis in children: immunopathological analysis and response to fluticasone propionate. Gastroenterology 2002;122(5):1216–25.

31. Arora AS, Perrault J, Smyrk TC. Topical corticosteroid treatment of dysphagia due to eosinophilic esophagitis in adults. Mayo Clin Proc 2003;78(7):830–5.

32. Aceves SS, Bastian JF, Newbury RO, et al. Oral viscous budesonide: a potential new therapy for eosinophilic esophagitis in children. Am J Gastroenterol 2007; 102(10):2271–9 [quiz: 2280].

33. Dohil R, Newbury R, Fox L, et al. Oral viscous budesonide is effective in children with eosinophilic esophagitis in a randomized, placebo-controlled trial. Gastroenterology 2010;139(2):418–29.

34. Konikoff MR, Noel RJ, Blanchard C, et al. A randomized, double-blind, placebo-controlled trial of fluticasone propionate for pediatric eosinophilic esophagitis. Gastroenterology 2006;131(5):1381–91.

35. Straumann A, Conus S, Degen L, et al. Budesonide is effective in adolescent and adult patients with active eosinophilic esophagitis. Gastroenterology 2010; 139(5):1526–37, 1537.e1.

36. Hurtado CW, Furuta GT, Kramer RE. Etiology of esophageal food impactions in children. J Pediatr Gastroenterol Nutr 2011;52(1):43–6.

37. Falk GW. Clinical presentation of eosinophilic esophagitis in adults. Gastroenterol Clin North Am 2014;43(2):231–42.

38. Desai TK, Stecevic V, Chang CH, et al. Association of eosinophilic inflammation with esophageal food impaction in adults. Gastrointest Endosc 2005;61(7): 795–801.

39. Sperry SL, Crockett SD, Miller CB, et al. Esophageal foreign-body impactions: epidemiology, time trends, and the impact of the increasing prevalence of eosinophilic esophagitis. Gastrointest Endosc 2011;74(5):985–91.

40. Alrazzak BA, Al-Subu A, Elitsur Y. Etiology and management of esophageal impaction in children: a review of 11 years. Avicenna J Med 2013;3(2):33–6.

41. Schoepfer AM, Safroneeva E, Bussmann C, et al. Delay in diagnosis of eosinophilic esophagitis increases risk for stricture formation in a time-dependent manner. Gastroenterology 2013;145(6):1230–6.e1–2.

42. Gentile N, Katzka D, Ravi K, et al. Oesophageal narrowing is common and frequently under-appreciated at endoscopy in patients with oesophageal eosinophilia. Aliment Pharmacol Ther 2014;40(11–12):1333–40.

43. Aceves SS, Newbury RO, Chen D, et al. Resolution of remodeling in eosinophilic esophagitis correlates with epithelial response to topical corticosteroids. Allergy 2010;65(1):109–16.
44. Lipka S, Keshishian J, Boyce HW, et al. The natural history of steroid-naive eosinophilic esophagitis in adults treated with endoscopic dilation and proton pump inhibitor therapy over a mean duration of nearly 14 years. Gastrointest Endosc 2014;80(4):592–8.
45. Dellon ES, Cullen NR, Madanick RD, et al. Outcomes of a combined antegrade and retrograde approach for dilatation of radiation-induced esophageal strictures (with video). Gastrointest Endosc 2010;71(7):1122–9.
46. Madanick RD, Shaheen NJ, Dellon ES. A novel balloon pull-through technique for esophageal dilation in eosinophilic esophagitis (with video). Gastrointest Endosc 2011;73(1):138–42.
47. Schoepfer AM, Gonsalves N, Bussmann C, et al. Esophageal dilation in eosinophilic esophagitis: effectiveness, safety, and impact on the underlying inflammation. Am J Gastroenterol 2010;105(5):1062–70.
48. Hirano I. Dilation in eosinophilic esophagitis: to do or not to do? Gastrointest Endosc 2010;71(4):713–4.
49. Peery AF, Shaheen NJ, Dellon ES. Practice patterns for the evaluation and treatment of eosinophilic oesophagitis. Aliment Pharmacol Ther 2010;32(11–12):1373–82.
50. Spergel JM, Book WM, Mays E, et al. Variation in prevalence, diagnostic criteria, and initial management options for eosinophilic gastrointestinal diseases in the United States. J Pediatr Gastroenterol Nutr 2011;52(3):300–6.
51. Lucendo AJ, Arias A, Molina-Infante J, et al. Diagnostic and therapeutic management of eosinophilic oesophagitis in children and adults: results from a Spanish registry of clinical practice. Dig Liver Dis 2013;45(7):562–8.
52. Dellon ES, Aderoju A, Woosley JT, et al. Variability in diagnostic criteria for eosinophilic esophagitis: a systematic review. Am J Gastroenterol 2007;102(10): 2300–13.
53. Liacouras CA, Wenner WJ, Brown K, et al. Primary eosinophilic esophagitis in children: successful treatment with oral corticosteroids. J Pediatr Gastroenterol Nutr 1998;26(4):380–5.
54. Rodrigo S, Abboud G, Oh D, et al. High intraepithelial eosinophil counts in esophageal squamous epithelium are not specific for eosinophilic esophagitis in adults. Am J Gastroenterol 2008;103(2):435–42.
55. Gonsalves N, Policarpio-Nicolas M, Zhang Q, et al. Histopathologic variability and endoscopic correlates in adults with eosinophilic esophagitis. Gastrointest Endosc 2006;64(3):313–9.
56. Stucke EM, Clarridge KE, Collins MH, et al. The value of an additional review for eosinophil quantification in esophageal biopsies. J Pediatr Gastroenterol Nutr 2015;61(1):65–8.
57. Blanchard C, Wang N, Stringer KF, et al. Eotaxin-3 and a uniquely conserved gene-expression profile in eosinophilic esophagitis. J Clin Invest 2006;116(2): 536–47.
58. Wen T, Stucke EM, Grotjan TM, et al. Molecular diagnosis of eosinophilic esophagitis by gene expression profiling. Gastroenterology 2013;145(6):1289–99.
59. Mavi P, Rajavelu P, Rayapudi M, et al. Esophageal functional impairments in experimental eosinophilic esophagitis. Am J Physiol Gastrointest Liver Physiol 2012;302(11):G1347–55.
60. Fox VL, Nurko S, Teitelbaum JE, et al. High-resolution EUS in children with eosinophilic "allergic" esophagitis. Gastrointest Endosc 2003;57(1):30–6.

61. Korsapati H, Babaei A, Bhargava V, et al. Dysfunction of the longitudinal muscles of the oesophagus in eosinophilic oesophagitis. Gut 2009;58(8):1056–62.

62. Nicodeme F, Hirano I, Chen J, et al. Esophageal distensibility as a measure of disease severity in patients with eosinophilic esophagitis. Clin Gastroenterol Hepatol 2013;11(9):1101–7.e1.

63. Martin Martin L, Santander C, Lopez Martin MC, et al. Esophageal motor abnormalities in eosinophilic esophagitis identified by high-resolution manometry. J Gastroenterol Hepatol 2011;26(9):1447–50.

64. Rieder F, Nonevski I, Ma J, et al. T-helper 2 cytokines, transforming growth factor beta1, and eosinophil products induce fibrogenesis and alter muscle motility in patients with eosinophilic esophagitis. Gastroenterology 2014;146(5):1266–77.e1–9.

65. van Rhijn BD, Oors JM, Smout AJ, et al. Prevalence of esophageal motility abnormalities increases with longer disease duration in adult patients with eosinophilic esophagitis. Neurogastroenterol Motil 2014;26(9):1349–55.

66. Colizzo JM, Clayton SB, Richter JE. Intrabolus pressure on high-resolution manometry distinguishes fibrostenotic and inflammatory phenotypes of eosinophilic esophagitis. Dis esophagus 2015. [Epub ahead of print].

67. Furuta GT, Kagalwalla AF, Lee JJ, et al. The oesophageal string test: a novel, minimally invasive method measures mucosal inflammation in eosinophilic oesophagitis. Gut 2013;62(10):1395–405.

68. Katzka DA, Geno DM, Ravi A, et al. Accuracy, safety, and tolerability of tissue collection by cytosponge vs endoscopy for evaluation of eosinophilic esophagitis. Clin Gastroenterol Hepatol 2015;13(1):77–83.e72.

69. Dellon ES, Rusin S, Gebhart JH, et al. Utility of a noninvasive serum biomarker panel for diagnosis and monitoring of eosinophilic esophagitis: a prospective study. Am J Gastroenterol 2015;110(6):821–7.

70. Subbarao G, Rosenman MB, Ohnuki L, et al. Exploring potential noninvasive biomarkers in eosinophilic esophagitis in children. J Pediatr Gastroenterol Nutr 2011; 53(6):651–8.

71. Sherrill JD, Rothenberg ME. Genetic and epigenetic underpinnings of eosinophilic esophagitis. Gastroenterol Clin North Am 2014;43(2):269–80.

72. Lu TX, Sherrill JD, Wen T, et al. MicroRNA signature in patients with eosinophilic esophagitis, reversibility with glucocorticoids, and assessment as disease biomarkers. J Allergy Clin Immunol 2012;129(4):1064–75.e9.

73. Zahm AM, Menard-Katcher C, Benitez AJ, et al. Pediatric eosinophilic esophagitis is associated with changes in esophageal microRNAs. Am J Physiol Gastrointest Liver Physiol 2014;307(8):G803–12.

Endoscopic Management of Anastomotic Esophageal Strictures Secondary to Esophageal Atresia

Michael A. Manfredi, MD[a,b,]*

KEYWORDS

- Esophageal atresia • Tracheoesophageal fistula • Esophageal stricture
- Esophageal dilation • Esophageal stenting • Intralesional steroid injection
- Endoscopic incisional therapy • Mitomycin C

KEY POINTS

- Esophageal dilation with balloon or savory dilators are equally safe and effective for the treatment of anastomotic strictures associated with esophageal atresia.
- Dilations should be performed every 2 weeks for 2 to 3 months before deeming a stricture refractory.
- Intralesional steroid therapy should be strongly considered as first-line therapy for refractory strictures.
- Other adjunct therapies, such as Mitomycin C, endoscopic incisional therapy, and esophageal stent placement, have some reported benefits; however, they also have more inherent risk.
- Nissen fundoplication should be considered if gastroesophageal reflux is suspected to be contributing to recurrent structuring.

INTRODUCTION

Esophageal atresia (EA) with or without tracheoesophageal fistula (TEF) is the most common congenital anomaly of the esophagus.[1] The overall incidence of EA/TEF ranges from 1 in every 2500 to 4500 live births. The first successful EA/TEF repair was performed by Dr Cameron Height in 1941. The technical goal of the surgery is to first divide the TEF very close to the trachea and then ligate it with nonabsorbable

Disclosure Statement: The author has nothing to disclose.
[a] Esophageal and Airway Atresia Treatment Center, Boston Children's Hospital, Boston, MA 02132, USA; [b] Pediatrics Harvard Medical School, Boston, MA 02115, USA
* 194 Corey Street, West Roxbury, MA 02132.
E-mail address: Michael.Manfredi@childrens.harvard.edu

sutures. Following TEF ligation, the EA is repaired through the creation of an anastomosis from the proximal esophageal pouch and the distal esophageal segment. The anastomosis is usually achieved in end-to-end fashion.[2,3]

Survival rates for patients with EA with or without TEF have improved greatly over the past 2 decades with technical advances in surgery as well as with critical care medicine. The most recent survival rates have ranged from 91% to 97%.[4–6] The survival rates for infants born full-term with no associated congenital anomalies have been of reported to approach 100%.[6,7] Nevertheless, despite high survival rates, patients with EA may deal with significant postoperative morbidity. **Box 1** lists the common morbidities associated with EA postsurgical repair both in the immediate postoperative period, as well as those that can occur later in a patient's life. In this review, we focus on the endoscopic management of esophageal strictures as the most common morbidity associated with EA repair.

ESOPHAGEAL STRICTURE
Pathophysiology and Incidence

The normal process of wound healing after creation of the esophageal anastomosis involves the creation of scar tissue. During the tissue remodeling phase of wound healing, fibroblasts promote wound contraction. Tissue contraction of open wounds is beneficial to close the injury; however, wound contraction in the setting of a circular end-to-end anastomosis creates narrowing. Therefore, it is quite natural to see a degree of narrowing at the site of the esophageal anastomosis after EA repair.

The reported incidence of anastomotic stricture after EA repair has varied in case series from as low as 9% to as high as 80%.[3,8–15] There are several factors implicated in the pathogenesis of anastomotic stricture. These include creation of the esophageal anastomosis under excessive tension, ischemia at the ends of the esophageal pouches, creation of the anastomosis with 2 suture layers, use of silk suture material, anastomotic leak, esophageal gap length greater than 4 cm (long gap EA), and postoperative gastroesophageal reflux.[16]

Esophageal Stricture Symptoms and Definitions

When a swallowed food bolus becomes too large to pass through the narrowed portion of the esophagus, symptoms of dysphagia will occur. Typical symptoms of

---

Box 1
Common morbidities associated with postsurgical esophageal atresia repair

Esophageal stricture

Esophageal leak or perforation

Anastomosis dehiscence

Recurrent tracheoesophageal fistula

Gastroesophageal reflux disease

Dysphagia

Esophageal dysmotility

Aspiration

Esophagitis

Barrett esophagus

Esophageal cancer

an esophageal stricture include feeding difficulties, coughing and choking during feeds, food impaction, and regurgitation of undigested material. In younger children, apnea may be a presenting symptom as well as feeding refusal. If a patient with EA develops any of these symptoms he or she should undergo a contrast fluoroscopy study and/or endoscopy to evaluate for a possible stricture. An esophageal stricture therefore is defined as an intrinsic luminal narrowing that leads to the patient becoming clinically symptomatic.

In older children and adolescents, an esophageal luminal diameter of 13 mm or smaller typically results in dysphagia to solids.[17] Dysphagia to liquids occurs when the esophageal diameter is even narrower. Typically, liquid dysphagia will occur with esophageal diameters of 5 mm or smaller; however, we have seen children drink normally with stricture diameters much smaller than this. Dysphagia to purées will occur generally when the esophageal diameter is 8 mm or smaller to 10 mm depending on the viscosity of the purée.

In adults, strictures are classified as simple or complex. A simple stricture is defined as one that is, short in length, focal, straight, and allows passage of an adult-diameter endoscope ($\approx$9 mm).[18,19] A complex stricture is classified as having one of the following characteristics: long in length (>2 cm), angulated, irregular, and or has a severely narrow diameter.[18,19] In general, simple strictures are more easily dilated and require fewer treatments to remediate the lumen size. Complex strictures are more likely to become refractory or recalcitrant.

In adults, a stricture is defined as refractory or recalcitrant when there is an inability to remediate the esophageal lumen to a diameter of 14 mm during 5 dilation sessions at 2-week intervals.[20,21] A recurrent stricture is defined as the inability to maintain a lumen patency for 4 weeks once the target diameter of 14 mm has been achieved.[20,21] An alternative definition of a refractory stricture is a stricture that requires ongoing dilation sessions (more than 7–10).[18]

There are no agreed on definitions for benign refractory strictures in pediatrics. It is our practice to follow the adult definitions; however, we modify the goal diameter based on the patient's age. For infants 6 months of age or younger, our goal lumen diameter to achieve is 10 mm. For infants older than 6 months and children to approximately the age of 7, we use a diameter of 12 mm. For older children approximately 7 years of age or older, we use the adult definition with a diameter of 14 mm.

In an attempt to better standardize and quantify strictures in children, Said and colleagues[22] developed an anastomotic stricture index (SI) defined as follows: $SI = \frac{(D-d)}{D} \times 100$, where D is the diameter of esophagus below the stricture and d is the diameter of the stricture. In this study, dilations were considered successful if the SI decreased to 10% or less. Parolini and colleagues[23] used the SI to classify strictures into mild (>0.1) and severe categories ($\geq$0.3). It is important to note that Parolini and colleagues[23] did not specify whether they measured the upper or lower esophagus in their calculation of the SI. Not surprisingly, both mild and severe groups were at increased risk of requiring esophageal dilations. A definition for a recalcitrant and recurrent pediatric stricture based on the SI has been proposed. A recalcitrant stricture would be a persistent SI greater than 10% after 5 dilation sessions, and a recurrent stricture would be an SI greater than 50% 4 weeks after SI less than 10% had been achieved.[9]

Nambirajan and colleagues[24] described an anastomotic index (AI) calculated as a ratio of the diameter of the upper pouch to the diameter of the anastomosis on contrast study. In this study, the AI did not predict the development of a recalcitrant stricture.

Recently, a new SI, the Esophageal Anastomotic SI (EASI), was described by Sun and colleagues.[25] In this study, the EASI was calculated at the time of postoperative contrast esophagram (5–10 days post anastomosis), and defined as follows: lateral $\frac{d}{D}$ + Anteroposterior $\frac{d}{D}$ 2. In this equation, d is the diameter of the stricture and D is the diameter of esophagus either below the stricture or above the stricture. The investigators concluded that EASI was more accurate using the diameter of the esophagus below the stricture as opposed to the calculations using the diameters above the stricture.[25] This is likely due the upper pouch generally being more dilated secondary to chronic obstruction in utero, as well as increased pressure in the upper esophagus secondary to increased resistance across the stricture area. In their study, an EASI of 0.30 or less highly correlated with requiring a course of dilatations.

Although all of the stricture indices show merit in standardizing stricture evaluation in pediatrics, further validation is required before any one can be accepted into clinical practice. In the meantime, it remains unclear whether these indices are clinically more useful than just estimating the stricture diameter. Indeed, it is possible that these indices may only prove useful for academic purposes. Furthermore, although estimating the size of the stricture is important, the patient's clinical symptoms should always be taken into account before starting any stricture therapy.

ESOPHAGEAL STRICTURE TREATMENT
Dilation

The cornerstone of esophageal stricture treatment is dilation. The goal of esophageal dilation is to increase the luminal diameter of the esophagus while also improving dysphagia symptoms. This is achieved through circumferential stretching and splitting of the scar tissue within the stricture.[19,26] Dilators can be characterized as mechanical (bougie) dilators or balloon-based dilators.

Mechanical (Bougie) Dilators

There are several different types of bougie-based dilators. Today, the most common types of bougie dilators used are guidewire based. These dilators are tapered cylindrical solid tubes made of polyvinyl chloride with a central channel to accommodate a guidewire.[27] These dilating tubes have varying lengths of tapering at the tip and also have radiopaque markers to allow for fluoroscopic guidance (eg, Savary-Gilliard dilators (Cook Medical, Bloomington, IN), American Dilators (CONMED, Utica, NY), and Safeguide (Medovations, Milwaukee, WI)).

There are also non-guidewire mechanical dilators that are tungsten weighted to allow for gravity assistance when the patient is in a seated position. The 2 commonly used non-guidewire bougie dilators are Hurst (Medovations, Milwaukee, WI) and Maloney dilators (Medovations, Milwaukee, WI). These 2 dilators differ by their tips. The Hurst dilators have a rounded blunt tip, whereas the Maloney dilators have a tapered tip.[27] Both dilators were designed for self-dilation at home.

Another type of mechanical dilator is the Tucker dilator (Medovations, Milwaukee, WI). These are small silicone bougies that are tapered at each end. There are loops on each end with a string attached to each end to allow for the dilator to be pulled antegrade or retrograde across strictures. These dilators are used when the patient has a gastrostomy tube. Tucker dilators can remain inside the patient for periodic serial dilations.

The basic technique of mechanical dilations involves the passage of a bougie dilator across the stricture. This results in both longitudinal shearing force as well as radial force on the stricture area. The goal of mechanical dilation is to pass serial bougie dilators of incremental size across the stricture site. Although fluoroscopy can be helpful to confirm your position as you pass the bougie dilator, it is not mandatory. It is generally recommended to use fluoroscopy in complex strictures.

Mechanical dilation is a tactile technique. As the bougie is advanced across the stricture site, it should be possible for the proceduralist to be able to feel a degree of resistance. The object is to feel and then overcome the resistance across the strictured area. Once moderate resistance is encountered with the bougie dilator, it is generally recommend passing no more than 3 consecutive dilators in increments of 1 mm in a single session for a total of 3 mm. Although there are no published studies, this consensus, known as the "rule of 3," is a well-established approach for mechanical dilations that is believed to improve safety and efficacy.[21,28]

Balloon Dilation

Balloons deliver equal radial force simultaneously across the entire length of the stricture. They are designed to pass through the endoscope with or without a guidewire. Through-the-scope dilation allows the endoscopist to directly visualize the stricture during and immediately after the dilation. A potential drawback for through-the-scope balloon dilation in EA stricture therapy is that it requires the use of an adult gastroscope, which has a minimum working channel of 2.8 mm. This size gastroscope can be difficult to use in younger infants weighing less than 10 kg.

In younger patients, the balloon can be passed over a guidewire under fluoroscopic guidance. This is performed by passing a 0.035-mm guidewire across the stricture through the endoscope working channel. A wire exchange under fluoroscopy is performed, leaving the wire in place as the scope is removed. The balloon is then passed over the wire.

Dilating balloons expand by the injection of liquid (eg, water, radiopaque contrast) under pressure using a handheld inflation device. A manometer on the device will measure the fluid pressure in the balloon to allow for accurate radial expansion force.[27]

Balloon dilators are designed to inflate to one set diameter or allow for sequential inflation to multiple sizes (typically 3 sizes per balloon). Multisized balloons will inflate to different sizes based on the amount of pressure infused into the balloon.

The basic approach to balloon dilation is to first estimate the size of the stricture. Once the size is estimated, the "rule of 3" can be applied to balloon dilators by choosing a balloon that will increase in size by increments of 1 mm in a single session for a total of 3 mm above the originally estimated stricture size. The balloon is advanced across the stricture either with endoscopic and/or fluoroscopic guidance. Ideally the balloon should be centered so that the middle of the balloon is centered across the stricture. Balloons are available with or without a wire.

The typical approach in our program is to have a wire across the stricture and typically into the stomach. The goal of the wire is to make certain that the tip of the balloon remains within the lumen of the esophagus. Having a wire across a complex stricture is recommended. If a complex stricture is encountered that is very narrow and/or torturous and a wire is not used, it is possible for the tip of the balloon to dissect through the esophageal wall.

Once the balloon is properly positioned, it can be inflated to the desired size. The optimal inflation time has not been established. Balloon inflation times of 30 to 60 seconds are generally accepted.[19] One recent study examined the effect of duration of balloon dilation by randomizing stricture patients into 2 groups.[29] The first group had balloon inflation times lasting only 10 seconds and the second group had balloon inflation times of 2 minutes. In this study, there was no significant difference in effectiveness of dilations in either group. Therefore, it appears that the act of inflation that tears the scar tissue is more important than the duration the balloon is inflated.

The use of fluoroscopy during balloon dilation is helpful. In the setting of a complex stricture, fluoroscopy is useful in advancing the wire and balloon safely across the stricture. In addition, inflating the balloon with contrast will allow the endoscopist to see if the stricture is being effectively dilated. It is useful to see the appearance of the stricture forming a waist around the balloon and the subsequent obliteration of a waist as the balloon is further inflated (**Fig. 1**). It is a practice of this author to use fluoroscopy frequently with our EA stricture dilations. In addition, there is the added benefit of using fluoroscopy to conduct a postdilation contrast study to evaluate for a postdilation esophageal leak or perforation.

Outcomes and Comparative Data

A recent systematic review analyzed 5 studies that looked at outcomes of balloon dilation in children with EA.[30] This study looked at total of 139 children with a total of 401 balloon dilation sessions. The reported success rate ranged from 70% to 100%, with approximately 3 dilation sessions per child.[22,31–34] The reported perforation rate for the combined studies was 1.8% following balloon dilation.[30] The reported success rate for bougie dilations in EA has been reported from 87% to 90% with mean number of 3.2 dilations per patient in both studies.[35,36] There was one reported esophageal perforation in the study with bougie dilation that was fatal to the patient. In a large study of bougie dilations in children (n = 107), the reported perforation rate was 0.9%. In this study, the stricture population was mixed, with most patients having caustic strictures.[37]

There have been several studies comparing the effectiveness of bougie dilation with balloon dilation. Lang and colleagues[34] retrospectively looked at patients with EA who underwent bougie dilation compared with balloon dilation. The balloon dilation group required fewer procedures compared with the bougie group: median 2.0 versus 8.5, respectively, $P = .002$. Jayakrishnan and colleagues[38] looked at technical success defined as being able to perform the dilation in 37 children (24 patients with EA). There

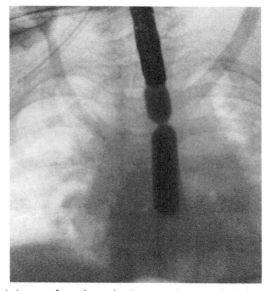

Fig. 1. Fluoroscopic image of esophageal stricture waist around the balloon.

were fewer technical failures in the balloon group compared with the bougie group (0/ 125 vs 4/88, $P<.02$). In addition, there were fewer perforations in the balloon group compared with the bougie group 1.6% versus 5.7% ($P = .1$).[38]

In adults, there have been 2 randomized controlled trials comparing bougie dilations with balloon dilations in benign esophageal strictures.[39,40] In these 2 studies, there was no significant difference in efficacy and safety. Therefore, it is generally recommended that the method of choice between balloon dilation and bougie depends on operator experience and comfort with the equipment. The only time that bougie dilation is completely contraindicated is in the setting of patients with epidermolysis bullosa. In this setting, the longitudinal sheering force may result in further damage to other segments of the esophagus.

TREATMENT THERAPIES FOR REFRACTORY STRICTURES

Once a stricture becomes refractory to esophageal dilation, there are several treatment therapies available as adjuncts to dilation therapy. These therapies are described as follows and should be considered before any surgical resection.

Intralesional Steroid Injection

The proposed mechanism of intralesional steroid injection in the treatment of esophageal strictures is to locally inhibit the inflammatory response, which in turn results in reduced collagen formation.[41] The efficacy of intralesional triamcinolone injection in peptic strictures has been shown by Ramage and colleagues[42] in a randomized double-blind placebo-controlled trial.[42] In this study, 2 (13%, 95% confidence interval [CI] 4%–38%) of 15 patients in the steroid group and 9 (60%, 95% CI 36%–80%) of 15 in the sham group required repeat dilation ($P = .021$). Those patients who received intralesional steroids were administered 4 quadrant injections of 0.5 mL of triamcinolone acetate (40 mg per mL) for total of 80 mg.

There have been multiple studies that have shown the benefit of intralesional steroids in reducing recurrent stricture formation. However, most reports are small uncontrolled studies evaluating strictures of diverse etiology.[43–46] Hirdes and colleagues,[47] in a multicenter double-blind placebo-controlled trial involving 60 patients with benign esophagogastric anastomotic strictures, reported no statistically significant decrease in frequency of repeat dilations with a median number of 2 dilations (range, 1–7) performed in the corticosteroid group versus 3 dilations (range, 1–9) in the control ($P = .36$). In addition, there was no improvement in dysphagia-free symptoms in each group; 45% of the patients remained dysphagia-free for 6 months in the triamcinolone group, compared with 36% of controls (relative risk, 1.26; 95% CI 0.68–2.36; $P = .46$).[47]

Potential complications of intralesional steroid therapy include adrenal suppression. Therefore, some investigators suggest surveillance for adrenal suppression[9]; however, this is currently not standard of care practice. In addition, there have been reports of increased *Candida* esophagitis.[47] Last, there has been one report of intralesional steroids contributing to the spontaneous rupture of a right aortic arch, presumably secondary to the steroids weakening the arterial wall.[9]

It is our group's practice to start intralesional steroid injections once a stricture is at its third or fourth dilation, if there has been no significant improvement in intraluminal diameter. We use triamcinolone acetate at a concentration of 10 mg/mL at a dose of 1 to 2/mg/kg per dose with a maximum dose of 80 mg. The injections are typically 4 quadrant; however, if the scar tissue is uneven, a preponderance of steroid will be injected at the site where the scar tissue is at its thickest.

Injection is typically recommended directly into the scar tissue; however, we also like to inject subcutaneously, just above the stricture, to allow for diffusion of the medication into the scar tissue area. The rationale behind this is that by directly injecting steroid into the scar tissue, you are more likely to extravasate steroid outside of the esophagus. This may potentially lead to increased risk of complications, as well as decreased effectiveness.

Our group typically will perform a combination of direct injection into the scar tissue and subcutaneous injection above the stricture. Typically patients will undergo anywhere from 1 to 3 steroid injection sessions in combination with dilation before considering additional adjunct therapy.

Mitomycin C

Mitomycin C is an antineoplastic agent that disrupts base paring of DNA molecules and inhibits fibroblast proliferation and reduces fibroblastic collagen synthesis by inhibiting DNA-dependent RNA synthesis. It also induces apoptosis at higher doses by suppressing cellular proliferation during the late G1 and S phases.[48] It has been proposed as an adjunct treatment to manage esophageal strictures.[49] Mitomycin C has been mainly placed topically in the literature; in addition, there are reports of injection of mitomycin C.[50]

There have been numerous descriptions of methods for topically applying mitomycin C. These have included soaking pledgets or cotton swabs and placing them topically on the stricture area; dripping mitomycin via an injection needle onto the affected area; and using a spray catheter. A recent publication described a novel approach that uses a microporous polytetrafluoroethylene catheter balloon.[51] The dose of mitomycin C used in these studies is also variable, ranging from 0.004 mg/mL to 1 mg/mL.[52]

A systematic review of the literature identified 11 publications using mitomycin C in children.[52] The results of the systematic review demonstrated complete relief of symptoms in 21 children (67.7%), with another 6 (19.4%) who had partial relief, and 4 with (12.9%) no benefit. There were no direct or indirect adverse effects of mitomycin C reported. The mean follow-up time for all of these studies was 22 months (range 6–60 months).[52] It is important to note that most of the literature on mitomycin C involves children with caustic strictures, and therefore results may not be applicable to anastomotic strictures. Even in this systematic review, 61% of the patients had caustic strictures and 22% had anastomotic strictures secondary to EA.[52]

A recent prospective study looking at 30 children with caustic strictures compared mitomycin C therapy to dilation therapy alone. Although this study was not blinded and does not appear to be randomized, the mitomycin C group did show a statistically significant improvement in dysphagia score ($P = .005$), and an improvement in the median interval between dilations. The mitomycin group required dilations every 10 weeks after treatment compared with the control group, which required dilations every 4 weeks.[53]

The largest published study to date of mitomycin C in patients with EA looked retrospectively at 21 patients.[54] In this study, 11 patients received mitomycin C topically, and were compared with 10 historical EA controls who received a minimum of 3 dilations. The mitomycin C group received a mean total of 5.4 dilations per patient (range 3–11) and 8 of 11 patients achieved a resolution of their strictures. These results were not significantly different from the control group, which may contradict enthusiastic case reports of the benefit of mitomycin C in patients with EA.[49,51,55–57] Of course, many of these studies lack strict definitions of recalcitrant strictures or criteria for success. Nevertheless, mitomycin C is still promising and likely should be considered a therapeutic modality in patients with recalcitrant strictures secondary to EA.

There is a hypothetical risk of secondary malignancy with mitomycin C, so this must be taken into account and should be discussed with the patient and parents before use.[58] There have been reports of de novo gastric metaplasia around the areas of the anastomosis in 2 of the 6 cases that received topical mitomycin C.[48] This author suggests that long-term follow-up with esophageal biopsies at the site of mitomycin C application should be performed. It is for the hypothetical risk of secondary malignancy with unproven efficacy that our group's preference is first a trial of triamcinolone injections before attempting mitomycin C therapy.

Stents

The use of temporary externally removable stents has been reported to provide an alternative or adjunctive means of preventing stricture formation by providing a continuous means of dilating the esophagus for prolonged periods of time. The 2 types of externally removable temporary stents currently available are self-expanding plastic stent (SEPS) and fully covered self-expanding metal stents (FCSEMS). The current SEPS on the market is made of a woven polyester mesh with a silicon membrane coating to prevent ingrowth of tissue (Polyflex; Boston Scientific Corporation, Marlborough, MA).[59] SEPS are packaged fully expanded and need to be manually loaded onto a delivery system before placement.

FCSEMS consist of a woven, knitted, or laser-cut metal mesh covered by a plastic or silicone membrane to prevent ingrowth.[59] Most FCSEMS are made of Nitinol, which is an alloy of nickel and titanium that has the properties of shape memory as well as super elasticity. Therefore, Nitinol stents have the ability to come packaged greatly compressed on a loading device and once deployed it will self-expand to its predetermined shape. Both SEPS and FCSEMS are deployed via a delivery device catheter over a guidewire under fluoroscopic guidance. However, FCSEMS are easier to place due to increased flexibility and smaller size of the delivery device, as well as the small compressed nature of the nondeployed stent.

There are currently no esophageal stents on the market designed for pediatric patients. The smallest esophageal stent currently available in the United States is the FCSEMS ALIMAXX-ES Fully Covered Esophageal Stent (Merit Medical Systems, South Jordan, UT) with a diameter of 12 mm and a length of 7 cm. This is why most stents placed in the esophagus of pediatric patients are airway stents (ie, Polyflex [Boston Scientific Corporation], AERO Fully Covered Tracheobronchial Stents [Merit Medical Systems], and Taewoong Niti-S Tracheobronchial Stents [Taewoong Medical, Goyang, South Korea]).

Airway stents range in diameter range from 8 mm to 20 mm and lengths ranging from 20 mm 80 mm. A drawback of airway stents is that they are more rigid than traditional esophageal stents, which in our experience leads to more ulceration to the esophagus and increase patient discomfort. An alternative to airway stents are biliary stents. There are several fully covered biliary stents on the market (ie, WallFlex [Boston Scientific Corporation], GORE VIABIL [Gore Medical, Flagstaff, AZ] and Taewoong Niti-S [Taewoong Medical]). Biliary stents are more flexible than airway stents, which we have found to cause less esophageal tissue injury, and to be associated with better patient comfort and tolerance. Biliary stents are limited only by their size, with available diameter sizes of 8 mm and 10 mm, and lengths of 40 mm, 60 mm, or 80 mm.

The use of removable stents to definitively treat benign esophageal strictures in adults has yielded mixed results, with a broad range of success rates from 12% to 80% for stricture resolution reflecting both retrospective and prospective study designs.[60–66] Relevant to our discussion may be the study by Barthel and colleagues,[61] which had the lowest success rate of 12% and looked primarily at anastomotic strictures.

In addition, a recent pooled analysis study of externally removable stents for benign esophageal strictures in adults (n = 232 patients) calculated a pooled success rate of externally removable stents in the treatment of refractory benign strictures to be 24.2%, with a pooled stent migration rate of 16.5% (77/468).[67] Other complications associated with stent placement in this population included chest pain (0.8%), granulation tissue (2.7%), ulceration (0.8%), nausea and retching (0.8%), stent-related perforation (1%), and stent-related stricture formation (0.2%).[67]

The pediatric data on stricture resolution after stent placement has been more promising, with success rates ranging from 50% to 86%[68–70]; however, most pediatric studies have been limited by small numbers, as well as mixed stricture populations. Our group has published the largest review to date of self-expanding stents for the treatment of anastomotic strictures with EA.[71] In our study, 23 patients with EA underwent a total of 40 stenting sessions. Both SEPS (n = 14) and FCSEMS (n = 26) were used. Procedural success was defined as requiring no additional therapy after stent removal at 30 days or more and at 90 days or more. The rate of stricture resolution for 30 days or more after final stent removal was 39% (9/23) and a 90-day success rate of 26% (6/23). We also found the mean duration of stent placement was 9.7 days (with a range of 2–30 days). Complications of stent placement in our population included migration (21% of SEPS and 7% of FCSEMS), granulation tissue (37% of FCSEMS and 0% of SEPS), deep tissue ulcerations (22% of FCSEMS and 0% if SEPS), as well as pain and retching (26% of FCSEMS and 23% of SEPS).[71]

The ideal duration of time a stent remains in place is unknown. In general, consensus is to leave the stent in place until inflammation has resolved, which is believed to reduce the risks of restricturing after stent removal. In the cases of severe adult strictures, the recommended duration varies from 8 to 16 weeks. In our study, the mean duration of time was 9.7 days, although our goal was to try to leave stents in place for 2 weeks.

Anecdotally, our group has noticed increased ulceration with longer stent duration. Therefore, our protocol is to keep patients in the hospital for the duration the stent is in place, using monitoring with periodic chest radiographs to assess for migration as well as for assessing the orientation of the stent to evaluate for erosion into the esophagus (**Fig. 2**A, B). We typically will endoscopically reevaluate a patient 1 week after the stent is placed to evaluate the tissue for any injury. At that time, we decide to leave the stent in place, replace it, or remove it completely.

It is our experience that patient symptoms often dictate stent removal, as many patients appear uncomfortable with the stent in place. It is also our experience that many children do not want to eat with the stent in place, so alternative means of receiving nutrition should be considered before placing the stent. Longer stent durations can be considered in patients with no discomfort; however, we strongly recommend evaluating the esophagus with chest radiographs and periodic endoscopy to ensure there is no evidence of significant tissue injury to the esophagus due to the stent (**Fig. 2**C).

The use of "dynamic stents," which are custom silicon stents attached to a nasogastric tube, has been proposed to be a useful treatment for strictures. In several published series, the reported healing of the strictures with intraluminal stents was 96%, 72%, and 69%, respectively.[72–74] In refractory anastomotic strictures due to EA, the dynamic stent has been used in 21 patients with a reported success rate of 81%.[75] The investigators of this study have hypothesized that the dynamic effect of food passage between the stent and the esophageal wall allows for the long-term improvement of esophageal patency.

Biodegradable stents (poly-L-lactide or polydioxanone) are a newer technology that has been under evaluation for benign strictures. In the largest study to date, there were

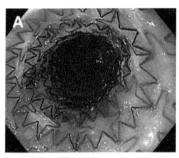
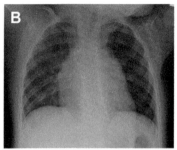
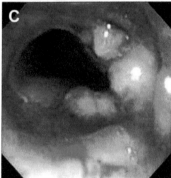

Fig. 2. (*A*) Endoscopic image of a fully covered self-expanding metal stent in the esophagus across a stricture. (*B*) Postprocedure radiograph 2 days later confirming proper stent position. (*C*) Endoscopic image of a deep esophageal ulceration caused by the distal edge of the stent eroding into the esophagus. This would later heal as a stricture.

9 (45%) of 20 patients dysphagia free at 6-month follow-up.[76] A pediatric study looking at 7 patients with caustic ingestion reported complete or partial benefit in 3 of 7 patients.[77] The reported stent migration rate is approximately 10%, and with stent degradation there is also a significant hyperplastic tissue response.[78] Biodegradable stents along with the other previously mentioned stents show promise, but still require further investigation before they should be considered for widespread use.

Incisional Therapy

Endoscopic electrocautery incisional therapy (EIT) has been reported as an alternative treatment for refractory strictures in a small number of adult series. There are variations in the EIT technique reported in the literature. The EIT technique involves the use of a needle knife to make incisions into a stricture at its most dense points. Typically, multiple radial incisions are made around the stricture site (**Fig. 3**). An electrosurgical generator applies a cut current to make the incision. Our approach is to make several incisions to the stricture site. The incisional therapy is then followed-up with balloon dilation. The balloon allows for preferential tearing along the incision site.

EIT therapy has shown promise in the treatment of refractory anastomotic strictures in a few adult series. Hordijk and colleagues[79] published a study of 20 patients with refractory anastomotic strictures and demonstrated that incisional therapy was safe and effective, especially in the treatment of simple, short strictures (<10 mm) that had previously proven refractory to bougie dilation. In a subsequent randomized prospective study, Hordijk and colleagues[80] evaluated 62 patients (31 in EIT group) and showed no difference in effectiveness between EIT and Savory dilations. Similarly,

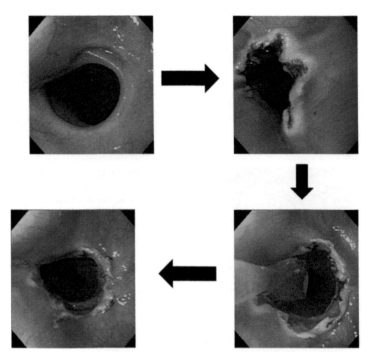

Fig. 3. Series of endoscopic images demonstrating EIT. First a series of radial incisions were made where the scar tissue was at its most dense, followed by balloon dilation to facilitate preferential tearing along the areas of prior incision.

Muto and colleagues[81] performed a retrospective study of 32 patients with refractory anastomotic strictures, and reported EIT to be safe and effective. In the study by Muto and colleagues,[81] the 6-month and 12-month patency rates were significantly different between the EIT group and the group receiving balloon dilation only (65.3% vs 19.8%, $P<.005$; 61.5% vs 19.8%, $P<.005$).

These results may support the findings of several smaller studies. In particular, Simmons and colleagues[82] retrospectively showed that 8 of 9 patients experienced a reduction in dysphagia symptoms and a reduced need for endoscopic dilations after incisional therapy. Also, Lee and colleagues[83] used a modified endoscopic incisional technique applying a transparent hood on the tip of the endoscope to enhance control and safety. In this study, 21 (87.5%) of 24 patients received only 1 EIT session and resumed eating solid meals and had no dysphagia. Three patients (12.5%) developed restricturing at a mean of 1.6 months.

Our own experience with EIT has shown similar promise. Specifically, we have reported on a total of 92 EIT sessions on 45 distinct strictures performed on 42 patients.[84] In our population, the most common stricture etiology was anastomotic secondary to EA (n = 40), although we also had patients with congenital (n = 4), and caustic strictures (n = 1). We categorized strictures in our population by the number of dilations done before EIT: nonrefractory ($\leq$4 dilations), refractory (5–9 dilations), or severe refractory ($\geq$10 dilations). In our study, 37.8% of the strictures were categorized as nonrefractory, 35.6% refractory, and 26.7% severe refractory. Average inner stricture diameter at the time of initial EIT was 7.7 mm (2–12 mm) and 93.3% were 1 cm or smaller in length. Procedural success was defined as requiring 5 or fewer dilations within 6 months of EIT and longer-term procedural success defined as requiring 6 or fewer dilations within 12 months.

Our reported experience suggests overall procedural success at 6 and 12 months may be 78% (32/41) and 64.5% (20/31), respectively. In addition, the 6-month procedural success rate based on stricture category has been 93.8% (nonrefractory), 92.3% (refractory), and 50% (severe refractory). The overall adverse event rate in our review was 9.8% with 4 major (4.4%) and 5 minor events (5.4%). All minor events required no intervention and patients were discharged home within 24 hours.[84] All major adverse events did not require surgery to seal the leak (2 sealed with nasal esophageal tube, 1 with endoscopic clip, and 1 with stent placement).[84]

In turn, we feel that EIT shows promise as a treatment option for pediatric refractory strictures and may be considered before surgical resection, even in severe cases. The complication rate, albeit low, is significant, and EIT should be considered only in experienced hands with surgical consultation. Further prospective longitudinal studies are needed to validate this treatment.

GENERAL APPROACH TO STRICTURE MANAGEMENT

The general recommendation for dilation in most patients with type C EA is that dilations should be started only when a patient become symptomatic. There have been several studies that showed no difference in outcomes between patients who were started on a routine dilation schedule compared with performing dilations when the patient is symptomatic.[24,85] We should point out that this applies to standard cases of EA in patients who have had an early surgical repair with minimal tension on the esophageal anastomosis. However, it is also important to note that infants may not become symptomatic for many months until the patient is transitioned to more solid foods. This is because the diameter of the esophagus needed to tolerate liquids (ie, breast milk or infant formula) is very small; therefore, there could be significant narrowing over the first few months that is not picked up until the patient has advanced his or her diet to more solid foods.

The symptomatic approach to dilation does not apply for patients with risk factors implicated in the pathogenesis of anastomotic strictures. Our approach for patients who are at higher risk for stricturing (ie, patients with long gap EA and patients who develop postanastomotic leaks), would be to start dilations before the patient becomes symptomatic. Routine dilations are typically started 3 to 4 weeks after esophageal anastomosis. Dilations typically occur every 1 to 2 weeks until the lumen maintains its patency. Dilations can then be spaced farther out once the diameter of the esophagus remains somewhat consistent.

All patients with EA postoperatively should be started on acid-blocking medicine. In general, H2 blockers can suffice for most patients with EA. If the patient is having issues with recurrent structuring, we would recommend switching the patient to a proton pump inhibitor. In patients with long gap EA or other high-risk esophageal anastomoses, we typically will start patients initially on a proton pump inhibitor to maximize acid suppression and minimize reflux injury. In patients who have recurrent stricturing and have documented reflux symptoms, and/or a hiatal hernia, a Nissen fundoplication should be considered to help decrease reflux and in turn hopefully reduce the rate of stricturing.

Once dilations are initiated, we consider starting adjunct therapy if no progress is made after the third dilation. Our group typically will start with triamcinolone injection for at least 2 to 3 sessions before attempting another therapy. If triamcinolone injection fails, we then move to mitomycin-C or stenting as the next approach. However, in strictures that lend themselves to incisional therapy (ie, stricture short in length, dense ring of scar tissue), we consider EIT as an alternative to mitomycin C, as well as instead of, or in addition to, stenting.

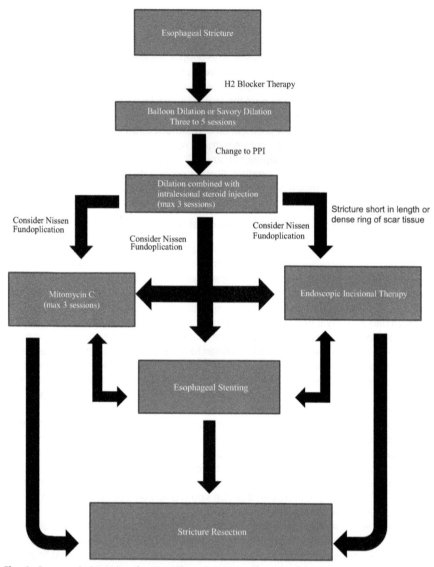

Fig. 4. Proposed algorithm for esophageal anastomotic stricture management in EA. Max, maximum; PPI, proton pump inhibitor.

Last, if all measures are unsuccessful, surgical stricture resection or interposition surgery should be performed. If a stricture is short in length, 1 cm or less stricture, resection should be strongly considered. **Fig. 4** lists a proposed algorithm for endoscopic management of esophageal strictures.

REFERENCES

1. Pinheiro PF, Simoes e Silva AC, Pereira RM. Current knowledge on esophageal atresia. World J Gastroenterol 2012;18:3662–72.

2. Achildi O, Grewal H. Congenital anomalies of the esophagus. Otolaryngol Clin North Am 2007;40:219–44.
3. Kunisaki SM, Foker JE. Surgical advances in the fetus and neonate: esophageal atresia. Clin Perinatol 2012;39:349–61.
4. Sfeir R, Bonnard A, Khen-Dunlop N, et al. Esophageal atresia: data from a national cohort. J Pediatr Surg 2013;48:1664–9.
5. Wang B, Tashiro J, Allan BJ, et al. A nationwide analysis of clinical outcomes among newborns with esophageal atresia and tracheoesophageal fistulas in the United States. J Surg Res 2014;190:604–12.
6. Sistonen SJ, Pakarinen MP, Rintala RJ. Long-term results of esophageal atresia: Helsinki experience and review of literature. Pediatr Surg Int 2011;27:1141–9.
7. Pedersen RN, Calzolari E, Husby S, et al. Oesophageal atresia: prevalence, prenatal diagnosis and associated anomalies in 23 European regions. Arch Dis Child 2012;97:227–32.
8. Baird R, Laberge JM, Levesque D. Anastomotic stricture after esophageal atresia repair: a critical review of recent literature. Eur J Pediatr Surg 2013; 23:204–13.
9. Levesque D, Baird R, Laberge JM. Refractory strictures post-esophageal atresia repair: what are the alternatives? Dis Esophagus 2013;26:382–7.
10. Rintala RJ, Pakarinen MP. Long-term outcome of esophageal anastomosis. Eur J Pediatr Surg 2013;23:219–25.
11. Konkin DE, O'Hali WA, Webber EM, et al. Outcomes in esophageal atresia and tracheoesophageal fistula. J Pediatr Surg 2003;38:1726–9.
12. Spitz L, Kiely E, Brereton RJ, et al. Management of esophageal atresia. World J Surg 1993;17:296–300.
13. Koivusalo AI, Pakarinen MP, Rintala RJ. Modern outcomes of oesophageal atresia: single centre experience over the last twenty years. J Pediatr Surg 2013;48:297–303.
14. Lain A, Cerda J, Canizo A, et al. [Analysis of esophageal strictures secondary to surgical correction of esophageal atresia]. Cir Pediatr 2007;20:203–8 [In Spanish].
15. Engum SA, Grosfeld JL, West KW, et al. Analysis of morbidity and mortality in 227 cases of esophageal atresia and/or tracheoesophageal fistula over two decades. Arch Surg 1995;130:502–8 [discussion: 8–9].
16. Harmon CM, Coran AG. Congenital anomalies of the esophagus. In: Coran AG, Caldamone A, Adzick NS, et al, editors. Pediatric surgery. 7th edition. Philadelphia: Elsevier; 2012. p. 893–918.
17. Pasha SF, Acosta RD, Chandrasekhara V, et al. The role of endoscopy in the evaluation and management of dysphagia. Gastrointest Endosc 2014;79:191–201.
18. Siersema PD. Treatment options for esophageal strictures. Nat Clin Pract Gastroenterol Hepatol 2008;5:142–52.
19. Lew RJ, Kochman ML. A review of endoscopic methods of esophageal dilation. J Clin Gastroenterol 2002;35:117–26.
20. Kochman ML, McClave SA, Boyce HW. The refractory and the recurrent esophageal stricture: a definition. Gastrointest Endosc 2005;62:474–5.
21. Siersema PD, de Wijkerslooth LR. Dilation of refractory benign esophageal strictures. Gastrointest Endosc 2009;70:1000–12.
22. Said M, Mekki M, Golli M, et al. Balloon dilatation of anastomotic strictures secondary to surgical repair of oesophageal atresia. Br J Radiol 2003;76:26–31.
23. Parolini F, Leva E, Morandi A, et al. Anastomotic strictures and endoscopic dilatations following esophageal atresia repair. Pediatr Surg Int 2013;29:601–5.

24. Nambirajan L, Rintala RJ, Losty PD, et al. The value of early postoperative oeso-phagography following repair of oesophageal atresia. Pediatr Surg Int 1998;13: 76–8.
25. Sun LY, Laberge JM, Yousef Y, et al. The esophageal anastomotic stricture index (EASI) for the management of esophageal atresia. J Pediatr Surg 2015;50:107–10.
26. Abele JE. The physics of esophageal dilatation. Hepatogastroenterology 1992; 39:486–9.
27. Siddiqui UD, Banerjee S, Barth B, et al. Tools for endoscopic stricture dilation. Gastrointest Endosc 2013;78:391–404.
28. Spechler SJ. AGA technical review on treatment of patients with dysphagia caused by benign disorders of the distal esophagus. Gastroenterology 1999; 117:233–54.
29. Wallner O, Wallner B. Balloon dilation of benign esophageal rings or strictures: a randomized clinical trial comparing two different inflation times. Dis Esophagus 2014;27:109–11.
30. Thyoka M, Timmis A, Mhango T, et al. Balloon dilatation of anastomotic strictures secondary to surgical repair of oesophageal atresia: a systematic review. Pediatr Radiol 2013;43:898–901 [quiz: 896–7].
31. Antoniou D, Soutis M, Christopoulos-Geroulanos G. Anastomotic strictures following esophageal atresia repair: a 20-year experience with endoscopic balloon dilatation. J Pediatr Gastroenterol Nutr 2010;51:464–7.
32. Johnsen A, Jensen LI, Mauritzen K. Balloon-dilatation of esophageal strictures in children. Pediatr Radiol 1986;16:388–91.
33. Ko HK, Shin JH, Song HY, et al. Balloon dilation of anastomotic strictures second-ary to surgical repair of esophageal atresia in a pediatric population: long-term results. J Vasc Interv Radiol 2006;17:1327–33.
34. Lang T, Hummer HP, Behrens R. Balloon dilation is preferable to bougienage in children with esophageal atresia. Endoscopy 2001;33:329–35.
35. Michaud L, Guimber D, Sfeir R, et al. Anastomotic stenosis after surgical treat-ment of esophageal atresia: frequency, risk factors and effectiveness of esopha-geal dilatations. Arch Pediatr 2001;8:268–74 [In French].
36. Serhal L, Gottrand F, Sfeir R, et al. Anastomotic stricture after surgical repair of esophageal atresia: frequency, risk factors, and efficacy of esophageal bougie dilatations. J Pediatr Surg 2010;45:1459–62.
37. Poddar U, Thapa BR. Benign esophageal strictures in infants and children: re-sults of Savary-Gilliard bougie dilation in 107 Indian children. Gastrointest Endosc 2001;54:480–4.
38. Jayakrishnan VK, Wilkinson AG. Treatment of oesophageal strictures in children: a comparison of fluoroscopically guided balloon dilatation with surgical bougin-age. Pediatr Radiol 2001;31:98–101.
39. Saeed ZA, Winchester CB, Ferro PS, et al. Prospective randomized comparison of polyvinyl bougies and through-the-scope balloons for dilation of peptic stric-tures of the esophagus. Gastrointest Endosc 1995;41:189–95.
40. Scolapio JS, Pasha TM, Gostout CJ, et al. A randomized prospective study comparing rigid to balloon dilators for benign esophageal strictures and rings. Gastrointest Endosc 1999;50:13–7.
41. van Boeckel PG, Siersema PD. Refractory esophageal strictures: what to do when dilation fails. Curr Treat Options Gastroenterol 2015;13:47–58.
42. Ramage JI Jr, Rumalla A, Baron TH, et al. A prospective, randomized, double-blind, placebo-controlled trial of endoscopic steroid injection therapy for recalci-trant esophageal peptic strictures. Am J Gastroenterol 2005;100:2419–25.

43. Kochhar R, Makharia GK. Usefulness of intralesional triamcinolone in treatment of benign esophageal strictures. Gastrointest Endosc 2002;56:829–34.
44. Kochhar R, Ray JD, Sriram PV, et al. Intralesional steroids augment the effects of endoscopic dilation in corrosive esophageal strictures. Gastrointest Endosc 1999;49:509–13.
45. Miyashita M, Onda M, Okawa K, et al. Endoscopic dexamethasone injection following balloon dilatation of anastomotic stricture after esophagogastrostomy. Am J Surg 1997;174:442–4.
46. Gandhi RP, Cooper A, Barlow BA. Successful management of esophageal strictures without resection or replacement. J Pediatr Surg 1989;24:745–9 [discussion: 9–50].
47. Hirdes MM, van Hooft JE, Koornstra JJ, et al. Endoscopic corticosteroid injections do not reduce dysphagia after endoscopic dilation therapy in patients with benign esophagogastric anastomotic strictures. Clin Gastroenterol Hepatol 2013;11:795–801. e1.
48. Michaud L, Gottrand F. Anastomotic strictures: conservative treatment. J Pediatr Gastroenterol Nutr 2011;52(Suppl 1):S18–9.
49. Uhlen S, Fayoux P, Vachin F, et al. Mitomycin C: an alternative conservative treatment for refractory esophageal stricture in children? Endoscopy 2006;38:404–7.
50. Spier BJ, Sawma VA, Gopal DV, et al. Intralesional mitomycin C: successful treatment for benign recalcitrant esophageal stricture. Gastrointest Endosc 2009;69: 152–3 [discussion: 3].
51. Heran MK, Pham TH, Butterworth S, et al. Use of a microporous polytetrafluoroethylene catheter balloon to treat refractory esophageal stricture: a novel technique for delivery of mitomycin C. J Pediatr Surg 2011;46:776–9.
52. Berger M, Ure B, Lacher M. Mitomycin C in the therapy of recurrent esophageal strictures: hype or hope? Eur J Pediatr Surg 2012;22:109–16.
53. Sweed AS, Fawaz SA, Ezzat WF, et al. A prospective controlled study to assess the use of mitomycin C in improving the results of esophageal dilatation in post corrosive esophageal stricture in children. Int J Pediatr Otorhinolaryngol 2015;79:23–5.
54. Chapuy L, Pomerleau M, Faure C. Topical mitomycin-C application in recurrent esophageal strictures after surgical repair of esophageal atresia. J Pediatr Gastroenterol Nutr 2014;59:608–11.
55. Chung J, Connolly B, Langer J, et al. Fluoroscopy-guided topical application of mitomycin-C in a case of refractory esophageal stricture. J Vasc Interv Radiol 2010;21:152–5.
56. Lakoma A, Fallon SC, Mathur S, et al. Use of mitomycin C for refractory esophageal stricture following tracheoesophageal fistula repair. European J Pediatr Surg Rep 2013;1:24–6.
57. Rosseneu S, Afzal N, Yerushalmi B, et al. Topical application of mitomycin-C in oesophageal strictures. J Pediatr Gastroenterol Nutr 2007;44:336–41.
58. Stocchi F, Carbone A, Inghilleri M, et al. Urodynamic and neurophysiological evaluation in Parkinson's disease and multiple system atrophy. J Neurol Neurosurg Psychiatry 1997;62:507–11.
59. Varadarajulu S, Banerjee S, Barth B, et al. Enteral stents. Gastrointest Endosc 2011;74:455–64.
60. Bakken JC, Wong Kee Song LM, de Groen PC, et al. Use of a fully covered self-expandable metal stent for the treatment of benign esophageal diseases. Gastrointest Endosc 2010;72:712–20.
61. Barthel JS, Kelley ST, Klapman JB. Management of persistent gastroesophageal anastomotic strictures with removable self-expandable polyester silicon-covered

(Polyflex) stents: an alternative to serial dilation. Gastrointest Endosc 2008;67: 546–52.

62. Dua KS, Vleggaar FP, Santharam R, et al. Removable self-expanding plastic esophageal stent as a continuous, non-permanent dilator in treating refractory benign esophageal strictures: a prospective two-center study. Am J Gastroenterol 2008;103:2988–94.

63. Fiorini A, Fleischer D, Valero J, et al. Self-expandable metal coil stents in the treatment of benign esophageal strictures refractory to conventional therapy: a case series. Gastrointest Endosc 2000;52:259–62.

64. Kim JH, Song HY, Choi EK, et al. Temporary metallic stent placement in the treatment of refractory benign esophageal strictures: results and factors associated with outcome in 55 patients. Eur Radiol 2009;19:384–90.

65. Pennathur A, Chang AC, McGrath KM, et al. Polyflex expandable stents in the treatment of esophageal disease: initial experience. Ann Thorac Surg 2008;85: 1968–72 [discussion: 73].

66. Repici A, Conio M, De Angelis C, et al. Temporary placement of an expandable polyester silicone-covered stent for treatment of refractory benign esophageal strictures. Gastrointest Endosc 2004;60:513–9.

67. van Halsema EE, van Hooft JE. Clinical outcomes of self-expandable stent placement for benign esophageal diseases: a pooled analysis of the literature. World J Gastrointest Endosc 2015;7:135–53.

68. Best C, Sudel B, Foker JE, et al. Esophageal stenting in children: indications, application, effectiveness, and complications. Gastrointest Endosc 2009;70: 1248–53.

69. Broto J, Asensio M, Vernet JM. Results of a new technique in the treatment of severe esophageal stenosis in children: poliflex stents. J Pediatr Gastroenterol Nutr 2003;37:203–6.

70. Zhang C, Yu JM, Fan GP, et al. The use of a retrievable self-expanding stent in treating childhood benign esophageal strictures. J Pediatr Surg 2005;40: 501–4.

71. Manfredi MA, Jennings RW, Anjum MW, et al. Externally removable stents in the treatment of benign recalcitrant strictures and esophageal perforations in pediatric patients with esophageal atresia. Gastrointest Endosc 2014;80:246–52.

72. Atabek C, Surer I, Demirbag S, et al. Increasing tendency in caustic esophageal burns and long-term polytetrafluorethylene stenting in severe cases: 10 years experience. J Pediatr Surg 2007;42:636–40.

73. De Peppo F, Zaccara A, Dall'Oglio L, et al. Stenting for caustic strictures: esophageal replacement replaced. J Pediatr Surg 1998;33:54–7.

74. Mutaf O, Genc A, Herek O, et al. Gastroesophageal reflux: a determinant in the outcome of caustic esophageal burns. J Pediatr Surg 1996;31:1494–5.

75. Foschia F, De Angelis P, Torroni F, et al. Custom dynamic stent for esophageal strictures in children. J Pediatr Surg 2011;46:848–53.

76. Repici A, Vleggaar FP, Hassan C, et al. Efficacy and safety of biodegradable stents for refractory benign esophageal strictures: the BEST (Biodegradable Esophageal Stent) study. Gastrointest Endosc 2010;72:927–34.

77. Karakan T, Utku OG, Dorukoz O, et al. Biodegradable stents for caustic esophageal strictures: a new therapeutic approach. Dis Esophagus 2013;26:319–22.

78. Tokar JL, Banerjee S, Barth BA, et al. Drug-eluting/biodegradable stents. Gastrointest Endosc 2011;74:954–8.

79. Hordijk ML, Siersema PD, Tilanus HW, et al. Electrocautery therapy for refractory anastomotic strictures of the esophagus. Gastrointest Endosc 2006;63:157–63.

80. Hordijk ML, van Hooft JE, Hansen BE, et al. A randomized comparison of electro-cautery incision with savary bougienage for relief of anastomotic gastroesopha-geal strictures. Gastrointest Endosc 2009;70:849–55.

81. Muto M, Ezoe Y, Yano T, et al. Usefulness of endoscopic radial incision and cut-ting method for refractory esophagogastric anastomotic stricture (with video). Gastrointest Endosc 2012;75:965–72.

82. Simmons DT, Baron TH. Electroincision of refractory esophagogastric anasto-motic strictures. Dis Esophagus 2006;19:410–4.

83. Lee TH, Lee SH, Park JY, et al. Primary incisional therapy with a modified method for patients with benign anastomotic esophageal stricture. Gastrointest Endosc 2009;69:1029–33.

84. Manfredi MA, Jennings R, Ngo PD, et al. Endoscopic electrocautery incisional therapy as a treatment for refractory pediatric esophageal strictures. Gastrointest Endosc 2014;79:AB140.

85. Koivusalo A, Pakarinen MP, Rintala RJ. Anastomotic dilatation after repair of esophageal atresia with distal fistula. Comparison of results after routine versus selective dilatation. Dis Esophagus 2009;22:190–4.

Moving?

Make sure your subscription moves with you!

To notify us of your new address, find your **Clinics Account Number** (located on your mailing label above your name), and contact customer service at:

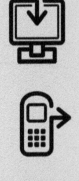

Email: journalscustomerservice-usa@elsevier.com

800-654-2452 (subscribers in the U.S. & Canada)
314-447-8871 (subscribers outside of the U.S. & Canada)

Fax number: 314-447-8029

Elsevier Health Sciences Division
Subscription Customer Service
3251 Riverport Lane
Maryland Heights, MO 63043

*To ensure uninterrupted delivery of your subscription, please notify us at least 4 weeks in advance of move.

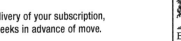

Printed and bound by CPI Group (UK) Ltd, Croydon, CR0 4YY

03/10/2024

01040492-0006